NONLINEAR ANALYSIS *for* HUMAN MOVEMENT VARIABILITY

T0312976

NONLINEAR ANALYSIS *for* HUMAN MOVEMENT VARIABILITY

NICHOLAS STERGIOU

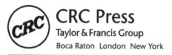

CRC Press
Taylor & Francis Group
Boca Raton London New York

CRC Press is an imprint of the
Taylor & Francis Group, an **informa** business

First published in paperback 2024

First published in 2016 by CRC Press
2385 NW Executive Center Drive, Suite 320, Boca Raton FL 33431

and by CRC Press
4 Park Square, Milton Park, Abingdon, Oxon, OX14 4RN

CRC Press is an imprint of Taylor & Francis Group, LLC

© 2016, 2024 Taylor & Francis Group, LLC

Library of Congress Cataloging-in-Publication Data

Names: Stergiou, Nicholas, editor.
Title: Nonlinear analysis for human movement variability / editor, Nicholas Stergiou.
Description: Boca Raton : Taylor & Francis, Taylor & Francis, a CRC title, part of the Taylor & Francis imprint, a member of the Taylor & Francis Group, the academic division of T&F Informa plc, 2016. | Includes bibliographical references and index.
Identifiers: LCCN 2015029283 | ISBN 9781498703321 (alk. paper)
Subjects: LCSH: Human locomotion. | Human mechanics. | Mathematical analysis.
Classification: LCC QP301 .N66 2016 | DDC 612.7/6--dc23
LC record available at http://lccn.loc.gov/2015029283

ISBN: 978-1-4987-0332-1 (hbk)
ISBN: 978-1-03-292063-4 (pbk)
ISBN: 978-1-315-37065-1 (ebk)

DOI: 10.1201/9781315370651

**Visit the Taylor & Francis Web site at
http://www.taylorandfrancis.com**

**and the CRC Press Web site at
http://www.crcpress.com**

Contents

Preface..vii
Editor xi
Contributors xiii

Chapter 1 Introduction 1
              John McCamley and Steven J. Harrison

Chapter 2 Time Series... 29
              Sara A. Myers

Chapter 3 State-Space Reconstruction... 55
              Shane R. Wurdeman

Chapter 4 Lyapunov Exponent.. 83
              Shane R. Wurdeman

Chapter 5 Surrogation 111
              Sara A. Myers

Chapter 6 Entropy 173
              Jennifer M. Yentes

Chapter 7 Fractals 261
              Denise McGrath

Chapter 8 Autocorrelation Function, Mutual Information,
              and Correlation Dimension 301
              Nathaniel H. Hunt

Chapter 9 Case Studies 343
              Anastasia Kyvelidou and Leslie M. Decker

Index..389

Preface

The entire creation is synthesized by essence and attributes, and has the need of Divine Providence, because it is not free of variability.

Maximus the Confessor (580–662)

Human movement variability can be defined as the typical variations that are present in motor performance and are observed across multiple repetitions of a task. This variability is inherent within all biological systems. It can also be observed quite easily as it is almost impossible for an individual, even an elite performer, to perform two identical actions of the same task. This has been described quite effectively as "repetition without repetition" since the repetition of an action involves unique and nonrepetitive neuromotor patterns. For example, when we play a game of throwing darts, we are unable to always hit the center. When we walk, if we observe our footprints on sand or in the snow, we will see that they never repeat themselves in the exact same fashion. When we stand quietly, especially if we close our eyes, we will observe that we continuously sway and are unable to remain completely still. The role of movement variability has attracted significant attention recently due to its relationship to pathology and performance.

Previous theoretical frameworks consider variability as an indicator of noise in the control system, and it has been quantified using traditional linear statistical measures (e.g., standard deviation). Such measures contain very limited information about how the motor control system responds to change either within or between individuals. Practically, linear measures are measures of centrality and, thus, provide a description of the amount or magnitude of the variability around a central point. This is accomplished by quantifying the magnitude of variation in a set of values independent of their order in the distribution. From this perspective, clinicians and scientists have believed that the mean is the "gold standard" of healthy behavior and that any deviation from this gold standard is error, or undesirable behavior, or the result of instability.

Recent literature from several disciplines and medical areas, including brain function and disease dynamics, however, has shown that many apparently "noisy" phenomena are the result of nonlinear interactions and have deterministic origins. As such, the measured signal, including its "noisy" component, may provide important information regarding the system that produced it. Therefore, new innovative clinical methods that use nonlinear mathematical analysis and investigate the temporal structure of variability have been proposed. These nonlinear methods are being used increasingly to describe complex conditions in which linear techniques for the analysis of variability have been inadequate, hence confounding scientific study and the development of meaningful therapeutic options. For example, nonlinear analysis of the temporal structure of the variability present has recently been used in research on heart rate irregularities, sudden cardiac death syndrome, blood pressure control, brain ischemia, epileptic seizures, and several other conditions. Such research allowed for better understanding of the complexity of these pathologies and eventually led to the development of better prognostic and diagnostic tools. Similarly, nonlinear analysis of the variability present in movement patterns generated as a result of motor-related disability provides a window into the neuromuscular status of the patient and insight into the complex strategies used to control movement and posture.

Our research team at the University of Nebraska, Omaha, have been pioneers in the investigation of human movement variability with nonlinear analysis and its investigative ability to develop critical prognostic and diagnostic tools for motor-related disabilities. Our annual workshop on movement variability is well attended by scientists and clinicians that come to Nebraska from all over the world. In addition, many scientists come to us for sabbaticals or to receive more extensive training. The editor and members of his scientific staff are routinely invited to conduct workshops and tutorials in conferences around the globe (i.e., Australia, Spain, Ireland, Germany, Portugal, Brazil, and many others). Through these experiences, we received countless requests for a comprehensive book on nonlinear analysis to study human movement variability.

We have finally decided to grant these requests and develop such a book. The organization of our book is as follows. After introductory chapters on dynamical systems and time series, we present a wide variety of nonlinear tools such as the Lyapunov exponent, surrogation, entropy, fractal analysis, and several others. Whenever possible, we include exercises with data analysis problems. Their solutions can be found in the complementary solutions manual. In addition, each chapter provides numerous examples from the literature and our research on how nonlinear analysis can be used to understand real-world applications. We believe that this will enhance the readers' understanding of the material presented in each section of the book. Finally, the book concludes with a chapter that presents numerous case studies in postural control, gait, motor control, motor development, and others to enhance comprehension. PowerPoint slides in each chapter are also provided for the same reason and also for assisting in a possible adaptation of this book as a course textbook. All the software used in this book is available to be downloaded freely from our website: http://www.unomaha.edu/college-of-education/biomechanics-core-facility/research/computer-codes.php

We believe that our approach will allow engineers, movement scientists, clinicians, and many others to develop the foundation necessary to utilize nonlinear analysis in their practices. Our book will offer the know-how that, along with the research capabilities provided, could leverage novel departures in the field of human movement variability research. The future may hold new advancements of our understanding of human performance, biomechanics, motor control, and motor learning, and, most importantly, of a variety of diseases and conditions that affect our nation's health.

This book is a result of the marvelous contributions of a select group of exceptional authors. They all worked extremely hard and with diligence, providing drafts on time and addressing all comments and revisions asked from them. On a personal note, they are all my students (either graduate students or postdocs), my academic children, and have worked with me for many years investigating the concepts presented in this book. Therefore, I am extremely proud about their progress and development demonstrated by their excellent chapters written for this book. However, at the same time I do not want to forget the contributions of numerous other graduate students and postdocs who have worked with me over the years on nonlinear analysis for human movement variability. Students such as Max Kurz, Joan Deffeyes, Naomi Kochi, Jessie Huisinga, Joshua Haworth, Dimitrios Katsavelis, Fabien Cignetti, Joseph Siu, Mukul Mukherjee, James Cavanaugh, Regina Harbourne, Srikant Vallabhajosula, and many others, who must forgive me for not mentioning their names here, have been instrumental in the development of the material presented in this book. I am blessed that I have worked with every single one of them. I am also blessed that I have been able to pass along to these students the knowledge that I acquired from my mentors at the University of Oregon where the ideas for this book were originally molded.

Our team has received significant financial support for the research on which this book is based. The NIH, NASA, U.S. Department of Education (NIDRR), NSF, VA, Nebraska Research Initiative, and many others, have consistently provided funds for our work and allowed us to progress with financial stability over the years. I am particularly grateful to the NIH and NIGMS for a COBRE P20GM109090 grant that supported the writing of this book.

Ramon Y. Cajal, the father of modern neurobiology, almost a hundred years ago wrote: "more than once I was hopelessly discouraged about my ability to pursue science." Such times have been aplenty in my career and in the development not only of this book but also in the investigation of a novel area of research that is different from traditional approaches. In these times, there is one certainty: that solace is needed around you to overcome even the highest of obstacles. This is why I am eternally grateful for my cornerstone, my wife Ann, my parents Jesus and Vaya, and my brother Dimitris, for their love, support, and constant encouragement.

MATLAB® is a registered trademark of The MathWorks, Inc. For product information, please contact:

The MathWorks, Inc.
3 Apple Hill Drive
Natick, MA 01760-2098, USA
Tel: 508-647-7000
Fax: 508-647-7001
E-mail: info@mathworks.com
Web: www.mathworks.com

Editor

Dr. Nick Stergiou is the distinguished community research chair in biomechanics and professor and director of the Biomechanics Research Building at the University of Nebraska at Omaha. He is also a faculty member in the Department of Environmental, Agricultural, and Occupational Health of the College of Public Health at the University of Nebraska Medical Center. His research focuses on understanding variability inherent in human movement, and he recently founded the first ever Center for Research in Human Movement Variability through a $10 million grant from the NIH/NIGMS. He is an international authority in the study of nonlinear dynamics and has published more than 200 peer-reviewed articles. Dr. Stergiou's research spans from infant development to older adult fallers and has impacted training techniques of surgeons and treatment and rehabilitation techniques of pathologies, such as peripheral arterial disease. He has received more than $20 million in personal funding from NIH, NASA, NSF, the NIDRR/U.S. Department of Education, and many other agencies and foundations. He also holds several patents and procured a private donation of $6 million to build the 23,000 sq. ft. Biomechanics Research Building that opened in August 2013. This is the first building on his campus exclusively dedicated to research.

Contributors

Leslie M. Decker
French Institute of Health and Medical
    Research
University of Caen Lower Normandy
Caen, France

and

Center for Research in Human
    Movement Variability
University of Nebraska at Omaha
Omaha, Nebraska

Steven J. Harrison
Center for Research in Human
    Movement Variability
University of Nebraska at Omaha
Omaha, Nebraska

Nathaniel H. Hunt
Department of Integrative Biology
University of California at Berkeley
Berkeley, California

and

Center for Research in Human
    Movement Variability
University of Nebraska at Omaha
Omaha, Nebraska

Anastasia Kyvelidou
Center for Research in Human
    Movement Variability
University of Nebraska at Omaha
Omaha, Nebraska

John McCamley
Center for Research in Human
    Movement Variability
University of Nebraska at Omaha
Omaha, Nebraska

Denise McGrath
School of Public Health, Physiotherapy
    and Population Science
University College Dublin
Dublin, Ireland

and

Center for Research in Human
    Movement Variability
University of Nebraska at Omaha
Omaha, Nebraska

Sara A. Myers
Center for Research in Human
    Movement Variability
University of Nebraska at Omaha
Omaha, Nebraska

Shane R. Wurdeman
Center for Research in Human
    Movement Variability
University of Nebraska at Omaha
Omaha, Nebraska

Jennifer M. Yentes
Center for Research in Human
    Movement Variability
University of Nebraska at Omaha
Omaha, Nebraska

1 Introduction

John McCamley and Steven J. Harrison

CONTENTS

Dynamical Systems...2
    Deterministic versus Stochastic 3
    Continuous versus Discrete...4
    Linear versus Nonlinear 5
    Growth Model and Its Limitations..5
    Logistic Map 6
    Bifurcation Diagram...10
    Chaos..12
Self-Organization 13
    Simple Examples of Self-Organization...15
    Self-Organization in Human Movement 18
    What Is the Cause of Self-Organization?..21
    Tell-Tale Signs of Self-Organization...22
Self-Organization and Complexity 23
    Self-Organized Criticality Hypothesis of Movement Variability......................24
Summary..25
References..26

Mathematics is the language with which God has written the universe.

Galileo Galilei (1564–1642)

The studies of the dynamical properties of systems have generally been restricted to reducing these systems to a linear approximation. The limitations that exist in such analysis have long been considered. In 1976 Robert May stated that many different situations from a variety of disciplines can be modeled and approximated by simple first-order difference equations. Then the investigation of the dynamical characteristics of these models entails the identification of constant equilibrium solutions and a linearized analysis to describe how stable they are when exposed to small perturbations. Unfortunately, the nonlinear dynamical features that are present have not been considered (May 1976).

The aim of this book is to consider the nonlinear dynamical features to be found in complex biological and physical systems, especially those characteristic to human movement. In this introductory chapter, we will set the stage for appreciating the relevance of nonlinear methods to the scientific study of complex systems. We will introduce key concepts that have motivated the development and application of nonlinear methods, including the notion of a dynamical system, and concepts such as chaos, nonlinear dynamics, self-organization, and complexity.

DYNAMICAL SYSTEMS

Early scientists believed that if it was possible to know all the possible aspects of a system, and through the laws of nature describe it and hence understand it, then it would be possible to know its future path (de Laplace 1902). Others, including James Maxwell (1831–1879), observed that systems exist with "sensitive dependence to initial data" (Hunt and Yorke 1993). In 1899, French mathematician Henri Poincaré (1854–1912) recognized that the laws of physics could not provide a complete understanding of the motion of celestial bodies (*three-body problem*); however, it was many years before people began to realize the importance of chaos, and how it applies to dynamical systems.

> A *dynamical* system is one which changes in time; what changes is the state of the system. The capitalist system is dynamical (according to Marx), while the decimal system is (we hope) not dynamical. A mathematical dynamical system consists of the space of states of the system together with a rule called the dynamic for determining the state which corresponds at a given future time to a given present state. Determining such rules for various natural systems is a central problem of science. Once the dynamic is given, it is the task of mathematical dynamical systems theory to investigate the patterns of how states change in the long run.
>
> **Hirsch (1984)**

The terms "dynamic" and "dynamical" are generally used to describe systems that evolve or change over time (Hirsch 1984; Thelen and Smith 1994; Crutchfield et al. 2010). Thelen and Smith (2006) are more specific. They apply the term "dynamic systems" to the systems of elements that change over time. "Dynamical system" is the more technical name they give to the mathematical equations that describe the time evolution of such systems with particular properties. The technical description is also favored by others. Hilborn (2000) attributes the term "dynamical systems theory" to the mathematical theory of dynamical systems, which have "a state space and a rule for the evolution of trajectories starting at various initial conditions." Crutchfield et al. (2010) also divide the definition of a dynamical system into a "state" and a "dynamic" part. Examples of dynamical systems exist all around (and within) us. They include astrological systems; chemical reactions; pendula; the economy (stock market); ecological systems (including plant and animal populations, cancer growth, and the spread of disease); and the human body (heart, brain, lungs). Studies of dynamical systems have led to the understanding of important concepts for biologists (Mpitsos and Soinila 1993). The way the variables of a dynamical system change over time can be described by a set of functions. These functions may be defined in continuous time by differential equations, or discrete time by difference equations. Within the realm of dynamical systems, there are many that will exhibit nonlinear characteristics. Among those nonlinear systems exists a subset of *chaotic*

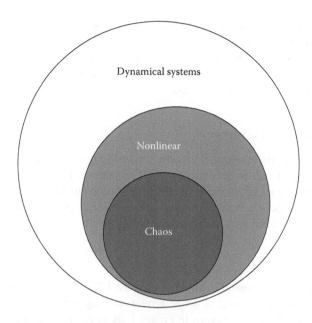

FIGURE 1.1   Not all nonlinear systems are chaotic, but all chaotic systems are nonlinear. Nonlinear systems are in turn a particular form of dynamical systems.

systems (Figure 1.1). Chaotic behavior exists in many seemingly simple systems such as the movement of a ferromagnetic beam buckled between two magnets under the effect of sinusoidal oscillations (Moon and Holmes 1979), a double pendulum (Richter and Scholz 1984), or a dripping tap (Shaw 1984). Chaos is often thought of in terms of noise within a system that is unpredictable in nature; however, its technical meaning is quite different. Not all nonlinear dynamical systems are chaotic, but all chaotic systems are nonlinear (Hilborn 2000). Chaos, and the important role it plays in understanding the dynamics of nonlinear systems, is discussed in more detail in a later section.

To understand the underlying properties of a dynamical system, it is necessary to understand the space that it occupies. The behavior of a dynamical system is ideally represented in a phase space, that is, in a space that contains dimensions sufficient to specify the state of the system. In subsequent chapters, methods for reconstructing phase spaces and quantifying the phase-space dynamics in terms of Lyapunov exponents and dimensions (Kantz and Schreiber 2004) will be introduced. The phase-space geometry of attractors can provide useful information about the dynamics of a system, and further understanding can be discovered through bifurcation analysis.

DETERMINISTIC VERSUS STOCHASTIC

Dynamical systems can be either deterministic or stochastic. A *deterministic* system is one that, given a current state, can only have one unique future state. A deterministic system is one in which the equations of the system, and the parameters describing the system, along with the initial conditions, describe the subsequent behavior of the system (Hilborn 2000). There is a one-to-one relationship, which is governed by a rule for the system. On the other hand a *stochastic* system can have more than one, perhaps many, future states for a given current state. These outcomes can occur according to some probabilistic process.

Continuous versus Discrete

A continuous measure is one that evolves continuously over time. The outcome is, thus, a function of time, for example, $x = f(t)$. Consider the children's story character Pinocchio, whose nose grows when he tells lies. We can create a function to describe the length of Pinocchio's nose over time. Let us say that his nose grows at 0.1 cm, multiplied by time in minutes, raised to the third power:

$$L = 0.1 \times t^3$$

When plotted this will appear as shown in Figure 1.2a. If the length of Pinocchio's nose is calculated (and grows) at discrete intervals, say at the end of each minute, then the length will grow as shown in Figure 1.2b. A discrete variable is measured at a particular point in time (as distinct from continuously) or it is something that is counted. The time intervals between drips from a tap can be considered discrete measurements. Discrete measures may often result from questionnaires. The difference between continuous and discrete measurements needs to be taken into account for many statistical analyses. It should be remembered that most measurements (especially digital ones) can only be taken at discrete intervals even if the system being measured is continuous.

Another discrete process is the way a bank pays interest on a savings account. The amount paid each period is based on the value at a discrete point in time, usually at the end of the period. This new value (unless a withdrawal is made)

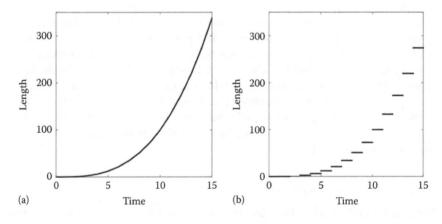

FIGURE 1.2 The length of Pinocchio's nose: (a) continuous growth and (b) growth using discrete measurements.

becomes the value on which the next payment is calculated. Populations may also grow in a discrete manner and are generally based on the annual changes in seasons.

The difference between continuous and discrete systems is important when conducting numerical analysis of chaotic processes (Mpitsos and Soinila 1993) with different nonlinear tools having a more suitable application to one or the other type of measure.

LINEAR VERSUS NONLINEAR

A *linear* function is one in which the outcome changes in direct proportion to the change in the input. A simple linear function can appear as:

$$Y = b + mX$$

where

b is the intercept
m is the slope
X is raised to the first power.

A plot of this function will be a straight line (Figure 1.3a). A linear system is governed by the paradigm that small changes to inputs lead to small changes in outcome. Not all functions appear as straight lines (Figure 1.3b). Functions of the form

$$Y = aX_n^2$$

are *nonlinear* since the right-hand side of the equation is not the equation of a straight line. Statistical tools for use with linear data are not meaningful when applied to nonlinear data. A new set of measures is necessary and these will be discussed in detail later in the text.

GROWTH MODEL AND ITS LIMITATIONS

Let us consider an initial bank deposit of $100 into a savings account. If the interest is 0.1 (10%) for a given period, at the end of the first period $10 will be added to the account. For the next period the deposit will be $110 (1.1*100) and at the end of this period $11 will be added and the total deposit will become $121 (1.1*1.1*100). This is an example of a growth model described by

$$X_n = r^n X_0$$

where

X_0 represents the initial deposit ($100)
r is the compounded interest rate (1.1)
n is the number of periods

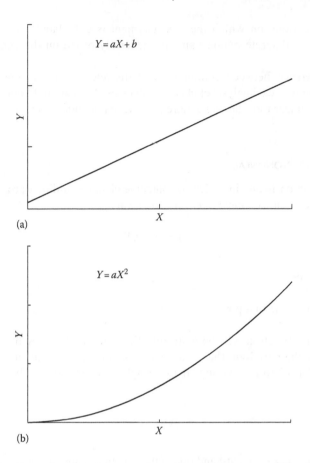

FIGURE 1.3   (a) Plot of a linear function and (b) plot of a nonlinear function.

An alternative way to write this function is

$$X_{n+1} = rX_n$$

For values of $r < 1$ the population will decay to zero over time (Figure 1.4a). For values of $r > 1$ such a system would soon grow to infinity (Figure 1.4b). This model is deterministic and linear, which can be seen if X_{n+1} is graphed against X_n (Figure 1.4c). A growth model of this form may not be realistic. Systems may be constrained whereby growth becomes limited at some point, such as when populations are limited by food sources or space, or when chemical reactions are limited by supply of reagents. In biological systems predators can provide further restriction on growth.

LOGISTIC MAP

To understand how a population is related to the population at a previous point in time, it must be able to grow, but this growth must also be limited. In 1976 biologist

R. May published a paper (May 1976) in which he introduced the "logistic" difference equation to describe the growth of populations:

$$N_{t+1} = N_t(a - bN_t)$$

In this function if $b = 0$ it becomes the previously described growth function, which will grow exponentially when $a > 1$. For $b \neq 0$ it produces a growth curve with a hump the shape of which can be changed by the parameter a. If the function is scaled such that $X = bN/a$, the resulting equation becomes

$$X_{t+1} = aX_t(1 - X_t)$$

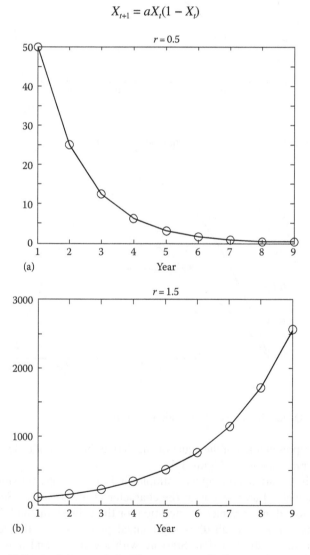

(a)

(b)

FIGURE 1.4 (a) For $r < 1$ the population decays to zero. (b) For $r > 1$ the population grows to infinity. *(Continued)*

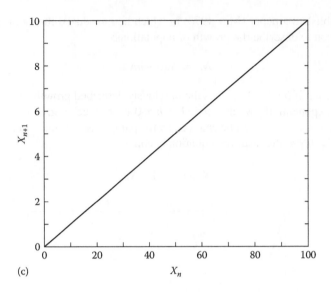

(c)

FIGURE 1.4 (*Continued*) (c) The growth model is linear.

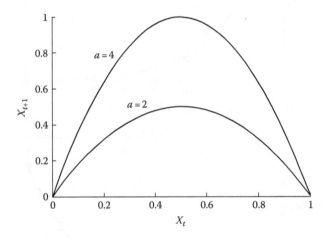

FIGURE 1.5 Quadratic curve of the equation $X_{t+1} = aX_t(1 - X_t)$ for $a = 2$ and 4.

A graphical representation of the equation, depicting the effect of different values of the parameter a, is shown in Figure 1.5.

While this equation may appear simple, it is not always possible to find a simple mathematical answer due to the character of the solutions. Solutions can, however, be found using numerical iteration, or the cobweb method. The cobweb method (Figure 1.6a through d) is a graphical plot to iterate the equation that requires a sketch of the function. Starting with a value X_0 and drawing a vertical line (Figure 1.6a: line 1), the corresponding value X_1 is found. The value X_1 can then be transferred to the horizontal axis of the graph by using a horizontal line (Figure 1.6a: line 2) and the diagonal line ($X_{t+1} = X_t$). Another vertical line (Figure 1.6a: line 3) will find the value of X_3. This process can be continued to show the growth of the population over time. May (1976) noted that as the value of a is increased, the outcome changes from a single value (Figure 1.6a) to oscillating between two values (Figure 1.6b). A further increase leads to a four-period oscillation (Figure 1.6c) and finally chaos (Figure 1.6d). Plots of these solutions are shown in Figure 1.7a through d, respectively.

In the one-dimensional form presented here the logistic equation has limited direct application to biological populations that generally involve interaction with other species and overlapping generations. The behavior of the logistic equation,

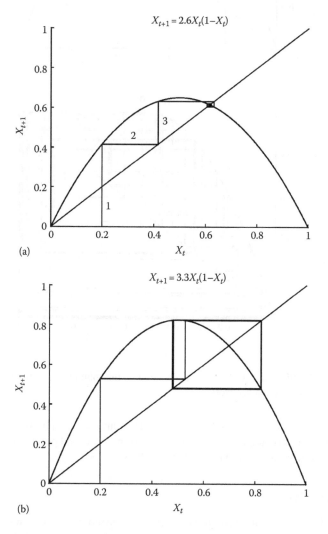

FIGURE 1.6 Cobweb plots showing (a) a single steady state; (b) the solution oscillates between two values. *(Continued)*

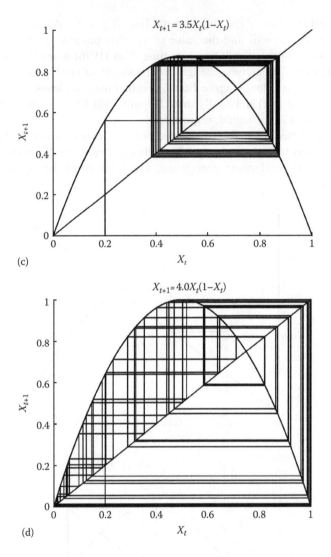

(c)

(d)

FIGURE 1.6 (*Continued*) Cobweb plots showing (c) the solution oscillations between four values; and (d) the solution is chaotic.

and other apparently simple nonlinear difference equations, can however account for many observations of apparently erratic fluctuations in animal populations as well as in other dynamical systems (May and Oster 1976).

BIFURCATION DIAGRAM

The transition from steady state to two- and four-period oscillations and to chaos is termed "bifurcations," and the point at which the number states or stability of the system changes is called a bifurcation point.

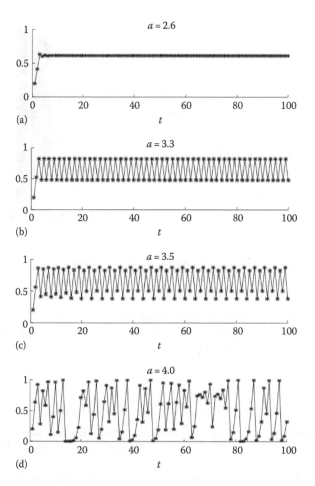

FIGURE 1.7 Plots showing solutions to the logistic equation: (a) steady-state; (b) period two oscillation; (c) period four oscillation; (d) chaos.

If the equation

$$X_{t+1} = aX_t(1 - X_t)$$

is numerically iterated and the values of X plotted after the transients have died out for successive values of a, and these values shown as a plot of X vs. a, then a *bifurcation diagram* (Figure 1.8) is generated. This diagram provides much useful information about the behavior of the system. The bifurcation diagram depicts the values of a when a period doubling (bifurcation) will occur and the broad areas of chaos interspersed with periodic windows. While not all nonlinear functions follow a period doubling route to chaos, those that do follow this pattern have been observed to follow mathematical rules (Feigenbaum 1978). Feigenbaum realized that the "rate of convergence" toward chaos is the same for different functions that exhibit bifurcations. If a_n is the value of a where period 2^n is "born" then: $\delta = (a_n - a_{n-1})/(a_{n+1} - a_n)$. Feigenbaum found

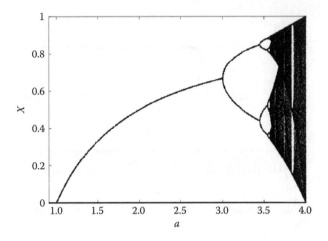

FIGURE 1.8 Bifurcation diagram for the function: $X_{t+1} = aX_t(1 - X_t)$.

that the value of δ is approximately the same for all values of n and for large value of n the value of δ approaches the same number for different functions. The value δ = 4.6692… has become known as the *Feigenbaum's number.*

CHAOS

In truth at first Chaos came to be, but next wide-bosomed Earth.

(From Hesiod, 750–650 BC, The Homeric Hymns and Homerica with English Translation by Hugh G. Evelyn-White (1914))

In violent order is disorder; and a great disorder is an order. These two things are one.

Wallace Stevens (1879–1955, "Connoisseur of Chaos")

One of the most well-known sets of equations to describe a chaotic system was developed by Edward Lorenz (1917–2008). He was trying to model particular weather patterns and, after simplifying equations for fluid dynamics, produced the following three coupled, differential equations (Lorenz 1963)

$$\frac{dX}{dt} = p(Y - X)$$

$$\frac{dY}{dt} = -XZ + rX - Y$$

$$\frac{dZ}{dt} = XY - bZ$$

with p, r, and b representing adjustable parameters.

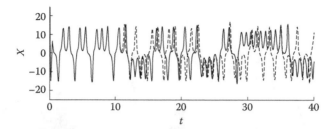

FIGURE 1.9 Solution to the Lorenz equations showing the effect of a small change in initial conditions: $p = 10$, $r = 24.5$, $b = 8/3$. Solid line: $X_0 = 10$, $Y_0 = 70$, $Z_0 = 19$. Dashed line: $X_0 = 10$, $Y_0 = 70$, $Z_0 = 19.001$.

Lorenz found (apparently almost by accident, and perhaps due to the computational limitations of the time) that the outcome of this set of equations is extremely sensitive to the initial conditions. Figure 1.9 shows how, when chaos exists, a small change in the initial value of Z (from 19 to 19.001) leads to large changes in the outcome after a short period of time. This sensitivity to initial conditions has become known as the butterfly effect (Lorenz 1972) and is a characteristic that exemplifies chaos.

Chaos theory has been applied to many fields of biological and nonbiological analysis. It has been used in systems ranging from psychology (Ayers 1997) to hydrology (Sivakumar 2000) and as a means to analyze the financial markets (Peters 1994). When a dynamical system displays sensitivity to its initial conditions, which lead to irregularity, it can be termed *chaotic* (Çambel 1993; Kaplan and Glass 1995; Williams 1997; Wiggins 2010). Such a system while appearing irregular is actually deterministic (Kaplan and Glass 1995); however, it is impossible to make long-term predictions for such a system. Kaplan and Glass (1995) add further to the definition of chaos, noting the same state is never repeated and that it is bounded. Often the equations that describe such behavior are deceptively simple as was shown in the previous section. Representation of system behavior in phase space provides a powerful basis for both visualizing and quantifying the dynamics of both nonlinear and chaotic systems (Figure 1.10). The concept of a phase space representation rather than a time or frequency domain approach is the hallmark of nonlinear dynamical time series analysis (Kantz and Schreiber 2004). In order to be bounded and unstable at the same time, a trajectory of a dissipative dynamical system has to live on a set of unusual geometric properties. Understanding if a system is chaotic, it may not provide the underlying laws that govern the system, but it will provide important information concerning whether the system is deterministic and the feasibility of making longer term prediction about future states of the system.

SELF-ORGANIZATION

One of the principal objects of theoretical research in any department of knowledge is to find the point of view from which the subject appears in its greatest simplicity.

J. Willard Gibbs (1839–1903) from Winfree (2001)

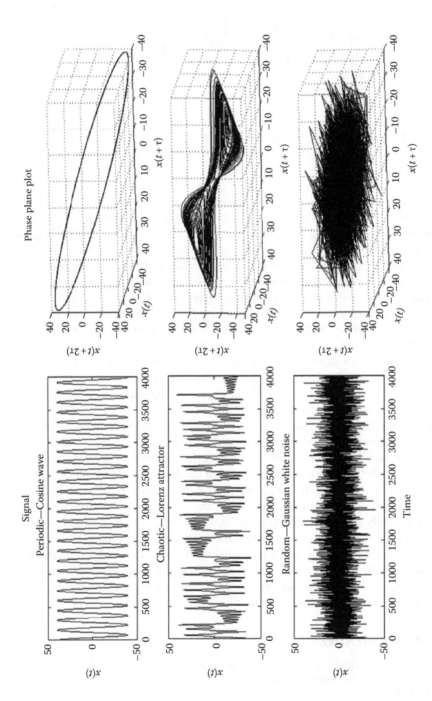

FIGURE 1.10 Phase space plots provide a means to geometrically show chaotic behavior which may not be readily apparent within a time series.

Organization in a system implicates the following property: the relationship between two components of the system is dependent upon the state of a third component (Ashby 1947). Self-organization can lead the system to change from an unorganized to an organized state. In other words, self-organization changes a system from having bad organization to having good organization (Ashby 1947). When a system establishes a state only because of the dynamical interactions among individual elements within the system, the state is self-organized (Bak 1997). This can only happen in natural systems when they are both complex and open to flux with the environment (Kugler and Turvey 1987; Thelen and Smith 1994; Kelso 1995). External processes do not cause self-organization, rather it is generated by components within the system (Haken 1977; Camazine et al. 2001; Thelen and Smith 2006). These systems are dynamical in nature (Bolender 2010), with many components interacting in nonlinear ways to produce highly complex, ordered behavior (Thelen and Smith 1994). The patterns that emerge are different from the elements that make up the system, and cannot be predicted solely from the characteristics of the individual elements (Thelen and Smith 1994).

The laws of physics cannot always describe the interactions that take place and lead to the observed patterns for biological systems (Camazine et al. 2001). When the nature of the connections, couplings, or interactions between components of a system changes and it results in a change, self-organization occurs, which enables the system dynamics to occupy a much smaller state space (Kauffman 1995). Self-organization results in increased complexity, which is "the amount of information the process stores in its causal states" (Crutchfield 2011).

SIMPLE EXAMPLES OF SELF-ORGANIZATION

> … and the thousands of fishes moved as a huge beast, piercing the water. They appeared united, inexorably bound to a common fate. How comes this unity?
>
> **Anonymous, seventeenth century from Shaw (1975)**

A quick Internet search of "bird flocking" results in amazing videos of great undulating masses of thousands of birds with global behavioral coordination. Where does this global coordination come from? Is there a leader or a group of leaders that are giving orders and communicating their plans to the group? No, there is no leader. The answer to the source of global coordination is that the flock self-organizes. In a school of fish, each individual bases its behavior not on the movement of the whole school of fish but rather on the movements of its neighbors. This simple rule for coupling individuals locally to the dynamic environment in a way that constrains the direction of animal motion has provided the basis for computer generated animations that reproduce many of the complex features evident in the flocking, swarming, and schooling behaviors found in nature (Reynolds 1987).

Perhaps the most well-known model of complex flocking behavior is the boids model. The behavior is based on only three simple (but nonlinear) rules that each boid follows locally. Each boid has interactions with the boids in its immediate vicinity, but they are not directly affected by the global behavior of the flock. The first rule is that the boid will change its heading in order to avoid collisions with the nearby boids. The second rule is that the boid will try to match the velocity with nearby boids. The third rule is that the boids will try to stay near to the center of mass of their nearby boids.

The advent of this model was a major breakthrough in the development of group behavior for flocking, herding, or schooling animals in air, on land, or in water, respectively (Lett and Mirabet 2008). It then becomes possible to generate complex flocking behavior without directly prescribing the path of each individual bird. This is akin to a dynamical systems theory of movement, wherein you do not store patterns but rather you store a simpler generative architecture that creates complex movements. Again, this model is an example of the organization of complexity from simplicity.

The potential of simple rules to produce self-organized complex dynamic patterns has been investigated through the systematic development of a class of models collectively referred to as cellular automata models (Wolfram 1984, 2002). Imagine a piece of graph paper on which the vertical axis is time. At the top of the graph paper the time is equal to 0 and increases as you go down the graph paper. For this top row at time equal 0 we have our initial condition. Each square in that row is a different cell and can have a state of either 0 or 1 (Figure 1.11).

The update rules define how the second step in time is dependent on the first. In this example of a simple one dimensional cellular automata, each cell at time $t + 1$ has a state that is dependent upon its value at time t and the states of its two nearest neighbors at time t. Again, this is a local interaction that, as we will see, leads to global emergent coordination patterns. Let's define how this update rule works.

We have already stated that the time evolution of each cell depends only on the previous state of itself and its two neighbors. This means the state of the cell is dependent upon the state of three cells at the previous time step. For these three cells there are eight combinations of what those states could have been (Figure 1.12):

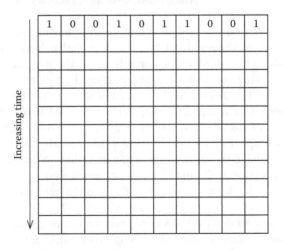

FIGURE 1.11   Cellular automata showing initial condition (top row).

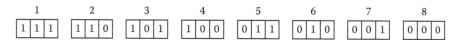

FIGURE 1.12 The eight possible combinations of states.

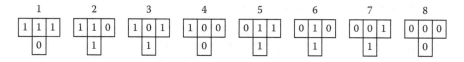

FIGURE 1.13 For each state an update rule must be defined.

And, for each of these eight combinations of what those states could have been in the previous time step, an update rule must define what the current state of the cell will be in the next time step (Figure 1.13):

For each one of these eight combinations we can define a rule by specifying what the next state of the cell will be depending on the previous cell and its two neighbors. Let us pick a specific instantiation of a rule by filling in a value of 0 or 1 for each question mark (Figure 1.14):

This rule can be stated by the outputs for each of the eight combinations—"01101110." Each rule is by convention stated in the base 10 version (decimal) of this binary format. This example (01101110) is 110 after we convert it from binary to decimal. With the base 10 convention, the update rules go from 0 ("00000000" in binary) to 255 ("11111111" in binary). If we take this rule and the initial conditions, we can begin to iterate the dynamics and see what global patterns emerge from this rule. The next five time steps are shown in the following. The three instances are highlighted. For example, "100" gives a "0" from combination number 4, "111" gives "0" from combination number 1, and "101" gives "1" from combination number 3. Notice that in this model of cellular automata the edges wrap around so that the cell to the right of the cell on the right edge is the cell on the left edge. Feel free to write in this page and finish the dynamics of the cellular automata shown (Figure 1.15).

The patterns become more apparent when you use more than 10 cells and when you use black cells for "1" and white cells for "0." Of course that would be a bit more cumbersome to do by hand. You can explore the different patterns that emerge from different update rules with the MATLAB® code included at the end of this chapter in the exercises. Here is a screenshot of the rule 110, the rule we iterated earlier (Figure 1.16).

1	2	3	4	5	6	7	8
1 1 1	1 1 0	1 0 1	1 0 0	0 1 1	0 1 0	0 0 1	0 0 0
0	1	1	0	1	1	1	0

FIGURE 1.14 Definition of the rule for the next state.

1	0	0	1	0	1	1	0	0	1
1	0	1	1	1	1	1	0	1	1
1	1	1	0	0	0	1	1	1	0
1	0	1	0	0	1	1	0	1	1
1	1	1	0	1	1	1	1	1	0
1	0	1	1	1	0	0	0	1	1

Increasing time →

FIGURE 1.15 First five steps of cellular automata model.

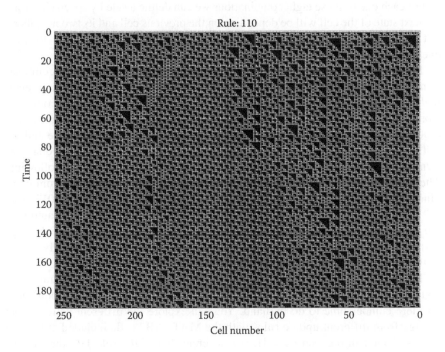

FIGURE 1.16 Screenshot of MATLAB® output for cellular automata rule 110.

SELF-ORGANIZATION IN HUMAN MOVEMENT

There are many examples of self-organization in nature (Camazine et al. 2001), both biological and nonbiological. In movement science, self-organization has been used to explain phenomena ranging from coordinated movements of limbs, body segments, and people, to the power law distributions of movement variability (Harrison and

Stergiou 2015). Perhaps the most well-known example of self-organization (as well as of the application of a dynamical systems approach) applied to an understanding of human movement is the Haken–Kelso–Bunz (HKB) model. The HKB model is a dynamical model of motor coordination. It was developed initially to describe the pattern of behavior observable in the simple task of rhythmically coordinating two fingers (Kelso 1981) but has since been applied to a wide range of motor coordination phenomena. The task involves simply oscillating your fingers in an antiphase pattern, such that one finger moves medially while the contralateral finger moves laterally and vice versa (see Figure 1.17a). If the required frequency of coordinated oscillation is increased, and you now slowly try to perform the task at a faster and faster rate, a curious phenomenon is observed. At a critical frequency you will observe your fingers

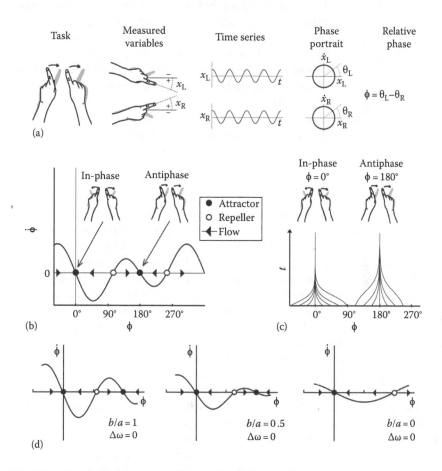

FIGURE 1.17   The dynamics of rhythmically coordinated finger movements. (Adapted from Harrison, S.J. and Stergiou, N., *Nonlinear Dyn. Psychol. Life Sci.*, 2015.) (a) Calculation of the collective variable relative phase. (b) The relative phase dynamics of the HKB equation. (c) From initial various initial conditions relative phase values are found to converge upon one of two stable states. (d) The relative phase dynamics of the HKB equation shown as a function of changes in the control parameter *b/a*.

spontaneously switch to an in-phase coordination pattern, such that both fingers are moving in the medial and lateral directions at the same time. In-phase refers to the fact that homologous (i.e., the same) muscles are involved at the same time. Antiphase (or alternatively out-of-phase) refers to the fact that nonhomologous muscles are involved at the same time in order to coordinate finger movements.

To model this phenomenon, Haken et al. (1985) developed the HKB model to capture the collective variable dynamics of this phenomenon. A collective variable is a variable that captures collective ordering or collective organization or a behavior. The collective variable identified for coordinated finger wiggling is relative phase (ϕ). As shown in Figure 1.17a relative phase is calculated by starting with the time series of the angle of oscillation of the component oscillators (i.e., fingers), and then calculating the phase of these oscillators. Here phase is simply defined in a space with dimensions of angle, and rate or change of angle (i.e., angular velocity). This phase space can be represented as a phase portrait in which we can calculate a phase angle (θ) for each oscillator. Relative phase is calculated as the difference in phase angle between the two phase angles. This collective variable captures in-phase coordination with a relative phase of $0°$ and antiphase coordination with a relative phase of $180°$.

The relative phase dynamics (i.e., how relative phase is constrained to change over time in this system) is captured by the following equation:

$$\dot{\phi} = \Delta\omega - a\sin(\phi) - 2b\sin(2\phi)$$

Here, $\dot{\phi}$ signifies differentiation with respect to time. The first term $\Delta\omega$ is used to denote the difference in intrinsic frequencies of the two oscillators in the model. For our present purposes $\Delta\omega$ is always 0. The parameters a and b are of key significance in the model. The ratio b/a acts as a control parameter in the model, such that changes in b/a are used to model changes in the collective frequency of oscillator movements. An increase in collective frequency is represented as a decrease in the ratio b/a. The relative phase dynamics for the equation, with $\Delta\omega = 0$ and $b/a = 1$, is shown in Figure 1.17b. Remembering that we are plotting relative phase against change in relative phase here, we can use this plot to graphically understand how the system will change over time given a particular initial value for relative phase. With reference for Figure 1.17b, if we start with a relative phase value of $45°$ we see that the rate of change of relative phase is negative, and as such the model predicts that the relative phase will change until it reaches $0°$ (i.e., in-phase coordination). Both $0°$ and $180°$ are referred to as stable fixed points or attractors. They represent states of coordination to which the system is organized to converge upon. This convergence can be seen in Figure 1.17c in which various initial relative phase values are seen to converge on either in-phase or antiphase coordination patterns. Note in Figure 1.17c that relative phase converges on the stable state at $0°$ faster than it does for the stable state at $180°$. The in-phase attractor at $0°$ is consequently said to have greater attractor strength. In Figure 1.17b both attractors and repellers are represented, capturing states the system is organized toward and away from respectively. This is captured by a vector field, with arrows shown to be pointing toward attractors, and away from repellers (Strogatz 1994). Here then we have graphically represented the two patterns that our fingers are drawn to when we coordinate them.

In Figure 1.17d we see the HKB equation plotted for three different values of the control parameter b/a. As we move from left to right across the plots, b/a decreases, and as such the frequency of finger coordination is modeled to decrease. As we decrease b/a (and increase finger oscillation frequency), a qualitative change in the relative phase dynamics is observed. At a critical frequency, one of the stable fixed points disappears. The antiphase attractor at 180° no longer exists. As this critical point is passed, a phase transition is said to have occurred, with the fingers transitioning from an antiphase to an in-phase coordination pattern. This particular phase transition represents a specific example of a bifurcation. We can now come to appreciate bifurcations as changes in number or type of fixed points in the dynamics of a system. You can see an animation of this by running the MATLAB program of the HKB model visualization found at the end of the chapter in the exercises.

The significance of the HKB equation, and of the dynamical systems approach more generally, is the discovered potential of simple models to capture multiple dimensions of biological phenomena and to produce nonobvious testable predictions. One such prediction in the case of the HKB model is hysteresis. We can see hysteresis in the case of coordinated finger movements if, after we transition from antiphase to in-phase coordination, we begin to decrease the frequency of coordination. If we do this we do not observe a transition back to antiphase as we move below the critical frequency. Rather the systems stays attracted to the continually stable in-phase mode of coordination.

What Is the Cause of Self-Organization?

Although the phenomenon of self-organization has been well characterized across myriad physical and biological systems, there are no widely agreed upon causes of self-organization. A general principle that does appear to apply across many of the identified instances of self-organization states that self-organization arises from a balance of competing processes. In the case of the HKB model the self-organized dynamics of coordinated finger movements are taken to arise from a balance of tendencies for competition and cooperation at the level of component oscillators. In the case of the simple growth model described earlier in this chapter, self-organization appears to arise from the interplay between positive and negative feedback. It will quickly become unsustainable in a natural system and require some form of limitation to keep the population in check. A graphical representation of a model with both positive and negative feedback is demonstrated with cellular automata. The iteration rules, in the context of density of ones and zeroes, have positive feedback (as the density of ones leads to more ones) and negative feedback (all ones may lead to zero). Positive and negative feedback loops are not readily apparent in the flocking behavior of birds. Positive feedback may be in the form of social interaction and protection from predation, whereas negative feedback may be as simple as getting too close so as to interrupt stable flight. In all cases, self-organization appears to be dependent upon the presence of nonlinear interactions between components of the system.

TELL-TALE SIGNS OF SELF-ORGANIZATION

There are multiple signatures you can look for in data to help identify if the system you are examining is self-organizing. The first sign is the existence of a control parameter and an order parameter, although they may not be a typically measured quantity. The control parameter should be something available for the experimenter to manipulate continuously. The order parameter should be a measured parameter that changes according to the control parameter. More specifically, continuous changes in the control parameter should move the system through critical points (also referred to as bifurcations, or phase transitions) in which the order parameter changes discontinuously. A classic example of a system with a control parameter and an order parameter is the logistic map that was described earlier. Let's revisit the logistic map to help us with these newer concepts we introduced.

The logistic map is defined by the following equation:

$$x_{t+1} = rx_t(1-x_t)$$

If you start this system with x between 0 and 1 and iterate it with the map, it can do many different things. The Figure 1.18 shows the behavior of the map after it has been iterated many times with r being held constant at various values. For smaller values of r, x will converge to a fixed point. For larger values of r, x will oscillate between 2, 4, 8, 16,... different values. At a certain value of r the logistic map displays chaotic dynamics. You can see in Figure 1.18 (and in Figure 1.8) that as the control parameter r is increased continuously, there are discontinuous changes in the order parameter (the periodicity of the system in this case).

While the logistic map only has a single variable and may not meet a strict definition of self-organization, coupled nonlinear iterative maps have been used to model cortical networks (Pashaie and Farhat 2009). These authors first developed mathematical models of each individual processing unit, and then coupled the resulting

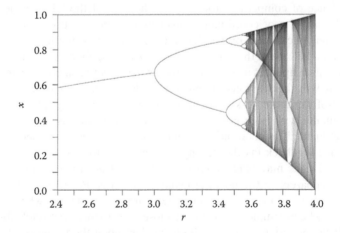

FIGURE 1.18 Bifurcation diagram for the logistic map.

complex elements using nonlinear couplings indirectly applied through the bifurcation parameters. They used the entropy of the activity of each element and the joint entropy between surrounding elements to quantify patterns of activity.

Another signature of a self-organizing system is the presence of multistability and hysteresis. A multistable system is one in which, for a single control parameter, there are multiple stable order parameters. Furthermore, multistability implies that noise in the system is sufficient to cause the system to switch between its multistable order parameters without any change in the control parameter. A similar situation is one of hysteresis. Hysteresis occurs when the value of the critical point (the point at which manipulation of a control parameter causes a bifurcation in the order parameter) depends upon the direction of change of the control parameter. A designed system that exhibits hysteresis is a thermostat that controls the temperature in one's house. If you set your thermostat to 72°F, it will cool the house if it detects temperatures above 72 and heat the house if it detects temperatures below 72. You do not want the heating and cooling to kick on often due to slight variations in the temperature so thermostats are built with hysteresis. Maybe the heat does not start until the temperature drops to 70 and the cooling does not start until the room temperature reaches 74. Interestingly, this is made possible by the addition of positive feedback. The simultaneous presence of positive and negative feedback in a system may not only produce self-organization and hysteresis, but is also the mechanism for chaos.

SELF-ORGANIZATION AND COMPLEXITY

> The laws of physics can explain how an apple falls but not why Newton, a part of a complex world, was watching the apple.
>
> **Bak (1997)**

Self-organization has been defined in many different ways by different people.

1. Self-organization is a process in which internal interactions of a system lead to the formation of patterns without any intervention by external processes (Haken 1977).
2. Self-organization is the spontaneous formation of patterns (Kelso 1995).
3. Self-organization is a process that leads to emergent patterns in a system of components (Camazine et al. 2001).
4. Self-organization is an "internally caused rise in complexity" (Shalizi et al. 2004).

We can see differences between these definitions but many commonalities as well. One interesting point to note here is that in the last definition—self-organization is a movement from lower complexity to higher complexity. In systems that have period doubling bifurcation cascades that lead to chaos, it has been demonstrated that complexity, by this definition, is maximized at the onset of chaos (Crutchfield 2011). Complexity is maximized in between complete order and disorder (Stergiou et al. 2006) (Figure 1.19). Thus, in systems that may exhibit chaos,

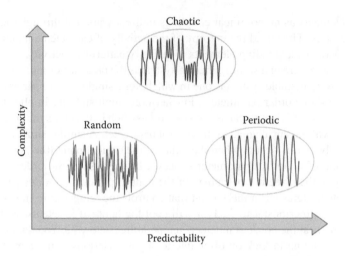

FIGURE 1.19 Chaotic systems lie between random and periodic systems in terms of predictability but are more complex than each of them.

self-organization is the movement, from order or disorder, toward the maximum complexity at the onset of chaos.

SELF-ORGANIZED CRITICALITY HYPOTHESIS OF MOVEMENT VARIABILITY

Another phenomenon that may be a product of self-organization is the presence of $1/f$ fractal scaling phenomenon movement variability. This fractal scaling (or power law, or $1/f$ noise) phenomenon arises in the variability of repeated performances of a task. It has been found in many phenomena that exist across many different time scales: heartbeat (Peng et al. 1993), finger tapping (Gilden et al. 1995), stride to stride fluctuations (Hausdorff et al. 1995), reaction times (Van Orden et al. 2003), self-esteem (Delignières et al. 2004), and more. The $1/f$ fractal scaling is where the spectral density as a function of the frequency obeys the following power law:

$$S(f) \approx \frac{1}{f^\beta}$$

In accordance with the definition, the value β can be found as the slope of a linear regression of the spectral density plotted against the frequency on a log–log plot, although more sophisticated methods have been developed as well (Peng et al. 1994; Wagenmakers et al. 2005).

One model for explaining this phenomenon is called self-organized criticality (Bak et al. 1987). In this model, the system requires no external manipulation of parameters but self-organizes to a critical point. An example of this behavior is found in a model of a sand pile. At each point in time, a grain of sand is dropped randomly on the sand pile. If the slope at that point is below a critical threshold, then the sand pile does not move and the slope at that point increases slightly. If the slope of the sand pile at that point goes beyond a certain threshold, then an avalanche is triggered, and sand is transferred down the slope. If the adjacent point down the slope is now above the threshold, then the avalanche continues. This system is attracted to have sand pile slopes exactly at the critical threshold (lower slopes build up and higher slopes decrease via avalanches). Thus, this system has a critical point as an attractor.

The sand pile model is a single instance of a class of self-organized criticality models. It leads to avalanche sizes and intervals between avalanches that obey a fractal power law. It has been proposed that this phenomenon is a source of natural complexity in nature (Bak et al. 1987), and that living systems will self-organize to this fractal scaling in order to be both creative and constrained in their behaviors (Van Orden et al. 2003).

SUMMARY

Dynamical systems theory, and complexity science more generally, has developed useful tools for analyzing and understanding the complex patterns to be found in measurements of biological and other systems. It has grown from the advances in understanding complex and nonlinear systems in physics and mathematics. In the case of movement patterns, this approach provides tools and techniques for investigating the dynamics of motor behavior that result from interactions between nervous system, body, and the surrounding environment in the performance of a particular task.

> When applied to human movement analysis "DST (dynamic systems theory) embraces the idea that the generation of movement patterns is multifactorial and that movement involves the coupling of the multiple degrees of freedom present in the human body."
>
> **Kurz and Stergiou (2004)**

This chapter has introduced the reader to important aspects of nonlinear analysis including dynamical systems, chaos, nonlinear dynamics, and complexity. It discussed the nonlinear dynamics of systems within and around us and how these can lead to chaos. The presence of chaos can be explained and understood though not always measured. Not all nonlinear systems are chaotic but all chaotic systems are nonlinear. Such systems transition from periodic to chaotic behavior and are highly sensitive to initial conditions.

The tools that exist to provide an understanding of the phase space geometry of nonlinear dynamical systems and for identifying and the presence of chaos will be discussed in detail in the succeeding chapters. Given the generality of the challenge of studying complex systems, new tools are continually being developed, and applied across a wide range of disciplines of scientific study. In some cases the nonlinear tools employed by movement scientists have originally been developed to meet the challenges of understanding and quantifying the dynamics of complex physical, chemical, neural, social, geologic, or economic systems. The methods introduced in this text are designed to account for (as opposed to average over) the complexity of the system under study. As such it is a reasonable expectation that when applied appropriately such measures may be more sensitive than their linear counterparts.

While the application and efficacy of the measures presented in this text do not require any particular theoretical commitments on the part of the scientist or clinician utilizing them, an understanding of dynamic systems theory provides a valuable perspective for interpreting them (see Harrison and Stergiou 2015). Dynamic systems theory also provides a starting point for investigating the hypothesis that observed behavior can be interpreted to be self-organized (Harrison and Stergiou 2015; Warren 2006). Biological and nonbiological systems often appear to create patterns in an apparently spontaneous manner without any external direction. It has been shown that the process of self-organization is a change from lower complexity to higher complexity, which in systems with period doubling bifurcation, is maximized at the onset of chaos. Self-organization is movement from order or disorder toward maximum complexity at the onset of chaos. For the movement scientist, the significance of the tools and techniques presented in this text is principally related to the hypothesis that the functionality of human movement (i.e., its stability and adaptability) is supported by both the complexity of the system, and principles of self-organization (Harrison and Stergiou 2015).

REFERENCES

Ashby, W.R., 1947. Principles of the self-organizing dynamic system. *Journal of General Psychology*, 37(2), 125–128.

Ayers, S., 1997. The application of chaos theory to psychology. *Theory & Psychology*, 7(3), 373–398.

Bak, P., 1997. How nature works: The science of self-organized criticality. *American Journal of Physics*, 65(6), 579.

Bak, P., Tang, C., and Wiesenfeld, K., 1987. Self-organized criticality: An explanation of the 1/f noise. *Physical Review Letters*, 59, 381–384.

Bolender, J., 2010. *The Self-Organizing Social Mind*, Cambridge, MA: MIT Press.

Camazine, S. et al., 2001. *Self-Organization in Biological Systems*, Princeton, NJ: Princeton University Press.

Çambel, A.B., 1993. *Applied Chaos Theory—A Paradigm for Complexity*, San Diego, CA: Academic Press Inc.

Crutchfield, J.P., December 2011. Between order and chaos. *Nature Physics*, 8, 17–24.

de Laplace, P.S.M., 1902. *A Philosophical Essay on Probabilities* (Trans.), London, U.K.: John Wiley & Sons.

Delignières, D., Fortes, M., and Ninot, G., 2004. The fractal dynamics of self-esteem and physical self. *Nonlinear Dynamics, Psychology, and Life Sciences*, 8(4), 479–510.

Feigenbaum, M.J., 1978. Quantitative universality for a class of nonlinear transformations. *Journal of Statistical Physics*, 19(1), 25–52.

Gilden, D., Thornton, T., and Mallon, M., 1995. 1/F noise in human cognition. *Science*, 267(5205), 1837–1839.

Haken, H., 1977. *Synergetics: An Introduction*, Berlin, Germany: Springer-Verlag.

Haken, H., Kelso, J.S., and Bunz, H., 1985. A theoretical model of phase transitions in human hand movements. *Biological Cybernetics*, 51(5), 347–356.

Harrison, S.J. and Stergiou, N., 2015. Complex adaptive behaviour and dexterous action. *Nonlinear Dynamics, Psychology, and Life Sciences*, 19(4), 345–394.

Hausdorff, J.M. et al., 1995. Is walking a random walk? Evidence for long-range correlations in stride interval of human gait. *Journal of Applied Physiology*, 78(1), 349–358.

Hilborn, R.C., 2000. *Chaos and Nonlinear Dynamics: An Introduction for Scientists and Engineers*, 2nd edn., Oxford, U.K.: Oxford University Press.

Hirsch, M., 1984. The dynamical systems approach to differential equations. *Bulletin of the American Mathematical Society*, 11(1), 1–64.

Hunt, B.R. and Yorke, J.A., 1993. Maxwell on chaos. *Nonlinear Science Today*, 3(1), 2–4.

Kantz, H. and Schreiber, T., 2004. *Nonlinear Time Series Analysis*, 2nd edn., Cambridge, U.K.: Cambridge University Press.

Kaplan, D. and Glass, L., 1995. *Understanding Nonlinear Dynamics*, New York: Springer.

Kauffman, S.A., 1995. *At Home in the Universe: The Search for Laws of Self-Organization and Complexity*, New York: Oxford University Press.

Kelso, J.A.S., 1995. *Dynamic Patterns: The Self-Organization of Brain and Behavior*, Cambridge, MA: MIT Press.

Kelso, J.A.S., 1981. On the oscillatory basis of movement. *Bulletin of the Psychonomic Society*, 18(2), 63.

Kugler, P.N. and Turvey, M.T., 1987. *Information, Natural Law, and the Self-Assembly of Rhythmic Movement: Resources for Ecological Psychology*, Hillsdale, NJ: Lawrence Erbaum Associates Inc.

Kurz, M.J. and Stergiou, N., 2004. Applied dynamic systems theory for the analysis of movement. In Stergiou, N., ed. *Innovative Analyses of Human Movement*, Champaign, IL: Human Kinetics, pp. 93–117.

Lett, C. and Mirabet, V., 2008. Modelling the dynamics of animal groups in motion. *South African Journal of Science*, 104(5–6), 192–198.

Lorenz, E.N., 1963. Deterministic nonperiodic flow. *Journal of the Atmospheric Sciences*, 20, 130–141.

Lorenz, E.N., 1972. Predictability: Does the flap of a butterfly's wings in Brazil, set up a tornado in Texas? *139th Meeting of American Association for the Advancement of Science*, Washington, DC. December 29, 1972.

May, R.M., 1976. Simple mathematical models with very complicated dynamics. *Nature*, 261, 459–467.

May, R.M. and Oster, G.F., 1976. Bifurcations and dynamic complexity in simple ecological models. *The American Naturalist*, 110(974), 573–599.

Moon, F.C. and Holmes, P.J., 1979. A magnetoelastic strange attractor. *Journal of Sound and Vibration*, 65(2), 275–296.

Mpitsos, G.J. and Soinila, S., 1993. In search of a unified theory of biological organization: What does the motor system of a sea slug tell us about human motor integration? In Newell, K.M. and Corcos, D., eds., *Variability and Motor Control*, Champagne, IL: Human Kinetics, pp. 225–290.

Pashaie, R. and Farhat, N.H., 2009. Self-organization in a parametrically coupled logistic map network: A model for information processing in the visual cortex. *IEEE Transactions on Neural Networks*, 20(4), 597–608.

Peng, C.K. et al., 1993. Long-range anticorrelations and non-Gaussian behavior of the heartbeat. *Physical Review Letters*, 70(9), 1343–1346.

Peng, C.K. et al., 1994. Mosaic organization of DNA nucleotides. *Physical Review E*, 49, 1685–1689.

Peters, E.E., 1994. *Fractal Market Analysis: Applying Chaos Theory to Investment and Economics*, New York, NY: John Wiley & Sons.

Reynolds, C.W., 1987. Flocks, herds and schools: A distributed behavioral model. In *ACM SIGGRAPH Computer Graphics*, ACM, New York, NY, pp. 25–34.

Richter, P.H. and Scholz, H.-J., 1984. Chaos in classical mechanics: The double pendulum. In Schuster, P., ed. *Stochastic Phenomena and Chaotic Behaviour in Complex Systems*, Bremen, Germany: Springer, pp. 86–97.

Shalizi, C., Shalizi, K., and Haslinger, R., 2004. Quantifying self-organization with optimal predictors. *Physical Review Letters*, 93, 2–5.

Shaw, E., 1975. Naturalist at large—Fish in schools. *Natural History*, 84, 40–46.

Shaw, R., 1984. *The Dripping Faucet as a Model Chaotic System*, Santa Cruz, CA: Aerial Press.

Sivakumar, B., 2000. Chaos theory in hydrology: Important issues and interpretations. *Journal of Hydrology*, 227(1–4), 1–20.

Stergiou, N., Harbourne, R., and Cavanaugh, J., 2006. Optimal movement variability: A new theoretical perspective for neurologic physical therapy. *Journal of Neurologic Physical Therapy*, 30(3), 120–129.

Strogatz, S.H., 1994. *Nonlinear Dynamics and Chaos: With Applications to Physics, Biology, Chemistry, and Engineering*, Reading, MA: Addison-Wesley Pub.

Thelen, E. and Smith, L.B., 1994. *A Dynamic Systems Approach to the Development of Cognition and Action*, Cambridge, MA: The MIT Press.

Thelen, E. and Smith, L.B., 2006. Dynamic systems theories. In Lerner, R.M. and Damon, W., eds. *Handbook of Child Psychology*, 6th edn., Vol. 1: Theoretical Models of Human Development, Hoboken, NJ: John Wiley & Sons, Inc., pp. 258–312.

Van Orden, G.C., Holden, J.G., and Turvey, M.T., 2003. Self-organization of cognitive performance. *Journal of Experimental Psychology: General*, 132(3), 331–350.

Wagenmakers, E.-J., Farrell, S., and Ratcliff, R., 2005. Human cognition and a pile of sand: A discussion on serial correlations and self-organized criticality. *Journal of Experimental Psychology: General*, 134(1), 108–116.

Warren, W.H., 2006. The dynamics of perception and action. *Psychological Review*, 113(2), 358–389.

Wiggins, S., 2010. *Introduction to Applied Nonlinear Dynamical Systems and Chaos*, 2nd edn., New York: Springer-Verlag.

Williams, G.P., 1997. *Chaos Theory Tamed*, Washington, DC: Joseph Henry Press.

Winfree, A.T., 2001. *The Geometry of Biological Time*, New York: Springer.

Wolfram, S., 1984. Universality and complexity in cellular automata. *Physica D: Nonlinear Phenomena*, 10(1–2), 1–35.

Wolfram, S., 2002. *A New Kind of Science*, Champaign, IL: Wolfram Media.

2 Time Series

Sara A. Myers

CONTENTS

What is a Time Series?...29
Some Examples of Time Series Data..32
Several Important Aspects of Time Series Data Analysis...34
    Length of the Time Series 35
    Sampling Frequency and Spectral Analysis...36
    Noise 41
    Filtering and Smoothing..42
    Resolution 45
    Stationarity..46
A General Note on Experimental Limitations of Time Series Data 49
Exercises 50
References..51

To see a world in a grain of sand,
And a heaven in a wild flower,
Hold infinity in the palm of your hand,
And eternity in an hour.

William Blake (1757–1827)

WHAT IS A TIME SERIES?

Time series is "simply a list of numbers assumed to measure some process sequentially in time" (Stergiou et al. 2004). Mathematicians have a more formal definition, that is, a set or a sequence of observations, with each one recorded at specific times, or at least sequentially (Brockwell and Davis 2002; Box et al. 2008). Time series are created from multiple sources for research purposes to understand various behaviors. For example, social scientists could collect graduation rates, physiologists record heart rates, economists study consumer spending, and climatologists examine weather patterns. Basically, any time observations are taken repeatedly over time, from any source or behavior, a time series is created.

A basic assumption of most time series analysis is that all time series inherently possess dependence between adjacent observations. In fact, this dependence is of interest because it reveals information about the source producing the behavior. In this way, time series analysis is essential for understanding human movement variability, because time series analysis reveals how the system evolves over multiple movement repetitions. To generate a time series, repeated measurements of some property of the system are made as the system varies in time. This may imply that time series data are essentially a list of numbers, but any list of numbers cannot be considered a time series. This chapter details what constitutes time series data and describes important specific considerations that should be kept in mind when working with time series data.

Consider the following two lists of numbers:

List A: 1, 2, 3, 4, 5
List B: 3, 1, 4, 2, 5

The average value for list A is 3; the average value for list B is 3. The range for list A is 4; the range for list B is 4. The standard deviation for list A is 1.58, and the standard deviation for list B is 1.58. Thus, the statistical descriptors of the two lists are the same—we cannot tell the difference between these two lists by these statistical measures. However, by examining the lists, it is easy to observe that they are not the same. The difference between the two lists is the order in which the numbers appear in the sequence, that is, to understand the difference between the two lists, we must examine these lists as ordered lists of numbers. To indicate an ordered list, we will use the notation [1, 2, 3, 4, 5] for list A, and [3, 1, 4, 2, 5] for list B. Further, to investigate the difference between these two lists, we would need an analysis technique that is sensitive to the order of the numbers in the list. In fact, the remaining chapters of this book discuss various methods of data analysis that quantify various aspects of the patterns formed by lists of numbers, based on the order in which the numbers appear in the sequence.

Time series data are a specific example of an ordered list of numbers, where time is the parameter that gives order to the list. For example, say every year on your daughter's birthday you measure her height, starting at age 5 until age 15. Her height in centimeters is [108, 115, 121, 128, 134, 140, 146, 152, 157, 161, 163]. Her age in years at each measurement is [5, 6, 7, 8, 9, 10, 11, 12, 13, 14, 15]. You can line them up, and each number in the top list is recorded at the same time as the corresponding one in the other list.

[108, 115, 121, 128, 134, 140, 146, 152, 157, 161, 163]
[5,   6,   7,   8,   9, 10, 11, 12, 13, 14, 15]

If you want to make a plot of height versus age, you will plot the pairs of corresponding numbers, that is, plot (5, 108), then plot (6, 115), then plot (7, 121), etc., because you will want to plot the first value, then plot the second value, then plot the third value, etc. (Figure 2.1).

Another way to record your daughter's age is to write the age at which she is 10 cm taller than the previous measurement. This ordered list would be age in years of [5.0, 6.5, 8, 9.5, 11.2, 13.1] and the corresponding height in cm is [108, 118, 128, 138, 148, 158]. This is also a time series. However, these readings were not taken at even time intervals. They are still time series data because they are an ordered list that is ordered based on time. Note that some analysis techniques

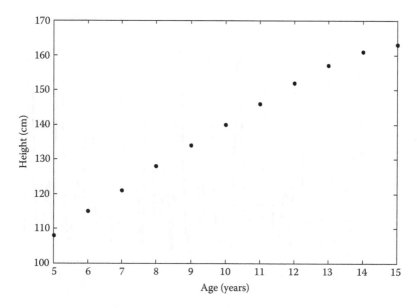

FIGURE 2.1 Plot of height versus age for a hypothetical girl. A time series is formed by the ordered list of how the girl's height changes with each year increase in age.

assume equal time intervals between data points (such as the spectral analysis technique to be discussed later), so be aware of which type of data you are analyzing. This is where the concepts of discrete versus continuous time series (discussed in Chapter 1) become important. Discrete time series are series in which observations are made in discrete sets, such as at specific, fixed time intervals (Brockwell and Davis 2002). The term "continuous data or continuous time series" is described in various ways depending on the source. According to Brockwell and Davis, continuous series are those in which observations are recorded continuously for a specific amount of time (Brockwell and Davis 2002). However, Warner describes continuous data as those with a true interval/ratio level of measurement, or data in which the difference between two values is meaningful (Warner 1998). Discrete time series is also described as a sampling of continuous time series at certain intervals (Box et al. 2008). Most time series, which are analyzed using techniques described in this book, are discrete time series, with observations made at equal intervals (Warner 1998; Brockwell and Davis 2002; Box et al. 2008). As the examples that follow will illustrate, even time series that appear continuous, when examined closely, are composed of individual data points.

Now that we have a definition of what a time series is, let us examine some human movement data, that is, a plot of the knee angle versus time during walking (Myers et al. 2013, 1692–1702; Figure 2.2). These data were collected by applying several reflective markers to different body segments on a subject's body, making a video of the subject while walking, and then identifying where the markers were located in each frame of the video. Because the cameras had been calibrated to measure distance in three-dimensional space, the position of the markers could be used to

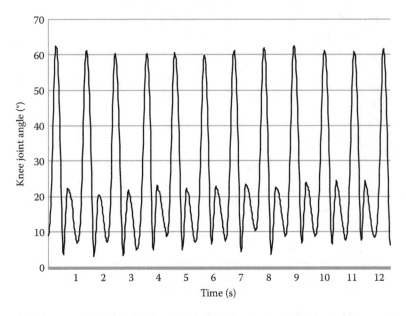

FIGURE 2.2　Plot of right knee flexion and extension angle versus time for a healthy older subject while walking.

calculate the position of the body segments in each frame, and knowing that, a knee angle could be calculated for each frame.

The time series plotted in Figure 2.2 is the knee angle calculated from each frame in the video, with the time at which the frame was acquired plotted on the x axis. If you zoom in on just 1.5 s of the data (Figure 2.3), you can see that the data are not actually a continuous line, but rather it is composed of individual points. In other words, the time series is not continuous, but rather it is discrete. If you count the dots in the 1.5 s of data, you will find that there are 90 points. This is because the camera acquiring the video was taking a picture about every 0.0167 s, or 60 frames/s (60 frames/s times 1.5 s = 90 data points). The Hertz, or Hz for short, is a common unit of measure for how many data points are acquired every second. In this example, the data were collected at 60 Hz.

SOME EXAMPLES OF TIME SERIES DATA

Time series analysis is useful in many different situations, whenever you are trying to describe the change of a system with time, that is, the dynamics of the system. For example, a psychologist had subjects fill out a survey once a day for 4 weeks, scoring the answers, and creating a time series that has 28 points (Fredrickson and Losada 2005). Astronomers have observed sunspot activity annually since 1700 by counting sunspots visible on the sun, creating a time series of length 314 (Figure 2.4; National Office of Oceanic and Atmospheric Administration 2013). Physiologists analyzed blood samples for luteinizing hormone every 10 min for 4 days, creating a time series 577 points long (Liu et al. 2007). Biomechanists interested in the gait function of patients with peripheral arterial disease analyzed the ankle flexion and

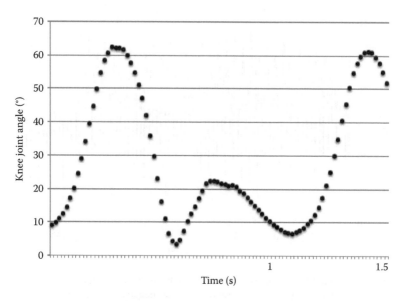

FIGURE 2.3 Expanded plot of right knee flexion and extension angle versus time for a healthy older subject while walking.

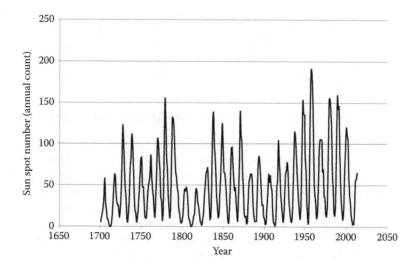

FIGURE 2.4 Plot of yearly sunspot activity data from National Office of Oceanic and Atmospheric Administration (2014) from 1700 until 2013. Analysis reveals that there is a cycle in sunspot activity, with activity maximizing about every 10.5 years.

extension angles captured by cameras taking 60 pictures/s for 45 s, resulting in a time series 2700 points long (Myers et al. 2009, 2011). Data from this experiment describe adjustments of the ankle with each step while walking on a treadmill. These adjustments are meaningful because they reflect the cooperative strategies of the locomotor system and are considered a marker of the system's health (Figure 2.5).

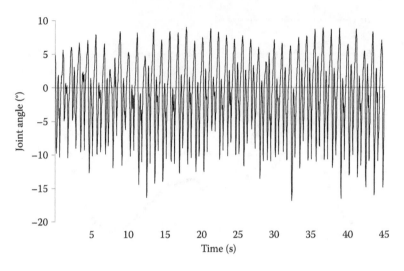

FIGURE 2.5   Ankle flexion and extension motion during walking in a patient with peripheral arterial disease. Plantarflexion is represented as negative values and dorsiflexion is shown with positive values. Data were collected at 60 Hz for 45 s, creating a time series that is 2700 data points long.

As you can see from this wide range of examples, there is no typical application of time series analysis. Scientists, engineers, and clinicians from many different disciplines use time series analysis to provide an understanding the dynamics of whatever system they are studying. While all these different applications may seem entirely unrelated, the methodology of the analysis overlaps considerably.

SEVERAL IMPORTANT ASPECTS OF TIME SERIES DATA ANALYSIS

While there are many varied uses for the analysis of time series data, there are some general aspects that are important regardless of the application, and these considerations are discussed in the following sections. Perhaps the most important initial consideration is the goal of the analysis. A general goal of all time series analysis is to understand the patterns in the data. How that understanding is to be used will influence the type of analyses that will be performed. The goals of time series analysis include forecasting, determining a transfer function for predictive purposes, describing a phenomenon or relationships between related time series, studying the effect of interventions on the time series, developing control schemes, and others (Warner 1998; Brockwell and Davis 2002; Box et al. 2008). Each of these purposes can be applied in varying domains from predicting the stock market, understanding weather patterns, or describing movement problems that result from pathology. Linear time series analysis methods assume observations are independent of past history. However, sequential observations of human movement are rarely independent of each other. This book acknowledges this fact and approaches human movement from this exact perspective that seems mostly lost in the current literature. Therefore, important features discussed here are centered on nonlinear algorithmical techniques to investigate human movement. However, regardless of the investigative approach, it is always essential to consider several fundamental issues of time series analysis. These include length of the time series, noise, resolution, stationarity and inherent periodicity, sampling frequency, spectral analysis, and filtering and smoothing. Each algorithm presented in this book has unique requirements, and many of these issues will be revisited in upcoming chapters. In the following section, we discuss these considerations as applicable for all algorithms.

LENGTH OF THE TIME SERIES

The length of the time series is often seen as a major limitation for the utilization of a certain types of analyses for time series data. In particular, for nonlinear analysis, the individuals (usually mathematicians) who have derived the formulas suggest that a certain number of data points are critical for performing the analysis. It is not that the nonlinear calculation with fewer data points than what they suggest cannot be done, but the problem is whether the answer received from using a shorter time series is really an accurate characterization of the dynamics of the system.

From a more intuitive perspective, you need a time series long enough to capture the essential dynamics of the system. As an example, consider the periodic behavior of the sunspot cycle. It takes over 10 years for the cycles to repeat. If you only record sunspot activity for 5 years, you would not be able to discover from your data that there is a 10-year cycle. If you collect 10 years, you will observe a complete cycle, but you would not know that the same pattern will be repeated. The more complete the cycles you have, the better your ability to characterize the dynamics, just as in estimating the population mean, the more samples you have from that population the better.

So how long is long enough? This depends on which analytical technique you want to use—some require more data than others. One mathematical rule of thumb is that you want a time series that is at least 10^D data points in length, where D is the dimensionality of the system. The dimensionality will be discussed later in the book, but for many systems of interest, it is probably at least three, and likely a bit higher, depending on the system that you are studying. So if the dimension of your system happens to be 6, you need 10^6 or 1,000,000 data points. However, whether or not it is practical to obtain such a time series is another important consideration. Let us say you are studying ecological time series data, such as the annual population of a certain species. You can only collect one data point per year, so a technique that requires 1,000,000 data points is clearly out of the question. Less stringent guidelines suggest having at least 5 and if possible 10 repetitions of the cycle to be able to understand the underlying dynamics (Warner 1998).

The problem with the discussion is that, while the inventor of certain technique can only guarantee the results if there are this large number of data points, the technique may be somewhat robust with respect to sample size and thus able to give reasonable results for a smaller number of data points. The big question, then, is how robust are the techniques for nonlinear analysis with respect to the length of the time series. This varies from one technique to the next, and even for a given technique, different algorithms can have different requirements. Also see the following discussion about sampling frequency as it relates to the length of the time series.

Sampling Frequency and Spectral Analysis

Sampling frequency is a critical consideration when dealing with time series data. It is a measure of how often you acquire a data sample, and thus, sampling frequency multiplied by the length of time that you sampled gives the number of data points in your time series. The sampling frequency needs to be high enough to capture the dynamics of the quickest changes in your system. For example, with the sunspot data (Figure 2.4), there is a cycle about every 10.5 years. So if you only sampled every 20 years, you would miss it. Even if you sampled every 10 years, that would not be enough to catch the cycle. The minimum frequency at which you need to sample in order to have a chance of obtaining periodic dynamics is twice the frequency of the fastest dynamics. This principle is known as the Nyquist sample theory. But this gives you only two data points for every cycle, so going up to a sampling frequency of about five times the fastest frequency is a good rule of thumb for periodic data. In human locomotion, the highest frequencies that occur during walking are less than 12 Hz. Thus, a 24 Hz sampling rate should be satisfactory; however, in reality, biomechanists usually sample at 5–10 times the highest frequency in the signal. Remember, if data are undersampled, the entire signal is not captured. If data are oversampled, more measurement noise could be introduced.

So how do you decipher what frequencies are in your data? One method is spectral analysis, which entails breaking down the biological signal into simple signals. The typical approach to analyzing data is to describe the data in terms of how they change over time, which is known as the time domain. An alternative approach arises in the form of data analysis in the frequency domain. This type of analysis presents data as a function of frequencies contained in the signal rather than a function of amplitudes over time. Frequency-domain analysis is used extensively to provide additional insights into healthy and pathological movement (Giakas et al. 1996; Giakas and Baltzopoulos 1997; Stergiou et al. 2002; Giakas 2004; Wurdeman et al. 2011; McGrath et al. 2012). More specifically, spectral analysis is a numerical technique to write your data as the sum of multiple discrete sine and cosine functions of different frequencies. There are many different frequency transforms available, but the most commonly used transform is the Fourier transform. This transform uses sums of sine and cosine functions to represent the more complex functions, in our case, signals of human movement. The plot of the power at each frequency is referred to as the power spectral density plot or simply the power spectrum.

Calculating the power spectrum is like shining light through a prism. Just as the prism shows the light has many component colors, the spectral analysis shows your data as many component wave functions. There are four characteristics of signals included in the sine and cosine waves that represent the signal. These are frequency, amplitude, vertical offset or shift off the baseline, and the phase angle, which indicates where the signal starts and shifts from right to left. Any signal, $h(t)$ is made up of these four characteristics. Equation 2.1 incorporates each of these variables:

$$h(t) = A_0 + A\sin(2\pi ft + \theta) \qquad (2.1)$$

but $2\pi f = \omega$, so another way to write Equation 2.1 is Equation 2.2:

$$h(t) = A_0 + A\sin(\omega t + \theta) \tag{2.2}$$

where
A_0 is the offset
A is the amplitude
f is the frequency
θ is the phase shift
ω is the angular velocity

Thus, if you know these characteristics, then you can write the equation for the signal.

To demonstrate how different frequencies contribute to a signal consider the following: a sine wave of 3 Hz, a cosine wave of 13 Hz, a sine wave of 30 Hz, and the sum of these three wave functions. The peak in the power spectrum corresponds to the frequency of the wave function in the time series (Figure 2.6a through c), and the time series that is a sum of three wave functions has three peaks, corresponding to the three frequencies which were added together (Figure 2.6d). The reason for wanting to divide your data into sine and cosine functions is because then you can see which frequencies are contributing the most to your data just by examining the peak positions. If the peak corresponding to 3 Hz is very high, then you likely have a 3 Hz component in your signal. If the 3 Hz component of your signal is the highest frequency that is significant, then you know you would need a sampling frequency of at least 6 Hz (2×3 Hz = 6 Hz) to be able to see it, but something more like 15 Hz (5×3 Hz = 15 Hz) would be best to define it better. For real data, determining the highest frequency can be a bit tricky, because often the signal approaches the baseline gradually without a clear cutoff point (Figure 2.7).

To examine the sampling frequency issue from another perspective, let us examine sampling a known signal at various frequencies (Figure 2.8). Each frame on the left side of Figure 2.8 shows the signal we are trying to sample in a solid black line, and the data that we actually sample in black dots, with a line connecting the dots. Each frame on the right side is the power spectrum calculated from the data that we sampled (from the black dots). The signal that we are trying to sample is the sum of two wave functions, one at 2 Hz and one at 3 Hz; it is the same data as in Figure 2.6d. In Figure 2.8a, the sampling frequency is 30 Hz—10 times the highest frequency in the signal we are trying to sample. The curve fits the data so well that the plot of the actual data can barely be seen. Moving down in Figure 2.8, the sampling frequency is reduced. At 6 Hz, the sampling rate is twice the highest frequency in the signal, and one can see from the power spectrum that the spectral analysis is just barely able to capture the highest frequency peak. However, examining the time series plot on the left, we see that the there are significant gaps where the sampled data do not match the signal of interest very well. The power spectrum contains all peaks that it should based on the original data. So, based on this spectral analysis, 6 Hz is the lowest sampling rate that is acceptable. At even lower sampling rates (Figure 2.8e), peaks show up in the power spectra that do not belong based on the known dynamics

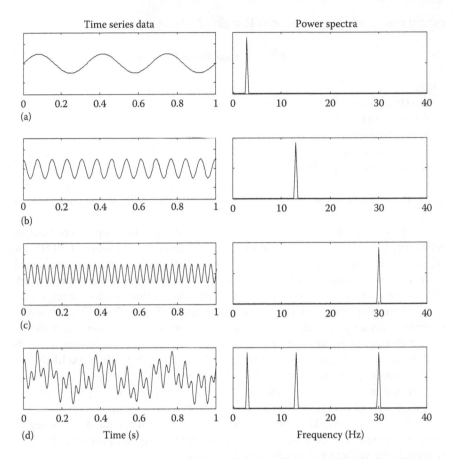

FIGURE 2.6 Time series data (left) and corresponding power spectra (right) for a sine wave of 3 Hz (a), a cosine wave of 13 Hz (b), a sin wave of 30 Hz (c), the sum of these three wave functions (d).

of the time series. This phenomenon is called aliasing and is the reason that you always need to have a sampling rate at least twice the highest frequency of interest in your time series.

Spectral analysis is a very powerful tool for finding periodic components in your data, and thus, it is widely used. But you should bear in mind that it is a mathematical technique to write your time series data as a sum of sine and cosine functions. The interpretation of the periodicity in your data depends on your understanding of the underlying mechanism, and what periodicity or lack thereof means in terms of the system you are studying. There are a number of software programs that will allow you to calculate the power spectrum of your data, but there are many subtleties, not discussed here (such as windowing, detrending, and zero-padding (Percival and Walden 1993; Stoica and Moses 1997; Huang et al. 1998; Beard 2003; Prabhu 2013), that can help you do a better job with the analysis. See Percival and Walden (1993), or any good digital signal processing textbook for a more in-depth discussion of

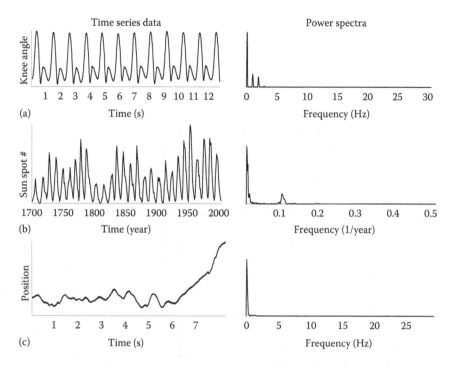

FIGURE 2.7 Time series data (left) and corresponding power spectra (right) for knee joint angle (a), sun spot number (b), and the front-to-back postural sway from infant sitting (c). Unlike the sine wave, determining the highest occurring frequency for actual data is not clear-cut. Here, the highest frequency is approximately 3 Hz for the knee joint angle, 0.1 Hz for sun spot number, and 1 Hz for the front-to-back postural sway.

spectral analysis. Or, for a more lighthearted introduction, see "Who Is Fourier? A Mathematical Adventure" (Sakakibara 1995).

   Much of the discussion so far has focused on acquiring sufficient data—the algorithms require long time series, and higher sampling frequencies ensure that higher frequency components are captured in the data. However, there are reasons not to just sample at the highest frequency possible. One limitation may just be storage space. If you sample at 10,000 Hz instead of 100 Hz, you have 100 times as much data to store. With computer memory being cheaper and cheaper, this is not the problem once was. But do not be confused by the requirement of many of the non-linear analysis algorithms for having a large number of data points, and think that you can crank up the sampling frequency to get the required number of data points. Remember that the reason you need all those data points is because you need to track the system over a long enough time that the dynamics of the system can be observed. For example, the sunspot data (Figure 2.6b) have a cycle of about 10.5 years. The data were acquired every year for over 307 years. One could gather data every day for 1 year and have an even longer time series (365 data points). But even though the time series is longer, it would not allow you to determine the 10.5-year cycle. This is because you need to let the system evolve for long enough time that the essential

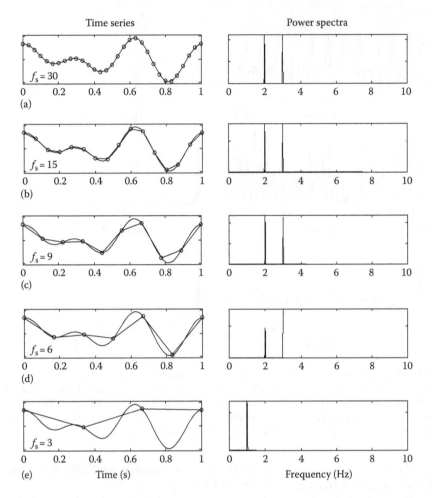

FIGURE 2.8 Time series data (left) and corresponding power spectra (right) for sum of a 2 and a 3 Hz wave function. Smooth plot of left side is the underlying signal; the black circles are data points sampled from the underlying signal, and the sampled data points are connected by black lines to show the time series that one would obtain if sampling at the frequencies indicated (a) 30 Hz, (b) 15 Hz, (c) 9 Hz, (d) 6 Hz, and (e) 3 Hz. The power spectra on the right side were calculated using the sampled data points. As the sampling frequency is reduced, the actual dynamics of the sample are lost in the signal, but until 3 Hz, all frequency peaks are still present. When sampled at 3 Hz, peaks at frequencies that are not part of the actual data begin to show up, which is called aliasing.

dynamics can be captured. Sampling every day does not tell you much about the 10.5-year cycle, because the system has not evolved significantly from one data sample to the next. In other words, the result you get today will be highly correlated with the result you get tomorrow. This concept will be elaborated further in the chapter that contains the discussion of the autocorrelation function (Chapter 8).

Noise

In any experimental measurement, there are always concerns about measurement error or contamination of what you are trying to measure with other information that you are not trying to measure. For example, let us assume that I am measuring the position of a simple pendulum as a function of time. The time series in Figure 2.9a represents the actual position of a pendulum bob. Random noise, representing measurement error, is plotted in Figure 2.9b.

Noise is particularly important for the nonlinear analyses. Often the assumption is made that the noise is "random" meaning that there is no correlation between noise at one data point and the noise at another data point. You may recall from physics that white light contains all colors of visible light and that the prism separates the light into component colors. The spectral analysis described here plays on the analogy between separating light into component colors based on frequency and separating time series data into wave functions (sine and cosine functions) with different frequencies. When random noise is broken down into a sum of sine and cosine functions, it has all frequencies that the time series can have represented. Thus, it is called "white" noise to emphasize that it has all frequencies, just as white light has

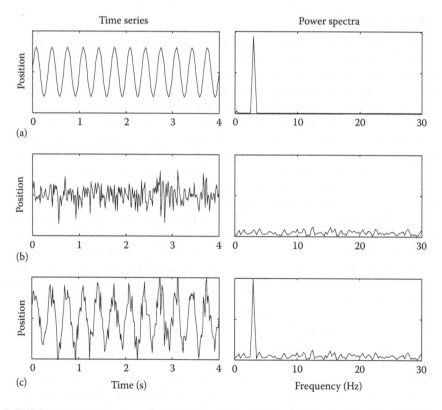

FIGURE 2.9   Sine function (a), white noise (b), and the sum of the sine function and white noise (c). The left side is the time series, and the right side is the power spectrum. The sine function represents the position of a pendulum bob.

all colors in it. The power spectrum of white noise is flat, as can be seen by look-ing carefully at the baseline in Figure 2.9b and comparing it to the zero baseline in Figure 2.9a. When the signal is contaminated by white noise, this is also seen in the power spectrum (Figure 2.9c).

However, there is no guarantee that the noise in an experiment will be white noise. For example, the AC power outlets into which data acquisition equipment is plugged are 60 Hz power in North America and many other parts of the world and 50 Hz in Europe. The equipment is designed to minimize the contamination of the output from this power line noise, but the result is not perfect, and so 60 Hz (or 50 Hz in Europe) is a common type of noise that can be seen in data acquired at 120 Hz (or 100 Hz in Europe) or higher sampling frequency (recall the requirement to sample at twice any given frequency to detect it). Thus, the problem with noise in nonlinear dynamics analysis is that you are trying to detect the dynamics of the system of interest, and the experimental data may be contaminated by a signal with unknown dynamics. As in any experiment, anything that can optimize the signal-to-noise ratio is beneficial. Additionally, some of the algorithms to be discussed in other chapters may be more robust to experimental noise than others.

FILTERING AND SMOOTHING

Experimental noise is a problem in time series analysis. As highlighted in the previ-ous section, interference from other biological signals, movement artifacts or high-frequency noise in our acquisition system contaminate the dynamics of our signal of interest. One approach commonly used to deal with these issues in time series analysis is filtering the data. "Filtering" comes from the analogy to light, where a color filter allows only certain wavelengths of light to pass. For example, a red filter absorbs green light, and allows the red light to pass through, so when you look through the filter, everything appears as shades of red. One might call a red filter a "red pass" filter, since red light is allowed to pass through it. Any operation that changes the data by reducing or amplifying components in either the time or frequency domain should be considered filtering. Another common term for filtering is "smoothing," which comes from the idea that data become smoother when fit to an equation such as polynomials or splines (more about this later) (Woltring 1985; Dohrmann et al. 1988; Vaughan et al. 1999; Giakas 2004). Whether the data should be filtered or not depends on the research question. When asking questions about movement variability, filtering and smoothing are avoided as much as possible. However, these operations are commonly performed in discrete point analyses, especially those that use differentiation with multiple calcu-lation steps such as joint torque and power calculations. Differentiation in this case is the calculation of velocity and acceleration from displacement data. This process pref-erentially amplifies higher frequencies. Thus, every time you differentiate, the noise becomes larger relative to the signal, so the measurement noise must be filtered to maintain the biological phenomenon. Velocities are noisier than positions and accel-erations are noisier than velocities. Position data must be smoothed before calculating velocities and accelerations. The first central difference method (of differentiation) is a type of smoothing: averaging. To check whether the proper smoothing was performed, the position, velocity, and acceleration should be graphed. The more filtering that is performed, or the more frequencies that are removed, the "smoother" the signal will be. However, this is exactly when you need to consider if you have missed any important true biological phenomena, especially high-frequency impact phenomena. This is notoriously the case with running related biomechanical data in the literature where kinematics are filtered with a cutoff below 6 Hz even though important high-frequency phenomena exist between 12 and 20 Hz (Giakas 2004). We believe that one of the reasons for the lack of a true understanding of the mechanisms behind running injuries is actually the massive contamination of the literature with inaccurate results which stifle scientific progress (Stergiou et al. 1999; Giakas 2004).

A common type of smoothing is using polynomials. In this method, the data are forced to fit a certain mathematical model. This is a poor method because there is limited control over what data are included or excluded, so it is likely that true data will be removed. A better method that is an extension of the idea of using polynomials to smooth is the spline. A spline function consists of a number of low-order polynomials that are pieced together. Cubic, or third order, and quartic, or fourth order, splines are the most popular for biomechanics applications. Another type of smoothing is digital filtering. Again, the basic premise of filtering in time series analysis is based on the idea of breaking up the measured signal into its various frequency components using the spectral analysis techniques discussed earlier, and then removing frequencies that are not of interest. Filtering is performed by setting a key frequency known as the cutoff frequency. The cutoff informs the filter to keep or remove subsequent or remaining frequencies. Filters also differ based on the operation used to change the frequency components, which is called the transfer function. The type of transfer function determines which frequencies are kept and which are filtered. Three different bands can be used in a transfer function, including a pass, transition, and stop. A pass preserves the specified frequency components, a transition band progressively decreases the power of the frequency components covered, and the stop band removes all remaining frequencies.

There are also different algorithms that can be implemented to correctly filter the data. Two of the most common implementations of this technique are the Butterworth filter, the critically damped filter, and the Jackson filter (Smith 2002). The algorithms will use the selected cutoff and contain different bands depending on what type of data are being smoothed. One can select whether to remove frequencies above a certain cutoff frequency, called a "low-pass" filter, because lower frequencies are allowed to pass through the filter. A "high-pass" filter would block low frequencies and allow high frequencies to pass through. A "band pass" or "notch pass" filter passes through frequencies in an intermediate range, while rejecting higher and lower frequencies. Because random noise is a high-frequency component of the measured signal, a low-pass filter is used to remove it. The cutoff frequency must be carefully selected to remove noise without removing the signal of interest. Figure 2.10b shows that a cutoff frequency above the three features of interest leaves them intact, but if the cutoff frequency is too low (Figure 2.10c and d), the peaks of interest are removed. It is important to select a cutoff frequency that will preserve most of the data of interest. Typically, a cutoff frequency that maintains 99% of the data is chosen. The roll-off is the transition between areas to maintain or smooth. The slope of the cutoff is the roll-off and this changes with the order of the polynomial. As the order is increased, the sharpness of the slope is increased and vice versa.

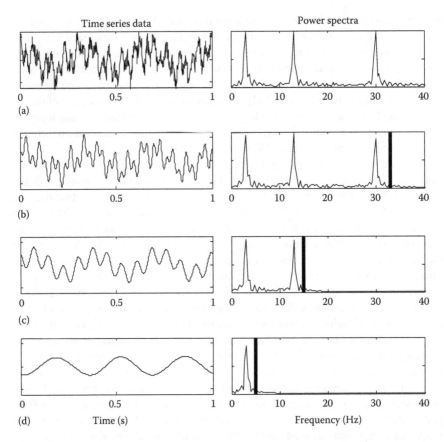

FIGURE 2.10 Time series left and power spectrum right: (a) unfiltered, (b) filtered using a cutoff frequency of 33 Hz, (c) filtered using a cutoff frequency of 15 Hz, and (d) filtered using a cutoff frequency of 5 Hz. The filter used was a "brick wall" filter (very high-order Butterworth filter), and cutoff frequency is indicated by vertical bar.

There are many decisions to be made when it comes to whether and how to filter data. Ultimately, the hypotheses and research questions should determine which filter should be implemented. One way to make sure that filtering is not altering the data in a way that changes the phenomenon is to filter interactively. This is important because a computer has no way to know when the filter being implemented is affecting the data. As the filter is being applied, the raw data should be graphed with the filtered data to make sure that phenomena are not being smoothed out of the data. A good starting point to know what not to filter is to think back to sampling theorem. Based on Nyquist sample theory, data under the Nyquist frequency should not be filtered. The discussion later regarding the potential biological importance of nonstationarity further emphasizes this point.

Filtering data is a very common method of data manipulation for many types of linear analyses. The problem is that most of the filtering techniques are based on statistically preserving the linear features of the data. These methods, such as

Butterworth filtering, were not designed to be used on data that will subsequently be analyzed using nonlinear techniques. Thus, there is no reason to believe that the nonlinear dynamics of the time series would still be intact after filtering, and in fact, one would expect that these methods would be counterproductive for nonlinear analysis (Rapp et al. 1993; Theiler and Eubank 1993). Some nonlinear filters have been developed, but again testing them on experimental data is problematic because the nature of the underlying attractor, if there is one, is unknown. Thus, it is likely the filter is distorting the underlying dynamics (Kantz and Schreiber 2003). Data previously described or seen as "noisy" have been shown in recent literature to have deterministic patterns and provide important information about the dynamics of the system. Filtering the time series can alter the embedding dimension needed to properly reconstruct the state space and can influence results of calculations of the time lag and others. In nearly all situations presented in this book, it is recommended that filtering be avoided (or at least be considered with extreme care) to capture the true dynamics of the system.

RESOLUTION

The concept of significant figures is probably familiar from high school. If a person's height is measured by comparing with the door frame, then the person might be measured to be about 72 in. (two significant figures). If a tape measure is used, the person's height might be measured as 72.75 in. (four significant figures). The more significant figures used, the more precision the measurement has, and the greater the number of figures that need to be recorded in the lab notebook. A similar issue arises when using computers for data acquisition in that different measurement techniques have different levels of precision associated with them. For example, if one is using video cameras to record knee angles, the resolution of the camera will limit the precision with which the knee position can be measured. If the knee position stored in the computer is examined, then after seeing 13.67485362842 stored as knee position for a given frame, it might be concluded that there are 13 significant figures. The problem is that typically the computer can store more significant figures than your measurement technique can provide. If one divides one (one significant figure) by three (one significant figure), your calculator will show 0.333333333, with as many three's as the screen will allow it to show. Doing division does not increase the number of significant figures in the result. Similarly, knee position of 13.67485362842 is limited by the pixel resolution of the camera, not by how many digits the computer can store. Some measurement techniques have better precision than others, so you need to be familiar with the limitations of the equipment being used.

The algorithms that have been developed for performing nonlinear analysis are often generated and tested by people who are not working with experimental data, but rather work with computer-generated time series. Computer programs are written to produce a time series based on known equations, the Lorenz equations, for example. The time series created in this manner has no noise, and precision as high as the computer is capable of storing. Experimental data, on the other hand, will likely be contaminated with some measurement noise and will only be able to measure the parameter of interest to a limited degree of precision. Why is a little round-off error a problem? A chaotic-behaving system is sensitive to small perturbations, frequently discussed in terms of sensitivity to initial conditions. Some of the algorithms used to study such systems may give different results depending on the precision of the data used. In fact, Lorenz discovered this property of chaotic systems when he entered the result of a previous calculation by hand into his computer and rounded it off as he entered it, only to find that the rounded off number gave dramatically different results in the calculation than the higher precision number that was not entered by hand on another run (Kerry 2008). In general, the significant digits should be used, as determined by the equipment measuring the phenomenon. It is recommended that you test the effect of rounding the data on the outcome value of the particular algorithm used to see how rounding may change the results. A detailed guide for testing the limitations of any particular algorithm can be found at the end of the chapter, which will guide decisions on the number of digits to use for time series analysis.

STATIONARITY

The concept of stationarity is, in vague terms, the requirement that there is statistical similarity of successive parts of a time series. It indicates that the mean and the variance should not change as a function of time in the time series. In Figure 2.11a,

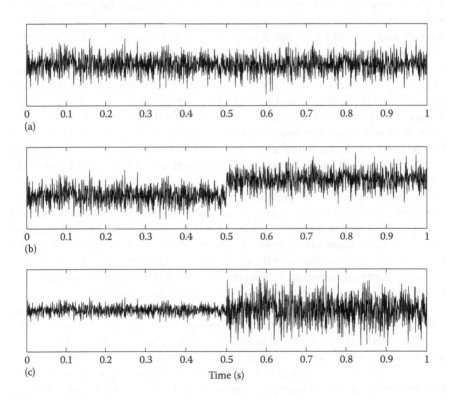

FIGURE 2.11 White noise time series data showing (a) stationarity, (b) nonstationarity due to change in mean, and (c) nonstationarity due to change in variance.

there is a stationary white noise time series, in Figure 2.11b, the time series is not stationary because the mean is different in the first half compared to the second half, and in Figure 2.11c, the time series is not stationary because the variance is different in the first half compared to second half. The sound of a cymbal clashing, if hit only once, is not stationary because the acoustic power of the clash, and hence, its variance diminishes with time.

The stationarity issue is perplexing because the exact nature of the stationarity required for nonlinear analysis is not clear. The stationarity requirement for the experimental data comes from an assumption commonly made by mathematicians in the derivation of the mathematical algorithms that are used for the nonlinear analysis. For example, Pincus assumes stationarity in the derivation of the algorithm for approximate entropy (Pincus 1991), and Wolf et al. assume stationarity in the derivation of the algorithm for maximum Lyapunov exponent (Wolf et al. 1985). There are nominally two types of stationarity for mathematicians, strong stationarity and weak stationarity. Strong stationarity requires all possible moments of ensembles (or shorter subsets) of time series data to be time invariant. In mathematics, a moment is, loosely speaking, a quantitative measure of the shape of a set of points. The first moment of the distribution of the random variable is the population mean. The second moment measures the width or distribution of a set of points in one dimension or in higher dimensions and can be represented as the shape of a cloud of points as it could be fit by an ellipsoid. Weak stationarity only makes this requirement for the mean and the autocorrelation function of time series data to be time invariant (Bendat and Piersol 2000). However, even weak stationarity is a difficult requirement to meet in experimental time-series data. For example, a sine function is not a stationary signal, since the mean for data that are near the bottom of a trough is not the same as the mean for data points that are near the top of a crest. Thus, none of the time series presented in this chapter, except for Figures 2.9b and 2.11a (white noise), would meet the requirement of stationarity.

Lack of stationarity or nonstationarity is often discussed as a limitation to other forms of nonlinear analysis. However, some authors have attempted to quantify nonstationarity of a time series as a useful measure in itself (Rieke et al. 2003; Cao et al. 2004; Chau et al. 2005; Makinen et al. 2005; Gourevitch and Eggermont 2007; Tong et al. 2007). For example, some of the debate about global climate change centers around the stationarity, or lack thereof, of climate-related variables (Karner 2002; Gagan et al. 2004; Mailhot et al. 2007). More specifically, nonstationarity may be inherent to biological systems and should actually be embraced and studied and not be considered as a limitation. Further, multiple researchers suggested that nonstationarities in physiological data may be the result of fractal properties, which has led to investigations of studying these long-term fluctuations in the data (Stanley 1971; Goldberger and West 1987; Meesman et al. 1993; Peng et al. 1993; Turcott and Teich 1993, 1996; Goldberger 1996; Viswanathan et al. 1997). Nonstationarity as a true physiological phenomenon can occur because such processes are more complex than the concept of homeostasis; instability or nonstationarity in the behavior demonstrate that the dynamics can occur over multiple timescales (Viswanathan et al. 1997; Pavlov et al. 2006). For example, in an electroencephalogram, the interspike intervals formed three distinct orbits during the hour before the occurrence of an epileptic seizure. In this case, nonstationarity in the data indicated the onset of a seizure (So et al. 1998). In the analysis of interbeat intervals of healthy individuals and individuals with congestive heart failure, the diseased population demonstrated greater inconsistency across multiple time scales. Even though the interbeat intervals of healthy individuals did change time scales, the behaviors displayed similar dynamics across those multiple scales, whereas individuals with congestive heart failure (CHF) were unable to regulate the interbeat intervals over particular time scales (Viswanathan et al. 1997). The concept of nonstationarity as a true biological phenomenon is supported by the fact that systems are under neurophysiological control and those control mechanisms, in the absence of disease, can regulate activity in many varying situations (i.e., time scales).

A commonly used technique to remove nonstationarity of time series data is to difference the data (Chatfield 2003). Differencing is the process of subtracting values between two data points to create a new point in a "differenced" series. Thus, a new time series is created, where the value at each point is found by subtracting the data at that time point from the next data point, resulting in a time series shorter by one than in the original time series. This procedure may be repeated multiple times, as necessary, until the data appear to be stationary. For example, investigators in our laboratory applied this technique to time series data from infant sitting postural control, and the approximate entropy was calculated before and after differencing. The results showed no benefit to differencing the data, as the approximate entropy was better correlated with developmental variables if no differencing was done. Our conclusion was that approximate entropy is robust to the requirement of mathematical nonstationarity (Deffeyes et al. 2007).

Another technique that can address the issue of nonstationarity is detrending. Briefly, detrending occurs before the application of a nonlinear algorithm, usually as a first step in the calculation process. A good example is detrended fluctuation analysis (DFA Chapter 7) that fits a power law to the series' average fluctuations across different scales (Viswanathan et al. 1997). These scales come in the form of box sizes and the least square line is fitted to the data in each box. The original data are detrended by subtracting the least square line of each window, which makes the time series stationary. This technique is described in more detail in Chapter 7. A note of caution, detrending must only be done if you are certain that the trend is not part of the dynamics of the signal. This would occur in the case of errors in measurement due to calibration, or drift from the equipment signal (Kantz and Schreiber 2003).

Some experimentalists have a more pragmatic concept of stationarity. The need for requiring a stationary time signal is that the underlying system dynamics must not change over the course of the data acquisition. If the system jumps from a chaotic behavior to a limit cycle behavior in the middle of the time series, clearly the system is nonstationary, and application of any of the nonlinear analysis algorithms discussed in this book would be problematic. However, the time series could potentially be divided into multiple stationary signals, evaluated, and compared. In this way, stationarity within signals is maintained and nonlinear algorithms can be implemented and used to describe differences between signals. There is also precedence for interpreting stationarity or lack thereof as a motor control technique to understand the dynamics of a system (Newell 1997; Stergiou et al. 2004).

An interesting description of stationarity is also provided by Small (2005). Small notices that the definition of stationarity is not the same for all systems. For linear systems, there is stationarity if all its moments (statistical descriptors) remain the same over time. A nonstationary system is then one that has some type of temporal dependence that arises from an external source. Thus, if we extend the definition of the system to include all such external sources, then the system is stationary. This reminds us of dynamical systems theory in which a system cannot be considered without its constraints, namely morphological, environmental, and biomechanical constraints.

Small (2005) also provides an interesting example to illustrate the earlier discussion, as he describes someone standing on the beach watching the ups and downs of the tide. This individual will describe this system as nonstationary. However, if the same individual considers the relative positions of the earth, the moon, and the sun, then he could determine that if all are studied together, he will have an approximately stationary system (Small 2005).

A GENERAL NOTE ON EXPERIMENTAL LIMITATIONS OF TIME SERIES DATA

One approach to understanding the effect of these limitations on your data as you are using any particular algorithm is to use computer-generated data from several systems with known dynamics, such as a sine function, the Lorenz equations, the Henon map, pseudorandom noise, and so forth, and manipulate them to have the same limitations (data length, resolution, etc.) as your experimental data. For example, you can round the data off to have a precision similar to the experimental data, add noise, and/or add a linear trend to increase nonstationarity, and then run the algorithm of interest on these different time series and observe if the result is consistent with expectations based on the system dynamics that generated the time series. One way to add noise is to use a pseudorandom number generator, such as the "randn" function in MATLAB®, to generate a random time series and then add that to clean computer-generated time series from a system with known dynamics. One issue is that the dynamics of the noise that may be contaminating the experimental data are not known. It may not be random. It could be periodic, as in the case of contamination with 60 Hz (or 50 Hz in Europe), or it could be chaotic, generated by a process that appears to be random but actually has some structure to it. Dealing with experimental limitations of time series data is one of the greatest challenges to successful application of nonlinear analysis algorithms to systems with unknown dynamics (Rapp 1994). However, by exploring the effect of each limitation, the dynamics of the time series can be understood much better and the benefits could outweigh the time expense. In closing, remember the following considerations when conducting time series analysis:

- *Length*: Make sure data are long enough to capture a minimum of 5–10 cycles of the phenomenon being studied; the more data present, the more likely the true dynamics have been captured in the signal.

- *Sampling frequency*: Sample at the correct rate of frequency at least 2 times, but not more than 10 times the highest frequency. This will make sure the entire signal is captured without adding noise to the signal. The frequency in the data is determined with a spectral analysis.
- *Noise*: Optimize the signal-to-noise ratio and be aware of how the nonlinear algorithm used is affected by noise.
- *Filtering and smoothing*: Be very cautious in filtering data intended to use for nonlinear analysis. If filtering must be done, ensure the cutoff is above the Nyquist frequency and perform the filtering interactively.
- *Resolution*: Determine how many significant digits to be used based on the precision of the equipment collecting the data. Test the effect of rounding the data on the outcome value of the nonlinear algorithm of choice.
- *Stationarity*: Nonstationarity may be an important biological measure in itself. Various techniques can be used to remove nonstationarity; however, these techniques may impact the dynamics of the signal. Some algorithms are affected by stationarity less than others.

EXERCISES

1. Define a time series.
2. What is a common unit of measure for how many data points are acquired every second?
3. How long does your data have to be?
4. Let {1, 5, 20, 2, 35} be the original time series. Create a differenced time series.
5. Competitive cyclists pedal with a cadence of about 90 cycles/min. What is the minimum sampling frequency you would need to estimate the cadence from knee flexion time series data? What would be a preferred sampling rate?
6. A physiologist measures the electrical signal from a research subject's muscle as he flexes his elbow using electromyography (EMG). Spectral analysis shows frequencies lower and higher than the range of interest. What sort of filter might the physiologist want to apply to the data to remove the unwanted low and high frequencies? Another researcher only wants to remove the high frequencies. What sort of filter should the second researcher apply?
7. For a period of 15 years an ornithologist measured the annual population of the white-faced scops owl living in a patch of forest, and found the following result: [11 13 15 16 15 17 19 22 21 21 24 27 26 28 29]. Make a time series plot of the data. Does it appear to be stationary? Difference the data and make a plot of the differenced time series. Does the differenced time series appear more stationary than the original time series?
8. If you have access to MATLAB, make a plot of a sine function from time 0 to 10 s. Sample at a frequency of 100 Hz, and make the sine function with a with a frequency of 0.5 Hz and amplitude of 5. Restrict the axes to 3–4 s, and −10 to +10 in sine amplitude.

9. Make a plot of a sine function from time 0 to 10 s, with a frequency of 0.5 Hz and add in Gaussian distributed random noise, with a mean of 0 and a standard deviation of 1.

10. Calculate the power spectra of both of the plots you made in questions #4 and #5.

REFERENCES

Beard, J. 2003. *The FFT in the 21st Century: Eigenspace Processing.* New York: Springer.

Bendat, J.S. and A.G. Piersol. 2000. *Random Data: Analysis and Measurement Procedures,* 3rd edn. New York: John Wiley & Sons.

Box, G.E.P., G.M. Jenkins, and G.C. Reinsel. 2008. *Time Series Analysis: Forecasting and Control,* 4th edn. Hoboken, NJ: John Wiley & Sons, Inc.

Brockwell, P.J. and R.A. Davis. 2002. *Introduction to Time Series and Forecasting,* 2nd edn. New York: Springer.

Cao, H.Q., D.E. Lake, M.P. Griffin, and J.R. Moorman. 2004. Increased nonstationarity of neonatal heart rate before the clinical diagnosis of sepsis. *Annals of Biomedical Engineering* 32(2): 233–244.

Chatfield, C. 2003. *The Analysis of Time Series: An Introduction,* 6th edn. Boca Raton, FL: Chapman & Hall/CRC Press.

Chau, T., D. Chau, M. Casas, G. Berall, and D.J. Kenny. 2005. Investigating the stationarity of pediatric aspiration signals. *IEEE Transactions on Neural Systems and Rehabilitation Engineering* 13(1): 99–105.

Deffeyes, J.E., R.T. Harbourne, S.L. DeJong, W.A. Stuberg, A. Kyvelidou, and N. Stergiou. 2007. Approximate entropy is robust to non-stationarity in analysis of infant sitting postural sway. Paper presented at *Proceedings of the 2007 American Society of Biomechanics Annual Meeting,* Stanford, CA.

Dohrmann, C.R., H.R. Busby, and D.M. Trujillo. 1988. Smoothing noisy data using dynamic programming and generalized cross-validation. *Journal of Biomechanical Engineering* 110(1): 37–41.

Fredrickson, B.L. and M.F. Losada. 2005. Positive affect and the complex dynamics of human flourishing. *American Psychologist* 60(7): 678–686.

Gagan, M.K., E.J. Hendy, S.G. Haberle, and W.S. Hantoro. 2004. Post-glacial evolution of the Indo-Pacific Warm Pool and El Niño-Southern Oscillation. *Quaternary International* 118: 127–143.

Giakas, G. 2004. Power spectrum analysis and filtering. In *Innovative Analysis of Human Movement,* 1st edn. N. Stergiou, ed., pp. 223–258. Champaign, IL: Human Kinetics.

Giakas, G. and V. Baltzopoulos. 1997. Time and frequency domain analysis of ground reaction forces during walking: An investigation of variability and symmetry. *Gait and Posture* 5(189): 197.

Giakas, G., V. Baltzopoulos, P.H. Dangerfield, J.C. Dorgan, and S. Dalmira. 1996. Comparison of gait patterns between healthy and scoliotic patients using time and frequency domain analysis of ground reaction forces. *Spine* 21(19): 2235–2242.

Goldberger, A.L. 1996. Non-linear dynamics for clinicians: Chaos theory, fractals, and complexity at the bedside. *Lancet* 347(9011): 1312–1314.

Goldberger, A.L. and B.J. West. 1987. Applications of nonlinear dynamics to clinical cardiology. *Annals of the New York Academy of Sciences* 504: 195–213.

Gourevitch, B. and J.J. Eggermont. 2007. A simple indicator of nonstationarity of firing rate in spike trains. *Journal of Neuroscience Methods* 163(1): 181–187.

Huang, N.E., Z. Shen, S. Long, M.C. Wu, H.H. Shih, Q. Zheng, N. Yen, C.C. Tung, and H.H. Liu. 1998. The empirical mode decomposition and the Hilbert spectrum for nonlinear and nonstationary time series analysis. *Proceedings of the Royal Society London A* 454: 903–995.

Kantz, H. and T. Schreiber. 2003. *Nonlinear Time Series Analysis*, 2nd edn. Cambridge, U.K.: Cambridge University Press.

Karner, O. 2002. On nonstationarity and antipersistency in global temperature series. *Journal of Geophysical Research-Atmospheres* 107(D20): 4415.

Kerry, E. May 23, 2008. Retrospective—Edward N. Lorenz (1917–2008). *Science* 320(5879): 1025.

Liu, P.Y., A. Iranmanesh, D.M. Keenan, S.M. Pincus, and J.D. Veldhuis. 2007. A noninvasive measure of negative-feedback strength, approximate entropy, unmasks strong diurnal variations in the regularity of LH secretion. *American Journal of Physiology-Endocrinology and Metabolism* 293(5): E1409–E1415.

Mailhot, A., S. Duchesne, D. Caya, and G. Talbot. 2007. Assessment of future change in intensity-duration-frequency (IDF) curves for southern Quebec using the Canadian regional climate model (CRCM). *Journal of Hydrology* 347(1–2): 197–210.

Makinen, V.T., P.J.C. May, and H. Tiitinen. 2005. The use of stationarity and nonstationarity in the detection and analysis of neural oscillations. *NeuroImage* 28(2): 389–400.

McGrath, D., T.N. Judkins, I.I. Pipinos, J.M. Johanning, and S.A. Myers. 2012. Peripheral arterial disease affects the frequency response of ground reaction forces during walking. *Clinical Biomechanics* 27(10): 1058–1063.

Meesmann, M., F. Gruneis, P. Flachenecker, and K.D. Kniffki. 1993. A new method for analysis of heart-rate-variability counting statistics of 1/f fluctuations. *Biological Cybernetics* 68(4): 299–306.

Myers, S.A., J.M. Johanning, I.I. Pipinos, K.K. Schmid, and N. Stergiou. 2013. Vascular occlusion affects gait variability patterns of healthy younger and older individuals. *Annals of Biomedical Engineering* 41(8): 1692–1702.

Myers, S.A., J.M. Johanning, N. Stergiou, R.I. Celis, L. Robinson, and I.I. Pipinos. 2009. Gait variability is altered in patients with peripheral arterial disease. *Journal of Vascular Surgery* 49(4): 924–931.

Myers, S.A., I.I. Pipinos, J.M. Johanning, and N. Stergiou. 2011. Gait variability of patients with intermittent claudication is similar before and after the onset of claudication pain. *Clinical Biomechanics* 26(7): 729–734.

National Office of Oceanic and Atmospheric Administration. 2013. Available from ftp://ftp.ngdc.noaa.gov/STP/SOLAR_DATA/SUNSPOT_NUMBERS/YEARLY, cited March 2008.

Newell, K.M. 1997. Degrees of freedom and the development of center of pressure profiles. In *Applications of Nonlinear Dynamics to Developmental Process Modeling*. K.M. Newell and P.M.C. Molenar, eds., pp. 63–84. Hillsdale, NJ: Erlbaum.

Pavlov, A.N., V.A. Makarov, E. Mosekilde, and O.V. Sosnovtseva. 2006. Application of wavelet-based tools to study the dynamics of biological processes. *Briefings in Bioinformatics* 7(4): 375–389.

Peng, C.K., J. Mietus, J.M. Hausdorff, S. Havlin, H.E. Stanley, and A.L. Goldberger. 1993. Long-range anticorrelations and non-Gaussian behavior of the heartbeat. *Physical Review Letters* 70(9): 1343–1346.

Percival, D.B. and A.T. Walden. 1993. *Spectral Analysis for Physical Applications*, 1st edn. Cambridge, MA: Cambridge University Press.

Pincus, S.M. March 15, 1991. Approximate entropy as a measure of system complexity. *Proceedings of the National Academy of Sciences of the United States of America* 88(6): 2297–2301.

Prabhu, K.M.M. 2013. *Window Functions and Their Applications in Signal Processing*, 1st edn. Boca Raton, FL: CRC Press.

Rapp, P.E. July–September 1994. A guide to dynamical analysis. *Integrative Physiological and Behavioral Science* 29(3): 311–327.

Rapp, P.E., A.M. Albano, T.I. Schmah, and L.A. Farwell. April 1993. Filtered noise can mimic low-dimensional chaotic attractors. *Physical Review E: Statistical Physics, Plasmas, Fluids, and Related Interdisciplinary Topics* 47(4): 2289–2297.

Rieke, C., F. Mormann, R.G. Andrzejak, T. Kreuz, P. David, C.E. Elger, and K. Lehnertz. May 2003. Discerning nonstationarity from nonlinearity in seizure-free and preseizure EEG recordings from epilepsy patients. *IEEE Transactions on Bio-Medical Engineering* 50(5): 634–639.

Sakakibara, Y. 1995. Introduction. In *Who is Fourier? A Mathematical Adventure*. Boston, MA: Language Research Foundation.

Small, M. 2005. *Applied Nonlinear Time Series Analysis*, 1st edn. Singapore: World Scientific Publishing.

Smith, S.W. 2002. *Digital Signal Processing: A Practical Guide for Engineers and Scientists*, 1st edn. Boston, MA: Newnes.

So, P., J. Francis, T. Netoff, B.J. Gluckman, and S.J. Schiff. 1998. Periodic orbits: A new language for neuronal dynamics. *Biophysical Journal* 74: 2776–2785.

Stanley, H.E. 1971. *Introduction to Phase Transitions and Critical Phenomena*. International Series of Monographs on Physics. New York, NY: Oxford University Press.

Stergiou, N., B.T. Bates, and S.L. James. 1999. Asynchrony between subtalar and knee joint function during running. *Medicine and Science in Sports and Exercise* 31(11): 1645–1655.

Stergiou, N., U.H. Buzzi, M.J. Kurz, and J. Heidel. 2004. Nonlinear tools in human movement. In *Innovative Analysis of Human Movement*. N. Stergiou, ed., pp. 63–90. Champaign, IL: Human Kinetics.

Stergiou, N., G. Giakas, J.B. Byrne, and V. Pomeroy. 2002. Frequency domain characteristics of ground reaction forces during walking of young and elderly females. *Clinical Biomechanics* 17(8): 615–617.

Stoica, P. and R.L. Moses. 1997. *Introduction to Spectral Analysis*, 1st edn. Upper Saddle River, NJ: Prentice Hall.

Theiler, J. and S. Eubank. October 1993. Don't bleach chaotic data. *Chaos* 3(4): 771–782.

Tong, S., Z. Li, Y. Zhu, and N.V. Thakor. 2007. Describing the nonstationarity level of neurological signals based on quantifications of time-frequency representation. *IEEE Transactions on Biomedical Engineering* 54(10): 1780–1785.

Turcott, R.G. and M.C. Teich. 1993. Long-duration correlation and attractor topology of the heartbeat rate differ for healthy patients and those with heart failure. *Proceedings of the Society of Photo-Optical Instrumentation Engineers*, Bellingham, WA.

Turcott, R.G. and M.C. Teich. 1996. Fractal character of the electrocardiogram: Distinguishing heart-failure and normal patients. *Annals of Biomedical Engineering* 24(2): 269–293.

Vaughan, C., B. Davis, and J. O'Connor. 1999. *Dynamics of Human Gait*. Cape Town, South Africa: Kiboho Publishers.

Viswanathan, G.M., C.K. Peng, H.E. Stanley, and A.L. Goldberger. 1997. Deviations from uniform power law scaling in nonstationary time series. *Physical Review E* 55(1): 845–849.

Warner, R.M. 1998. *Spectral Analysis of Time-Series Data*. New York: Guilford Press.

Wolf, A., J.B. Swift, H.L. Swinney, and J.A. Vastano. 1985. Determining Lyapunov exponents from a time series. *Physica* 16D: 285–317.

Woltring, H.J. September 1985. On optimal smoothing and derivative estimation from noisy displacement data in biomechanics. *Human Movement Science* 4(3): 229–245.

Wurdeman, S.R., J.M. Huisinga, M. Filipi, and N. Stergiou. 2011. Multiple sclerosis affects the frequency content in the vertical ground reaction forces during walking. *Clinical Biomechanics* 26(2): 207–212.

3 State-Space Reconstruction

Shane R. Wurdeman

CONTENTS

Introduction 55
Geometric Objects in a Space 56
The Lorenz Attractor 58
Embedding Dimension 61
Time Lag 62
False Nearest Neighbor Method 66
Autocorrelation and Average Mutual Information 70
Practical Issues 72
Problems with Finding an Embedding Dimension 75
Problems with Finding a Time Lag 77
Embedding Dimensions Used in Previous Studies 80
Summary 80
Exercises 81
References 81

> The despotism of tradition (custom) is everywhere the standing hindrance to human advancement.
>
> **John Stuart Mill (1806–1873)**

INTRODUCTION

A time series can be used to reconstruct the attractor of the underlying dynamic process. State-space reconstruction from a time series is a powerful approach for the analysis of the complex, nonlinear systems that appear ubiquitous in the natural and human world. This is a very important step in identifying the structural characteristics of a time series. It is also necessary in calculating the Lyapunov exponent, the correlation dimension, and other nonlinear tools.

However, before this is completed, to help the reader better conceptualize this procedure, some examples using geometric objects are presented. These examples will help introduce a general concept for the reconstruction of the state-space, where the structural characteristics of a time series are embedded and many of the nonlinear tools are applied.

GEOMETRIC OBJECTS IN A SPACE

There are two geometric objects in the left panel of Figure 3.1. What are they? This question can be answered in various ways, because there are numerous ways to describe these objects. One way to describe these objects is by their dimension, but there are also several ways to define a dimension. Here, dimension means a measure to describe the size of an object: length, width, and height.

The object at the top left of Figure 3.1 looks like a circle, which has a dimension of two because the size of a circle can be described by its width and height. How about the object at the bottom left of Figure 3.1? It looks like a line, whose size can be described only by its length, and therefore has a dimension of one. But are they really a circle and a line? If an observer changes position to examine these objects, these objects may be neither a circle nor a line. If the observer slightly moves to the left or to the right, then a cylinder with a dimension of three may be discovered instead of a circle. Also, if the line is examined from above or below, then a square with a dimension of two may be discovered (Figure 3.1).

What can we learn from these examples? The true shapes of those objects are revealed when they are examined in a higher-dimensional space or where the dimensionality is equal to the true dimension of the objects. But what does this have to do with the nonlinear analysis of a time series? Consider that a time series is also an object in a space and just in the same way as with the geometric objects, the time series can be observed in a higher-dimensional space. Then, it is possible to capture the true structure of the time series that may be hidden in a lower-dimensional space. For example, in Figure 3.2, two time series are examined in a lower- and a higher-dimensional space. Interestingly, these two time series have a similar standard

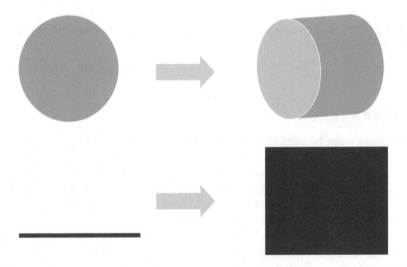

FIGURE 3.1 Top left: An object that looks like a circle with a dimension of two. Bottom left: An object that looks like a line with a dimension of one. Top right: A cylinder with a dimension of three. The same object as in the top left seen from a different angle. Bottom right: A square with a dimension of two. The same object as in bottom left seen from above or below.

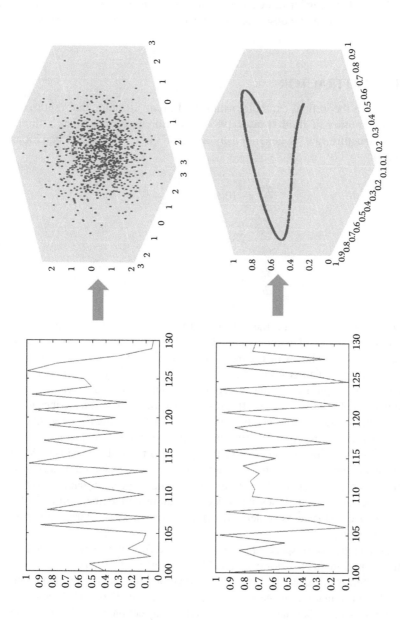

FIGURE 3.2 Top: Time series 1. A deterministic time series. Mean = 0.59; standard deviation = 0.30. Bottom: Time series 2. Random time series. Mean = 0.50; standard deviation = 0.29. Linear measures cannot distinguish between time series 1 and time series 2. The attractors seen in the three-dimensional space clearly show their differences in structure.

deviation and mean (top: 0.59 ± 0.30; bottom: 0.50 ± 0.29). However, these linear statistical measures fail to differentiate between the two time series, because there is more in the structure of these time series. This can be assessed when the two time series are observed in a higher-dimensional space. As soon as their true structure or their dynamic behavior can be observed, specific tools can be utilized to assess their differences.

THE LORENZ ATTRACTOR

Let us examine a theoretical example, using the Lorenz attractor that represents the convective motion of fluid (Fraser 1989). The Lorenz attractor has a three-dimensional structure and is generated by a set of three differential equations (Equation 3.1):

$$\frac{dx}{dt} = -10(x - y)$$

$$\frac{dy}{dt} = 28x - y - xz \qquad (3.1)$$

$$\frac{dz}{dt} = xy - 2z$$

These equations provide us with the values for the X, Y, and Z coordinates. Thus, we have three sequences of numbers called $X(t)$, $Y(t)$, and $Z(t)$. The plots of each of these sequences are shown in Figure 3.3a through c. All three sequences can be plotted together in a three-dimensional plot (Figure 3.3d). Each point in this three-dimensional graph also defines a vector and contains the three values from the coordinates (X, Y, and Z; Figure 3.4). This vector is the state that describes what is going on with the system at a specific time. For example, at time $t = t_1$, we have a vector ($X(t_1)$, $Y(t_1)$, $Z(t_1)$) representing the state of the system at time t_1 (Figure 3.4). A visual representation of the behavior of the system in the state-space is called a state-space plot or phase-space plot. A phase space can be considered as a special case of state-space, and, in general, the term is used to describe a mechanical system where state-space consists of all possible values of position and momentum variables (the first derivative and successive derivatives). However, these two terms are often used interchangeably.

We have seen that a state-space can be reconstructed from the variables $X(t)$, $Y(t)$, and $Z(t)$ from the Lorenz attractor example. The sequences of $X(t)$, $Y(t)$, and $Z(t)$ or state-space vectors were generated by known equations for the system. However, in biological data, equations to generate vectors are not available. Only a scalar sequence of observations is usually available. In the next section, we will see how to reconstruct the state-space from a scalar time series.

Question: How do we reconstruct the state-space? What do we need for the reconstruction of the state-space?

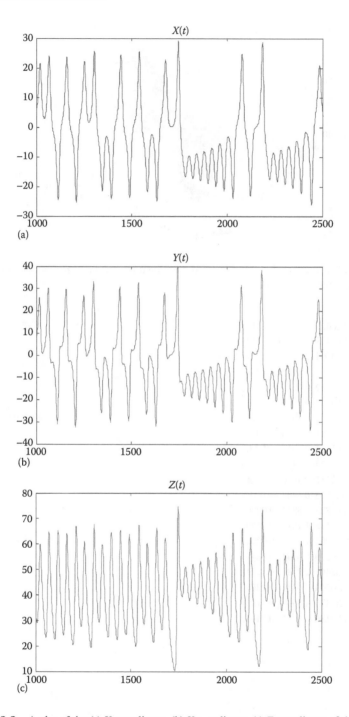

FIGURE 3.3 A plot of the (a) *X* coordinate, (b) *Y* coordinate, (c) *Z* coordinate of the Lorenz time series generated by known differential equations. (*Continued*)

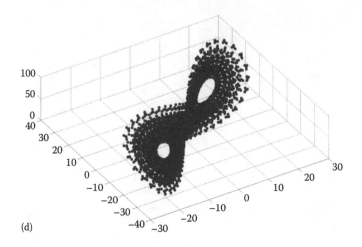

(d)

FIGURE 3.3 (*Continued*)   (d) A three-dimensional plot of the Lorenz attractor generated by known differential equations.

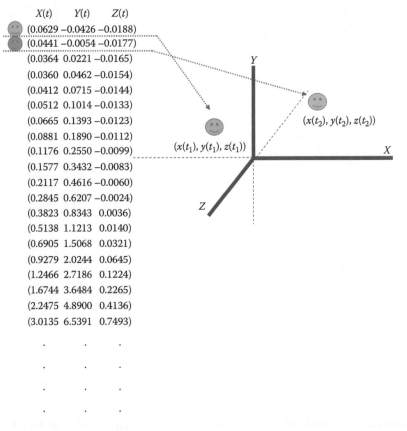

FIGURE 3.4   Each point in the three-dimensional graph defines a vector and contains three values from each coordinate (X, Y, and Z).

EMBEDDING DIMENSION

What is needed is a "transformation" of a single sequence in time into a higher-dimensional space. This transformation provides increased information that increases the uniqueness of the object being analyzed. This kind of transformation is called embedding, and the goal is to create a state-space where the structure of a given system is embedded. From the example of geometric objects discussed earlier, it was observed that an object will have multiple dimensions. Each dimension represents a unique characteristic of the object. As an example to further explain multidimensionality, consider three separate cylinders (Figure 3.5). If these objects are only considered in three dimensions, then we do not have enough unique information to realize any differences between the objects. However, if another dimension is added, such as color, then it is possible to observe that one of the cylinders is different. Then, a fifth dimension may be needed to further distinguish between the first two objects (e.g., texture). In order to fully analyze all the characteristics of the object, the space that contains the object will need to be unfolded into the number of dimensions that contain the object's true structure, which presents its unique identity. For our purposes, the object is the emergent attractor from the time series. If the dimension of the space that contains the true structure of the object can be identified correctly, then it is possible to observe the actual shape of the object. The dimension of the space that contains the true structure of this system is called the embedding dimension, and it is the minimum number of variables required to form a valid state-space from a given time series.

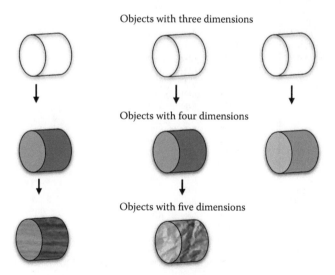

FIGURE 3.5 Dimensionality can be thought of different characteristics that uniquely identify an object. The three cylinders could be considered equivalent in three dimensions (top), but as further dimensionality is added (e.g., color and texture), differences in the three objects can be observed.

TIME LAG

Now, let us move on to actually reconstructing a state-space with an example. Let a time series be represented by a sequence of $\{f(1), f(2), \ldots, f(N)\}$, where $f(1)$, $f(2)$, and $f(N)$ represent first, second, and Nth data point, respectively. An actual reconstruction of the state-space requires a great amount of data points, but for the sake of this illustration, let us use a sequence of observations that has 30 data points ($N = 30$). Suppose we want to reconstruct the state-space with embedding dimension of three. We can do as described in the following example.

Example 3.1 (Figure 3.6)

First, take the data points from $f(1)$ to $f(28)$ and set this sequence called $X(t)$ aside. Next, take data points from $f(2)$ to $f(29)$ and set this sequence called $Y(t)$ next to $X(t)$. Finally, we take data points from $f(3)$ to $f(30)$ and set this sequence called $Z(t)$ next to $Y(t)$. Now, a matrix with 28 rows and 3 columns has been created.

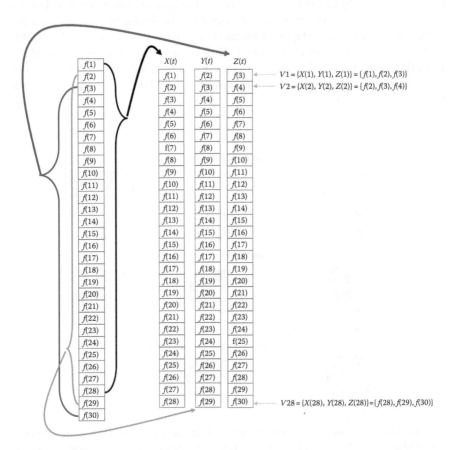

FIGURE 3.6 Reconstruction of the state-space from a scalar time series represented by a sequence of $f(1), f(2), \ldots, f(30)$. Time lag = 1.

The first row of this matrix is defined as vector V1, the second row as vector V2, and the last row as vector V28. Thus, 28 vectors have been created, whose elements consist of three numbers each from $X(t)$, $Y(t)$, and $Z(t)$. Therefore, V1 contains $X(1)$ that is $f(1)$, $Y(1)$ that is $f(2)$, and $Z(1)$ that is $f(3)$. V2 contains $X(2)$ that is $f(2)$, $Y(2)$ that is $f(3)$, and $Z(2)$ that is $f(4)$ and so forth. But is this the only way to reconstruct the state-space?

Example 3.2 (Figure 3.7)

Let us take the same time series $\{f(1), f(2),..., f(N)\}$ and reconstruct the state-space in a different manner. This time, take the data points from $f(1)$ to $f(24)$ and call it sequence $X(t)$. Then, take the data points from $f(4)$ to $f(27)$ and call it sequence $Y(t)$. Finally, take the data points from $f(7)$ to $f(30)$ and call it sequence $Z(t)$. Again, a matrix with three columns has been created. However, this matrix now has only 24 rows.

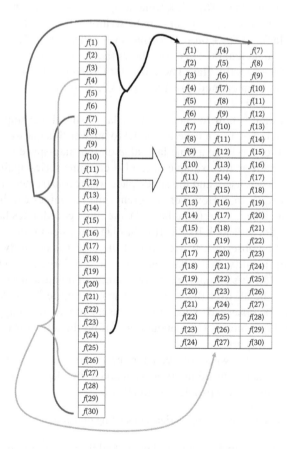

FIGURE 3.7 Reconstruction of the state-space from the same scalar time series represented by a sequence of $f(1), f(2),..., f(30)$. Time lag = 3.

What is the difference between Examples 3.1 and 3.2? In Example 3.1, the first vector $V1$ has $\{f(1), f(2), f(3)\}$. In Example 3.2, the same vector has $\{f(1), f(4), f(7)\}$. Suppose an available scalar time series is X-coordinate values generated by the Equation 3.1 for the Lorenz attractor, that is, $\{0.0629, 0.041, 0.0364, 0.0360, 0.0412, 0.0512, 0.0666, 0.0881,...\}$ (Figure 3.4). Then, $\{f(1), f(2), f(3)\} = \{0.0629, 0.0441, 0.0364\}$ for Example 3.1 and $\{f(1), f(4), f(7)\} = \{0.0629, 0.0360, 0.0665\}$ for Example 3.2.

Each vector contains three data points, but the indices are different. The difference in the indices of the data points in Example 3.1 for $V1$ is 1 ($2 - 1 = 1$, $3 - 2 = 1$), while the difference in the indices of the data points in Example 3.2 for $V1$ is 3 ($4 - 1 = 3$ and $7 - 4 = 3$). This difference in the indices is called the time lag. In fact, $Y(t)$ and $Z(t)$ can be rewritten in terms of $X(t)$ and the time lag. Example 3.1: we had $\{(X(t_1), Y(t_1), Z(t_1)\} = \{f(1), f(2), f(3)\}$. We can rewrite this as $\{f(1), f(2), f(3)\} = \{(X(t_1), X(t_1 + 1), X(t_1 + 2 \times 1)\}$. Example 3.2: we had $\{(X(t_1), Y(t_1), Z(t_1)\} = \{f(1), f(4), f(7)\}$. We can rewrite this as $\{f(1), f(4), f(7)\} = \{(X(t_1), X(t_1 + 3), X(t_1 + 2 \times 3)\}$. In general, a state-space with three dimensions can be written as $\{(X(t_i), Y(t_i), Z(t_i)\} = \{(X(t_i), X(t_i + 1 \times \text{time lag}), X(t_i + 2 \times \text{time lag})\}$. A state-space with m dimensions (i.e., m-dimensional state-space) can then be written as $\{(X(t_i), X(t_i + 1 \times \text{time lag}), X(t_i + 2 \times \text{time lag}),..., X(t_i + (m - 1) \times \text{time lag})\}$, where $i = 1, 2,..., N - (m - 1) \times$ time lag and $N =$ data length. This also shows the number of state vectors created is equal to $N - (m - 1) \times$ time lag. Therefore, for Example 3.1, $30 - (3 - 1) \times 1 = 28$ state vectors have been created. For Example 3.2, $30 - (3 - 1) \times 3 = 24$ state vectors have been created.

Now, the question is how to choose a time lag. Using the examples, which one is correct, a time lag of 1 or a time lag of 3? To answer this question, the effect of having too small or too large a time lag value on the state-space needs to be considered. Let us examine the example of the Lorenz time series again (Figure 3.3). The sequence $X(t)$ was used, and the state-space was reconstructed with an embedding dimension equal to 3. However, different time lag values can be used. When a small time lag value is used (time lag = 1), the three coordinates have very close values, and the plot will look like a straight diagonal line (Figure 3.8a). The true structure cannot be observed. It is clear that the object is not fully unfolded into its proper dimensionality. What happens when a very large time lag value (time lag = 30) is used? In this case, an excessive folding of an attractor is observed and state vectors will be all over the embedding space (Figure 3.8b). Again, the true structure cannot be observed. Thus, it is necessary to choose an appropriate time lag (time lag = 11), which is large enough to unfold the attractor but also not too large or too small (Figure 3.8c).

We have seen so far what we need for the reconstruction of the state-space, namely, an appropriate embedding dimension and a time lag. The next question we would like to discuss is how to actually find them.

Question: How do we find an appropriate embedding dimension?

One general method to find an appropriate embedding dimension involves calculations of some dynamic invariant, such as the correlation dimension or the Lyapunov

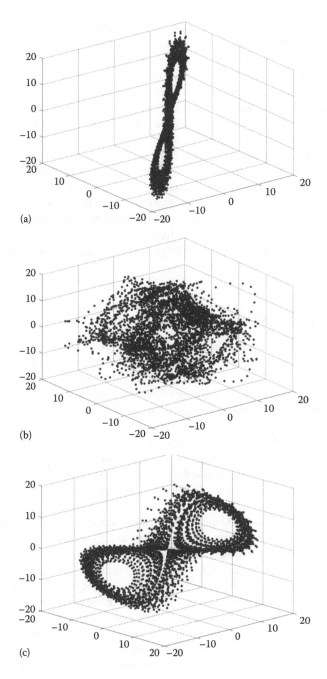

FIGURE 3.8 (a) The effect of different time lag values on the Lorenz attractor. When the time lag value is too small (time lag = 1), an attractor is not fully unfolded. (b) When the time lag value is too large (time lag = 30), state vectors are all over the embedding space. (c) When the time lag value is appropriate (time lag = 11), the attractor is fully unfolded but there is no excessive folding.

exponent for successive embeddings (Wolf et al. 1985). Choose the dimension as an appropriate embedding dimension where no changes in the dynamic invariant are observed. If the dynamic invariant is independent of the dimension, then this dimension can be considered large enough to unfold the dynamics of the attractor. However, one of the drawbacks of this approach is the cost of computing dynamic invariants for increasing dimensions. The computational cost can be expensive since many nonlinear tools, which require the reconstruction of the state-space, require a large amount of data points. Furthermore, there are cases where this approach did not work. Dynamic invariants could become independent at a dimension that is slightly greater than the dimension of the attractor, but this dimension may not be large enough to unfold the dynamic behavior of the attractor. The following section introduces the false nearest neighbor algorithm, which is the most commonly used method for finding an embedding dimension (Abarbanel 1996; Kennel et al. 1992; Stergiou et al. 2004). This approach is based on eliminating false projections that can occur when the dimension is not large enough to unfold the dynamics of the attractor.

FALSE NEAREST NEIGHBOR METHOD

Here, again, the same concept as in Figure 3.1 can be used to better illustrate how this is performed. Let us assume that there are a couple of data points in a space and, at this point, they seem to lie on a line (Figure 3.9a). They all look like they are close to each other or like they are close neighbors to each other. However, if they are observed in a higher-dimensional space, the data points are actually on a circle and only data point 1 and data point 3 are true neighbors (Figure 3.9b). Data point 2 is far from data point 1 and data point 3 and not a true neighbor to them. Data point 2 is a false nearest neighbor in a lower dimension. These data points in an m-dimensional space are expressed as a vector with m elements (Figure 3.10a). In one higher-dimensional space $m + 1$, they can be expressed as a vector with $m + 1$ elements (Figure 3.10b).

How do we determine whether those vectors are true or false nearest neighbors? We need to find out how far apart they are by calculating Euclidean distances in state-space. First the nearest neighboring state vector called $V(t)^{NN}$ for each state vector $V(t)$ needs to be identified (Figure 3.10a). Then, the distance between these vectors at m-dimensional space needs to be calculated (Figure 3.10c). This distance can be written as $\|V(t) - V(t)^{NN}\|$. The next step is to move up to a higher-dimensional space $m + 1$ and calculate the distance between these vectors written as $\|\hat{V}(t) - \hat{V}^{NN}(t)\|$ (Figure 3.10d). If these two vectors are true neighbors, then the difference in the distances between these vectors at m and at $m + 1$ (i.e., $\|\hat{V}(t) - \hat{V}^{NN}(t)\| - \|\hat{V}(t) - \hat{V}(t)\,NN\|$) should remain near constant. But if they are false nearest neighbors, then the difference in the distances should increase. This can be observed by examining the rate of separation between them. The rate of separation can be calculated by taking the ratio of the difference in the distances between the vectors at dimension m and dimension $m + 1$ to the distance of these two vectors at dimension m. If this ratio is beyond a certain threshold value called R_{tol}, the vector

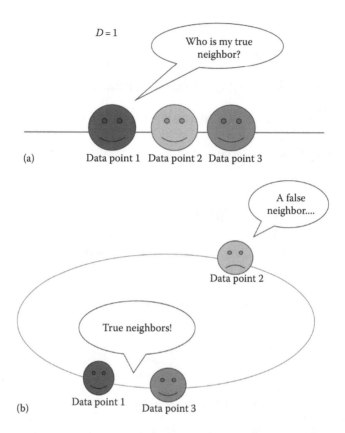

FIGURE 3.9 (a) Data points 1, 2, and 3 on a line. They all look like true neighbors. (b) Looking at data point 1, 2, and 3 from a higher-dimensional space reveals data point 2 is a false neighbor.

is a false neighbor. This threshold value is arbitrary; Abarbanel (1996) suggests the value of 15:

$$\frac{\left\|\hat{V}(t)-\hat{V}^{NN}(t)\right\| - \left\|V(t)-V^{NN}(t)\right\|}{\left\|V(t)-V^{NN}(t)\right\|} > R_{tol} \tag{3.2}$$

For a data set with short length, Kennel et al. (1992) presented an alternative equation to find a false nearest neighbor by using

$$\frac{\left\|\hat{V}(t)-\hat{V}^{NN}(t)\right\| - \left\|V(t)-V^{NN}(t)\right\|}{\sigma} > A_{tol} \tag{3.3}$$

where A_{tol} is a threshold value. Abarbanel (1996) recommends an arbitrary value of 2 for A_{tol}.

Let us examine this calculation with R_{tol} using a numerical example. In the two-dimensional space ($m = 2$), there is a vector at time t, $V(t) = [1.6180\ 8.000]$ and its neighbor

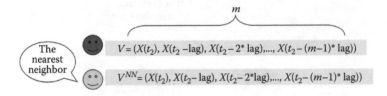

Example: Dimension of space = 2

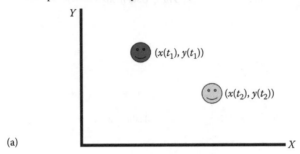

(a)

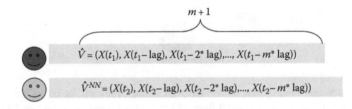

Example: Dimension of space = 3

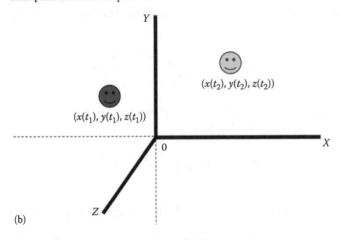

(b)

FIGURE 3.10 (a) In an m-dimensional space, a vector contains m elements. (b) In an $m + 1$ dimensional space, a vector contains $m + 1$ elements. *(Continued)*

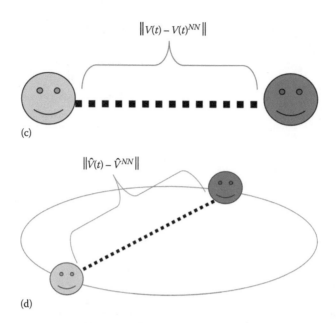

FIGURE 3.10 (*Continued*) (c) The distance between a vector and its neighbor in the *m*-dimensional space (d) The distance between the vector and its neighbor in the *m* + 1-dimensional space.

$V^{NN}(t) = [0.7885\ 5.7462]$. In a higher-dimensional space of $m = 3$, these vectors will be expressed as $\hat{V}(t) = [1.6180\ 8.000\ 0.354]$ and $\hat{V}^{NN}(t) = [0.7885\ 5.7462\ 45.408]$. The distance between the two vectors in the two-dimensional space is

$$\|V(t) - V^{NN}(t)\| = \sqrt{(1.6180 - 0.7885)^2 + (8.000 - 5.7462)^2} = 2.4016$$

while in the three-dimensional space, the distance is

$$\|\hat{V}(t) - \hat{V}^{NN}(t)\| = \sqrt{(1.6180 - 0.7885)^2 + (8.000 - 5.7462)^2 + (0.354 - 45.408)^2}$$

$$= 45.1180$$

Thus, the value obtained by using Equation 3.2 is

$$\frac{\|\hat{V}(t) - \hat{V}^{NN}(t)\| - \|V(t) - V^{NN}(t)\|}{\|V(t) - V^{NN}(t)\|} = 17.7864$$

which is greater than $R_{tol} = 15$. Therefore, these two vectors are false nearest neighbors.

In this way, every point on the trajectory is examined to calculate how many nearest neighbors are false neighbors, and the percentage of false nearest neighbors to true nearest neighbors is computed at different dimensional spaces. The percentage of false nearest neighbors should drop at a higher-dimensional space as the dynamics

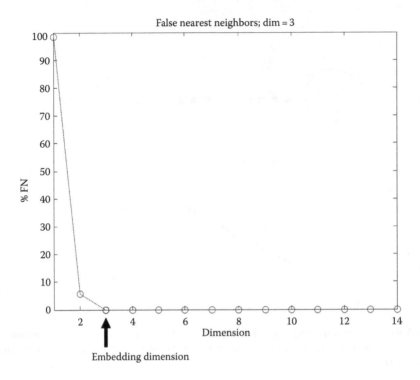

FIGURE 3.11 The percentage of false nearest neighbors for the Lorenz attractor. The percentage of false nearest neighbors hit zero when the dimension is three.

of the attractor are being unfolded. Figure 3.11 is the plot of the percentage of false nearest neighbors versus embedding dimension for the well-known Lorenz attractor. The value of the dimension where the percentage of false nearest neighbors reaches a minimum value around 0 is considered as the dimension that is large enough to describe the dynamics of the system. That dimension is selected as the embedding dimension. In this case, the proper dimension would be 3, which we expected a priori as the Lorenz attractor is generated with three equations.

Question: How do you find the time lag?

AUTOCORRELATION AND AVERAGE MUTUAL INFORMATION

As mentioned earlier, the time lag value should be neither too small nor too large, but what does this mean? Each state-space contains the information of the system at a specific time. For example, a vector $X(t_i)$ should contain the information about the system at time $= t_i$, and $X(t_i + \text{time lag})$ should contain the information about the system at time $= t_i + \text{time lag}$. Therefore, finding an appropriate time lag means to find the time lag value that gives new information about the system, which could not be obtained from the previous state-space. If the time lag value is too small, then the information that the state-space at time $t = t_i + \text{time lag}$ offers is almost the same as the information we obtained from the previous state-space at $t = t_{i-1}$. No new information is given from that state-space.

On the other hand, if the time lag is too large, $X(t_i + \text{time lag})$ offers different information that could be obtained from $X(t_i)$. However, these two vectors $X(t_i)$ and $X(t_i + \text{time lag})$ are highly independent, and a lot of information may be lost between them. So the time lag that gives just the "right" amount of information about the system needs to be identified.

What is needed here is to quantify the relationship between $X(t_i)$ and $X(t_i + \text{time lag})$. A correlation function can be used to measure their relationship. How dependent is the current state-space on the previous state-space? Or how well are they related to each other? One such correlation function that measures dependency among data points is the autocorrelation function calculated with Equation 3.4:

$$r(k) = \frac{\sum_{i=1}^{N-k}(x_i - \bar{x})(x_{i+k} - \bar{x})}{\sum_{i=1}^{N}(x_i - \bar{x})^2} \tag{3.4}$$

The time lag can be selected when the autocorrelation drops to $1/e$ or 0 (Figure 3.12; Sprott 2003). However, the autocorrelation function measures linear dependency and not nonlinear dependency among data points, something that is critical to our approach not only in this chapter but in the entire book. To measure nonlinear dependency in a time series, average mutual information can be used (Fraser 1989; Fraser and Swinney 1986). Average mutual information can be thought of as the nonlinear

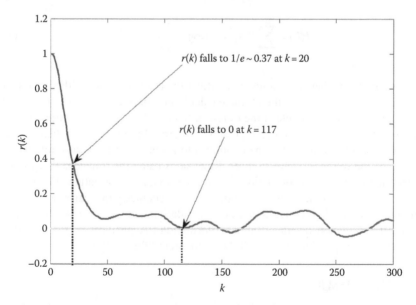

FIGURE 3.12 When calculating time lag using the autocorrelation function, the time lag is either selected as the point when the function drops to either $1/e$ or 0. In the figure using the Lorenz attractor, this would yield either a time lag of 20 or 117.

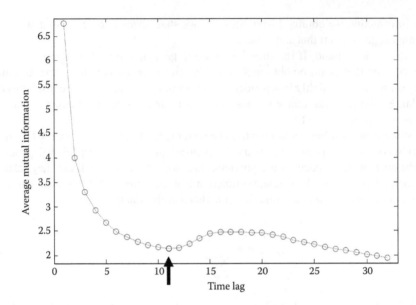

FIGURE 3.13 The first minimum average mutual information for the Lorenz attractor is at 11, which is the time lag value to be used for the reconstruction of the state-space.

version of the autocorrelation function (Equation 3.5). We select the first minimum of the average mutual information as the time lag (Figure 3.13). An illustrative example is provided for the reader in Figure 3.14a through d:

$$I(k) = \sum_{t=1}^{n} P(x_t, x_{t+1}) \log_x \frac{P(x_t, x_{t+k})}{P(x_t)P(x_{t+k})} \tag{3.5}$$

The choice of time lag can dramatically affect the attractor shape, although it is not certain that this will impact the ultimate calculations derived from the attractor. We can see this with our example of the Lorenz attractor. We can see the attractor generated from the known differential equations (Figure 3.15, top left). We then use only a single equation from the Lorenz equations to generate a time series, followed by reconstruction of the attractor in three dimensions using the time lags that we have determined through autocorrelation and average mutual information (Figure 3.15). This helps to observe the influence on the attractor geometry that can result from the different time lag choices based on linear calculation (autocorrelation) compared to nonlinear calculation (average mutual information). A justification for time-delay reconstruction is provided through Takens' theorem (Takens 1981).

PRACTICAL ISSUES

So far, the reconstruction of the state-space has been explained. In addition, how to find an embedding dimension and time lag that are required for the reconstruction of the state-space has been presented. However, are there any issues that should be

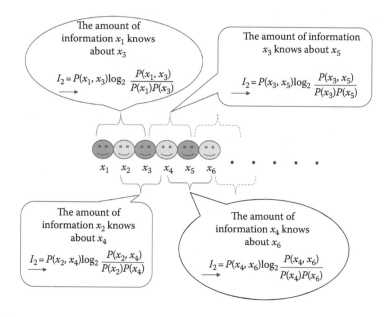

(a)

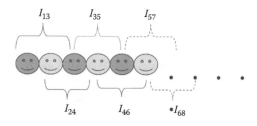

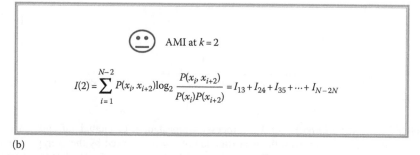

(b)

FIGURE 3.14 (a) The mutual information is calculated for every point with a time lag of $k = 2$. (b) The average mutual information is calculatevd across the time series for a time lag of $k = 2$. *(Continued)*

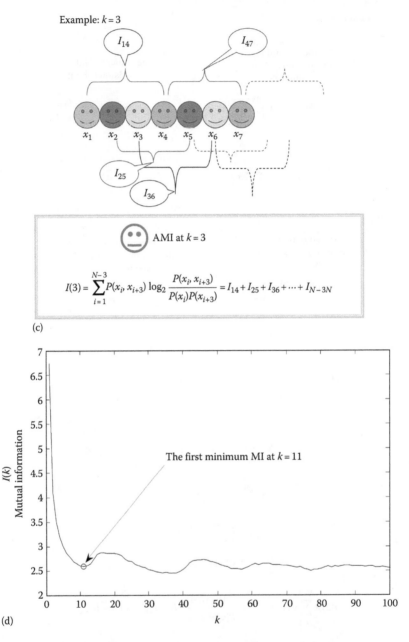

(c)

(d)

FIGURE 3.14 (*Continued*) (c) The process is repeated, with mutual information now calculated for every point with the next time lag of $k = 3$, followed by the average mutual information for time lag $k = 3$. (d) The average mutual information (I) is calculated for numerous time lag (k) values. In this example, it was calculated to $k = 100$. A plot is then made of $I(k)$ against k. The time lag is obtained by determining the first minimum mutual information, which corresponds to $k = 11$ for this example.

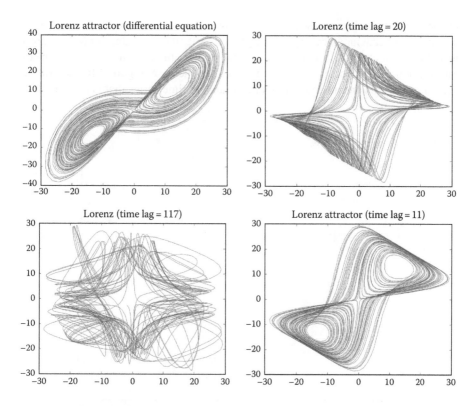

FIGURE 3.15 Comparing reconstructed Lorenz attractors using time lags of $k = 20$ (autocorrelation function dropped to 0), $k = 117$ (autocorrelation function dropped to $1/e$), and $k = 11$ (average mutual information) with the attractor generated from the Lorenz equations. The linear calculation to time lag (i.e., autocorrelation) results in overdistortion of the attractor whereas the nonlinear calculation (average mutual information) preserves more of the true geometry.

considered when the false nearest neighbor algorithm and average mutual information are applied to biological time series?

PROBLEMS WITH FINDING AN EMBEDDING DIMENSION

In the previous section, we explained that the embedding dimension should be greater than the dimension of the attractor so that the embedded data may approximate the true structure of the underlying attractor. But does this mean if there is no upper limit on an embedding dimension that can be used? Is it appropriate to use an embedding dimension of 15 to the data where the true embedding dimension is 3? There is a warning against such use of an unnecessarily high embedding dimension because such practice tends to decrease the density of the points on the attractor, thereby enhancing the effect of the noise present in the data (Sprott 2003).

Noise is not the only issue, however, when excessively high embedding dimensions are chosen. As mentioned earlier, the embedding dimension is selected when the percentage of false nearest neighbors drops to 0 or is closest to 0. Usually, there is a convergent behavior at lower percentage levels after the percentage of false nearest neighbors gets close to 0. However, with noisy data, the percentage of false nearest neighbors may decrease at first but may then increase. Figure 3.16a shows the percentage of false nearest neighbors for a random time series that is in fact white

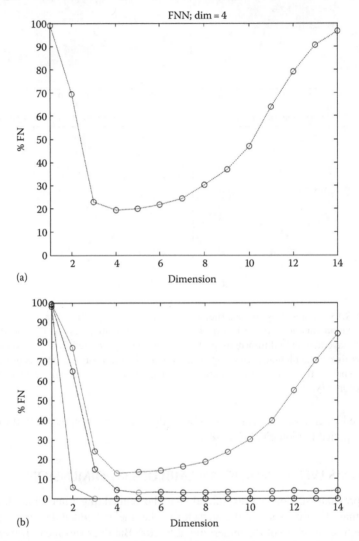

(a)

(b)

FIGURE 3.16 (a) The percentage of false nearest neighbors for a random time series, which drops at first and then goes up again without being close to 0. (b) The percentage of false nearest neighbors for the Lorenz attractor with different noise levels. The bottom dotted line indicates the percentage of false nearest neighbors for the noise-free data. The middle dotted line indicates the percentage of false nearest neighbors for the Lorenz attractor with a noise level of $L/R_A = 0.1$. The top dotted line indicates the percentage of false nearest neighbors for the Lorenz attractor with the noise level of $L/R_A = 0.5$. R_A is the size of the attractor, and L indicates the range of uniformly distributed random numbers.

noise. Figure 3.16b shows the percentage of false nearest neighbors for the Lorenz attractor with different levels of white noise. Here, the level of noise expressed as L/R_A is defined as a fraction of the root mean square of the size of the attractor (R_A) to random numbers uniformly distributed in $[-L\ L]$. The percentage of false nearest neighbors for the Lorenz attractor with zero noise level $L/R_A = 0$ is expressed in the bottom dotted line in Figure 3.16b, and it gives the value of embedding dimension equal to 3. However, as the noise level increases to $L/R_A = 0.1$ as expressed in the middle dotted line, the embedding dimension increases to 5. Finally, when the noise level increases to $L/R_A = 0.5$ expressed in the top dotted line, the result is similar to what we observed with the random time series. In higher embedding dimensions, the influence of noise in the percentage of false nearest neighbors increases clearly, showing that using an unnecessarily large embedding dimension is not a proper procedure. This highlights the importance of taking time and exercising caution to properly set up equipment and procedures to minimize noise entering the data through proper sampling rates and experimental design. The percentage of false nearest neighbors could potentially be used as an additional visual aid in determining how much noise is present in the data.

PROBLEMS WITH FINDING A TIME LAG

If a time lag of 1 is found using the average mutual information, what does it mean? It means that the first independent point occurs at time lag = 1, and there is no correlation among the data points. Figure 3.17 shows the average mutual information for a random time series with the first minimum average mutual information

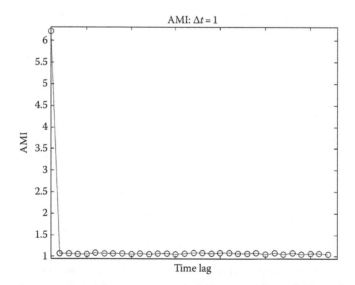

FIGURE 3.17 The first minimum average mutual information for a random time series (white noise) is at one, which indicates there are no correlations among the data points.

occurring at time lag = 1. Therefore, if in all the experimental data sets the time lag is 1, then it can be said that the data are very noisy. However, some additional checking is needed.

There are cases where no "first independent point" for a time series is found since all the data points are strongly correlated to each other. Let us think about a real experimental situation. What happens to a time lag if the data are sampled at an unnecessarily high frequency? In this case, there are strong correlations among the data points, and there may be no first independent point found or it may occur at a very large time lag. For example, Figure 3.18a shows the power spectrum of a time series of the horizontal displacement of the surgical instrument tip, which was originally collected incorrectly at a sampling frequency of 1000 Hz from a subject who performed surgical needle passing using daVinci™ Surgical System (Intuitive

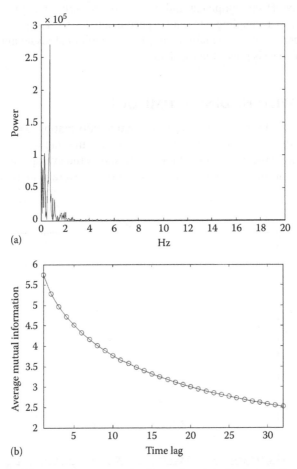

(a)

(b)

FIGURE 3.18 (a) The power spectrum of a time series of the horizontal displacement of the surgical instrument tip, which was originally collected at a sampling frequency of 1000 Hz from a subject who performed surgical needle passing using daVinci Surgical. (b) No first minimal average mutual information was found for the original data sampled at 1000 Hz. *(Continued)*

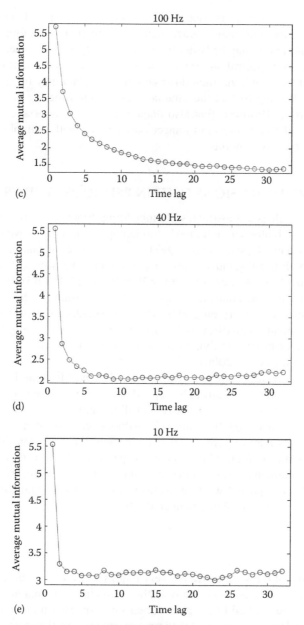

FIGURE 3.18 (*Continued*) The first minimum average mutual information for the data resampled at (c) 100 Hz is 22, (d) 40 Hz is 6, (e) 10 Hz is 5.

Surgical, Inc., Sunnyvale, CA). No first independent point was found for this original data because of strong correlations among the data points (Figure 3.18b). However, the first minimum average mutual information was found by downsampling the data. Downsampling the data gave a time lag value of 22 at 100 Hz (Figure 3.18c), 6 at 40 Hz (Figure 3.18d), and 5 at 10 Hz (Figure 3.18e), respectively.

If commercial software is used, it may return a time lag = 1 only because it cannot find the first minimum average mutual information. Therefore, when a time lag = 1 is identified, it may be better to examine the data again to see if that value is appropriate. If a spectral analysis of the data identifies the sampling frequency that was used was too high, then downsampling the data may be an option with subsequently retrying to find the time lag. A different time lag value may seem more appropriate. However, this also demonstrates the importance of correctly sampling your data and does not unnecessarily increase the sampling frequency just to obtain more data points.

EMBEDDING DIMENSIONS USED IN PREVIOUS STUDIES

The following values are estimates of embedding dimension (m) found in previous studies with biological data. In rhythmic upper extremity movements, m was found to be around 4 (Mitra et al. 1997). In lower extremity movements during locomotion with healthy individuals, m was found to be around 5–6 (Dingwell and Cusumano 2000; Miller et al. 2006; Wurdeman et al. 2013). For body sway during sitting postural control, m was found to be around 5–6 (Cignetti et al. 2011; Harbourne and Stergiou 2003), while for standing postural sway, m was found to be around 8–10(Riley and Clark 2003; Riley et al. 1999; Schmit et al. 2005, 2006). For heart rate dynamics, m was found to be around 7–14 (Andres et al. 2006; Casties et al. 2006).

This list is certainly not exhaustive but indicative. It should be mentioned here that these values are strongly dependent on the task and the population. Specifically, in locomotion, an embedding dimension of 5–6 may be adequate for healthy individuals, but the nature of a pathological movement with increased random elements may require a higher dimension. Furthermore, different measures, such as the motion of the ankle compared to the hip, may have different embedding dimensions. Consider transtibial amputees where the sound ankle motion has been reported with an average dimension of 5 and the hip motion having a dimension of 7 (Wurdeman et al. 2013).

SUMMARY

Reconstruction of the state-space is a very important procedure in terms of doing nonlinear time series analysis. Many of the nonlinear tools that are presented in later chapters are applied in a higher-dimensional space. An embedding dimension and time lag are required for the reconstruction of the state-space. There are several different algorithms to find an embedding dimension and time lag, but we presented the most commonly used methods—the false nearest neighbor algorithm to find an embedding dimension and the mutual information to find a time lag. We also described situations where some caution should be exercised using these tools. Since the reconstruction of the state-space is fundamental, each step should be carefully considered as a preparation for the application of nonlinear tools.

EXERCISES

1. Generate a time series using the following equations. Reconstruct the state-space for $X(t)$ using the embedding dimension = 2 and time lag = 1. Identify the state vectors 10 and 20. Plot the two-dimensional state-space plot for this time series:

$$X(t+1) = Y(t) + 1.0 - 1.4 * X(t)^2$$

$$Y(t+1) = 0.3 * X(t)$$

2. Repeat problem 1 with time lag = 5. Also state your observations.
3. Find the embedding dimension and time lag of a sine wave. Reconstruct the state-space for this time series and make a two-dimensional state-space plot.
4. What happens to the time lag if the sampling frequency is unnecessarily high? Explain.

REFERENCES

Abarbanel, H.D.I. (1996). *Analysis of Observed Chaotic Data*. New York: Springer-Verlag.

Andres, D.S., I.M. Irurzun, J. Mitelman, and E.E. Mola. (2006). Increase in the embedding dimension in the heart rate variability associated with left ventricular abnormalities. *Applied Physics Letters*, 89:144111.

Casties, J.F., D. Mottet, and D. Le Gallais. (2006). Non-linear analyses of heart rate variability during heavy exercise and recovery in cyclists. *International Journal of Sports Medicine*, 27(10):780–785.

Cignetti, F., A. Kyvelidou, R.T. Harbourne, and N. Stergiou. (2011). Anterior-posterior and medial-lateral control of sway in infants during sitting acquisition does not become adult-like. *Gait Posture*, 33(1):88–92.

Dingwell, J.B. and J.P. Cusumano. (2000). Nonlinear time series analysis of normal and pathological human walking. *Chaos*, 10(4):848–863.

Fraser, A.M. (1989). Reconstructing attractors from scalar time series: A comparison of singular system and redundancy criteria. *Physica D*, 34(3):391–404.

Fraser, A.M. and H.L. Swinney. (1986). Independent coordinates for strange attractors from mutual information. *Physical Review A*, 33(2):1134–1140.

Harbourne, R.T. and N. Stergiou. (2003). Nonlinear analysis of the development of sitting postural control. *Developmental Psychobiology*, 42(4):368–377.

Kennel, M.B., R. Brown, and H.D.I. Abarbanel. (1992). Determining minimum embedding dimension using a geometrical construction. *Physical Review A*, 45:3403–3411.

Miller, J.M., N. Stergiou and M.J. Kurz. (2006). An improved surrogate method for detecting the presence of chaos in gait. *Journal of Biomechanics*, 39(15):2873–2876.

Mitra, S., M.A. Riley, and M.T. Turvey. (1997). Chaos in human rhythmic movement. *Journal of Motor Behavior*, 29(3):195–198.

Riley, M.A., R. Balasubramaniam, and M.T. Turvey. (1999). Recurrence quantification analysis of postural fluctuations. *Gait & Posture*, 9:65–78.

Riley, M.A. and S. Clark. (2003). Recurrence analysis of human postural sway during the sensory organization test. *Neuroscience Letters*, 342:45–48.

Schmit, J.M., D. Regis, and M.A. Riley. (2005). Dynamic patterns of postural sway in ballet dancers and track athletes. *Experimental Brain Research*, 163:370–378.

Schmit, J.M., M.A. Riley, A. Dalvi, A. Sahay, P.K. Shear, K.D. Shockley, and R.Y.K. Pun. (2006). Deterministic center of pressure patterns characterize postural instability in Parkinson's disease. *Experimental Brain Research*, 168:357–367.

Sprott, J.C. (2003). *Chaos and Time Series Analysis*. Oxford, U.K.: Oxford University Press.

Stergiou, N., U.H. Buzzi, M.J. Kurz, and J. Heidel. (2004). Nonlinear tools in human movement. In: N. Stergiou (ed.), *Innovative Analyses of Human Movement*. Champaign, IL: Human Kinetics, pp. 63–90.

Takens, F. (1981). Detecting strange attractors in turbulence. In: D.A. Rand and L.-S. Young (eds.), *Dynamical Systems and Turbulence, Lecture Notes in Mathematics*, Vol. 898. New York, NY: Springer-Verlag, pp. 366–381.

Wolf, A., J.B. Swift, H.L. Swinney, and J.A. Vostano. (1985). Determining Lyapunov exponents from a time series. *Physica D*, 16:285–317.

Wurdeman, S.R., S.A. Myers, N. Stergiou. (2013). Transtibial amputee joint motion has increased attractor divergence during walking compared to non-amputee gait. *Annals of Biomedical Engineering*, 41(4):806–813.

4 Lyapunov Exponent

Shane R. Wurdeman

CONTENTS

Introduction 83
What is Chaos? 84
Lyapunov Exponents 85
Definition of the Spectrum of Lyapunov Exponents 89
Different Algorithms to Compute Lyapunov Exponents 94
Wolf et al. Algorithm 94
    Procedure 95
Rosenstein et al. Algorithm 100
    Procedure 101
Comparing the Two Algorithms 104
Summary 107
Exercises 107
References 108

> There is a self-satisfied dogmatism with which mankind at each period of its history cherishes the delusion of the finality of existing modes of knowledge.
>
> **Alfred North Whitehead (1861–1947)**

INTRODUCTION

As the search for the evidence of deterministic chaos has become popular in many different fields of science such as biology, ecology, economy, engineering, and medicine (Schaffer 1985; Mees and Sparrow 1987; Goldberger et al. 1990; Hassell et al. 1991; Peel and Speight 1994; Aguirre and Aguirre 1997; Piccoli and Weber 1998), attention has been given to methods to detect and quantify chaos (Gollub et al. 1980; Brandstater et al. 1983; Guckenheimer and Buzyna 1983; Malraison et al. 1983; Swinney 1983). The calculation of Lyapunov exponents has been one of the most popular methods used to detect the presence of chaos in dynamical systems and has been used for the analysis of various biological systems such as human gait (Buzzi et al. 2003; Stergiou et al. 2004; Yoshino et al. 2004; Kurz and Stergiou 2007; Smith et al. 2010; Decker et al. 2011), postural sway (Timmer et al. 2000; Harbourne and Stergiou 2003; Donker et al. 2007; Lamoth et al. 2009; Kyvelidou et al. 2010; Lamoth and van Heuvelen 2012), and handwriting (Longstaff and Heath 1999).

Lyapunov exponents carry their namesake from the Russian mathematician, mechanist, and physician Aleksander Lyapunov (1857–1918). He was a student of the famous mathematician Pafnuty Chebyshev, and he also became famous himself for the development of the stability theory of a dynamical system. He developed numerous methods beginning in 1899 referred to as Lyapunov methods. These methods make it possible to define the stability of sets of ordinary differential equations. Before getting into the details of Lyapunov exponents, let us begin our discussion by defining what a chaotic system is.

WHAT IS CHAOS?

There is no universal definition of chaos; however, we can identify certain properties that chaotic systems should have. First, a chaotic system is an aperiodic deterministic system, which means literally the system is without periodicity. In nature, such systems are prevalent. Turbulent flow patterns are one such example (Lorenz 1963). In fact, Edward Lorenz, a pioneer of chaos, discovered a property of chaos while he was studying turbulent flow patterns, which can be very irregular at one instance but can display well-organized behaviors at another instance. This property is called sensitive dependence on initial conditions which came to be known as "the butterfly effect" (Gleick 1987).

This property of sensitive dependence on initial conditions is often regarded as one of the signatures of chaos. For example, look at two trajectories of a dynamical system in phase space (Figure 4.1a). Let $x(0)$ be the initial condition for a trajectory and $x'(0)$ be its neighbor on another trajectory. The $x(0)$ and $x'(0)$ are separated by a very small distance of $\delta x(0)$ (Figure 4.1b). The initial condition of $x(0)$ generates the trajectory $x(t)$ and $x'(0)$ generates another trajectory $x'(t)$, where t is time. If the separation of the two trajectories expressed as $\delta x(t) = |x'(t) - x(t)|$ grows exponentially as time progresses, then there is sensitive dependence on initial conditions (Figure 4.1c and d). Now can we conclude that the system is chaotic? Before making that conclusion, we need to consider another property.

Sensitive dependence on initial condition is one of the main features of chaos. However, it is not a unique characteristic to chaotic systems. Sensitive dependence on initial conditions can also occur in linear systems. For example, let us examine a simple system that can be described with a linear equation of $X_{n+1} = 1.5X_n$ (Figure 4.2). Let the first initial condition $x(0) = 0.1$ and the second initial condition $x'(0) = 0.08$. Then, the initial separation is $\delta x(0) = |0.1 - 0.08| = 0.02$. After 30 iterations, the trajectories $x(t)$ and $x'(t)$ diverge exponentially, and the distance becomes $\delta x(30) = |12,783 - 10,227| = 2,556$. The distance of the two trajectories grew apart 127,800 times more than the original separation (Figure 4.2). However, this system is not chaotic. The difference is that this linear system is not bounded while chaotic systems are bounded. Sensitive dependence on initial conditions brings about chaos only if a system has bounded trajectories so that it will not expand to infinity. A system with linear dynamics has either sensitive dependence on initial condition or bounded trajectories, but it cannot have both of these properties at the same time. On the other hand, a system with chaotic dynamics has both sensitive dependence on initial conditions and bounded trajectories. In summary, for a system to be chaotic, it must be (1) deterministic, (2) aperiodic, (3) sensitive to initial conditions, and (4) bounded.

LYAPUNOV EXPONENTS

As mentioned earlier, the Lyapunov exponent can quantify chaos. It measures the rate at which nearby orbits converge or diverge. Let us again examine two trajectories in phase space, which have initial separation of $\left|\delta x(0)\right|$ and divergence of the trajectories $\left|\delta x(t)\right|$ after t time steps. The $\left|\delta x(t)\right|$ can be approximated by $e\lambda^t\left|\delta x(0)\right|$,

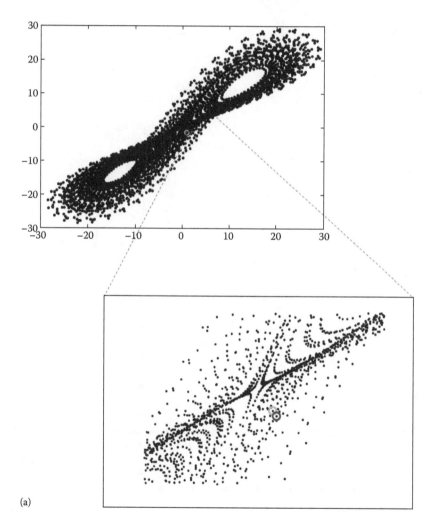

(a)

FIGURE 4.1 (a) Two initial conditions are randomly selected on the Lorenz attractor.

(*Continued*)

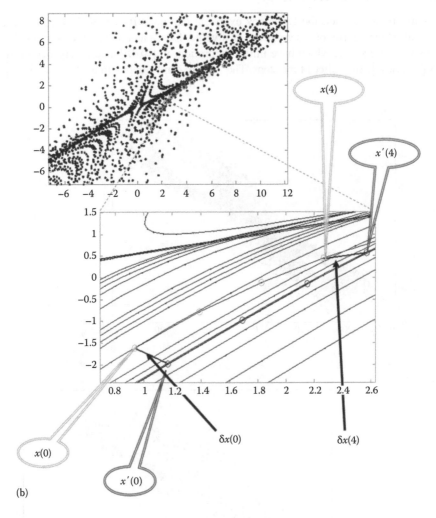

FIGURE 4.1 (*Continued*)   (b) Top: Two trajectories generated by the initial conditions after 10 steps. Bottom: Enlarged two trajectories generated by the initial conditions after four steps.   (*Continued*)

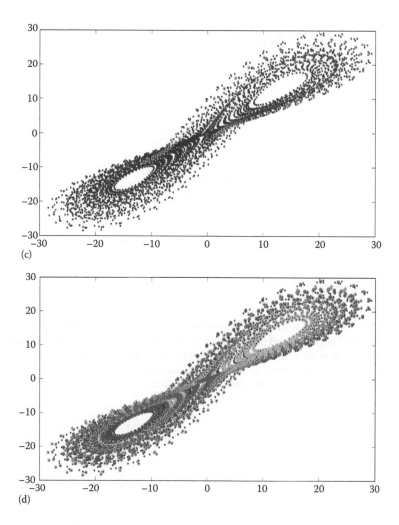

FIGURE 4.1 (*Continued*)   (c) Two trajectories after 50 steps. (d) Two trajectories experience exponential separation.

where λ is the Lyapunov exponent and e is the mathematical constant ($e \approx 2.72$). If $\lambda = 0$, $e^{\lambda t} = e^0 = 1$, then $|\delta x(0)| = |\delta x(t)|$, and there is neither convergence nor divergence of the trajectories. If λ is positive, then $|\delta x(t)|$ will have exponential growth, and the two trajectories will experience exponential separation. If λ is negative, then $|\delta x(t)|$ will have exponential decay, and the trajectories will have exponentially fast convergence. Figure 4.3 shows a plot of $\ln|\delta x(t)|$ versus t for two trajectories for the Lorenz system. The slope of a least squared fitted line on a curve represents the Lyapunov exponent λ. Because the distance between the two trajectories varies along the attractor depending on the strength of the exponential convergence

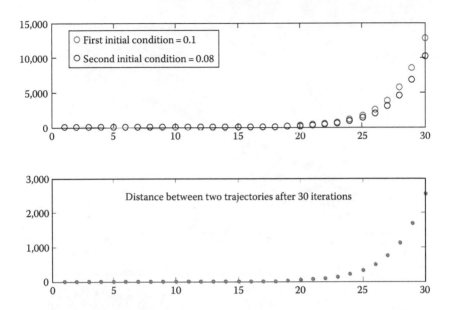

FIGURE 4.2 Sensitive dependence on initial conditions in a linear system. Top: The values of the first initial condition and the values of the second initial conditions for 30 iterations. The graph shows how the trajectories starting at very close distance can move apart after only 30 iterations. Bottom: The graph shows how the distance between two trajectories generated by the first and second initial conditions can grow apart.

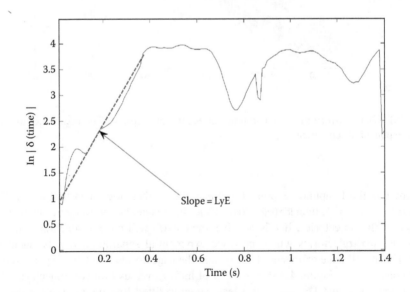

FIGURE 4.3 A plot $\ln\langle d(i)\rangle$ versus t for the Lorenz attractor. The slope of a dotted fitted line to the linear scaling region is the Lyapunov exponent.

or divergence, the curve is rather bumpy. Furthermore, the separation of the two trajectories cannot grow further apart than the diameter of the attractor, and therefore, there are plateau regions in the plot.

Here, we have only examined one Lyapunov exponent for the system. However, it is important to mention that there are as many Lyapunov exponents as the number of dimensions required to fully and uniquely describe the system. If the dimension of the state space is three, then there are three Lyapunov exponents. If the dimension of the state space is four, then there are four Lyapunov exponents and so on. This is called the spectrum of Lyapunov exponents.

DEFINITION OF THE SPECTRUM OF LYAPUNOV EXPONENTS

In m-dimensional phase space, we can create a small m-dimensional sphere of initial conditions. We will use the Rossler equations and subsequent attractor to demonstrate. As time evolves, the sphere evolves into an ellipsoid which has m principal axes (Figure 4.4). Let $\delta_i(t)$, $i = 1, 2,..., m$ be the length of ith principal axis of the ellipsoid, and $\delta_i(0)$ be called an initial separation vector. Then $\delta_i(t)$ is approximated by $e^{\lambda_i t}|\delta_i(0)|$, or

$$|\delta_i(t)| \approx e^{\lambda_i t}|\delta_i(0)| \tag{4.1}$$

Now, if we isolate $e^{\lambda_i t}$,

$$\frac{|\delta_i(t)|}{|\delta_i(0)|} \approx e^{\lambda_i t} \tag{4.2}$$

Next, we can solve for λ_i,

$$\ln \frac{|\delta_i(t)|}{|\delta_i(0)|} \approx \ln e^{\lambda_i t} \tag{4.3}$$

$$\ln \frac{|\delta_i(t)|}{|\delta_i(0)|} \approx \lambda_i t \tag{4.4}$$

$$\lambda_i \approx \frac{1}{t} \ln \frac{|\delta_i(t)|}{|\delta_i(0)|} \tag{4.5}$$

Since λ_i is the ith Lyapunov exponent, and $i = 1, 2,..., m$, we have m different Lyapunov exponents, $\lambda_1, \lambda_2,..., \lambda_m$. Figure 4.5 shows the case where $m = 3$, and the system has three Lyapunov exponents. Each principal axis of the ellipsoid expands or contracts at a rate given by a corresponding Lyapunov exponent, and thus, the rate of separation can be different for various orientations of the initial separation vector.

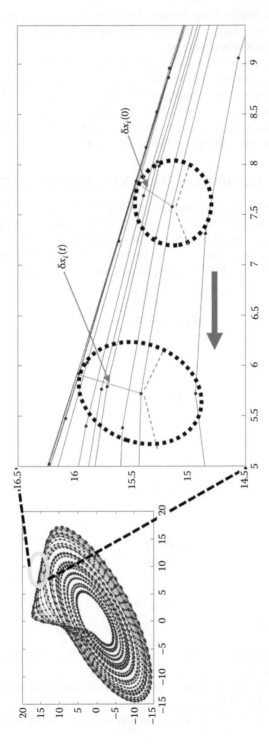

FIGURE 4.4   The chaotic Rossler system. A small m-dimensional sphere (in this case, $m = 3$) evolves into an ellipsoid with $m = 3$ principal axes.

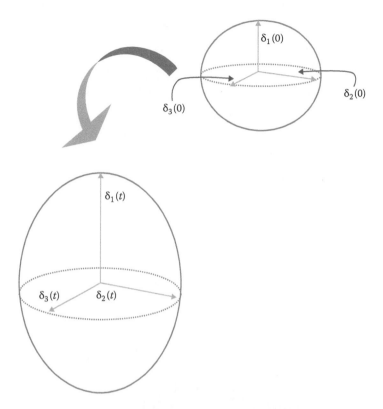

FIGURE 4.5 A three-dimensional sphere evolves into an ellipsoid with three principal axes. The length of each principal axis represents a Lyapunov exponent. This system has three Lyapunov exponents.

Since Lyapunov exponents may depend on a trajectory, computation of the Lyapunov exponents should be done by averaging over many different points on the same trajectory or the limit of Equation 4.5:

$$\lambda_i \approx \lim_{t \to \infty} \frac{1}{t} \ln \frac{|\delta_i(t)|}{|\delta_i(0)|} \tag{4.6}$$

Now, as the principal axis of the ellipsoid expands at a rate of $e^{\lambda_1 t}$, at the same time the area defined by the first two principal axes is growing as $e^{(\lambda_1 + \lambda_2)t}$ (Figure 4.6). Similarly, the volume defined by the first three principal axes is growing as $e^{(\lambda_1 + \lambda_2 + \lambda_3)t}$. Thus, the first j exponents are defined by the long-term exponential growth rate of a j-volume element, $e^{(\lambda_1 + \lambda_2 + \cdots + \lambda_j)t}$. This is the spectrum of Lyapunov exponents, where λ_1 is the largest Lyapunov exponent. Importantly, any continuous time-dependent dynamical system without a fixed point will have at least one zero exponent. The axes that are expanding will have positive exponents while

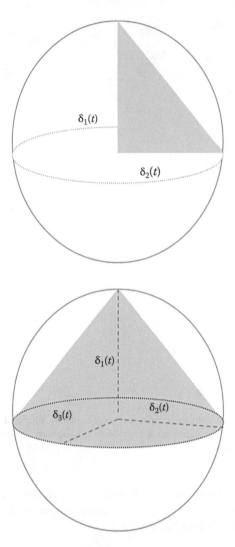

FIGURE 4.6 Top: As the principal axis of the ellipsoid expands at a rate of $e^{\lambda_1 t}$, at the same time the area defined by the first two principal axes is growing as $e^{(\lambda_1 + \lambda_2)t}$. Bottom: The volume defined by the first three principal axes is similarly growing as $e^{(\lambda_1 + \lambda_2 + \lambda_3)t}$.

those contracting will have negative exponents. The sum of Lyapunov exponents must be negative in a dissipative system, that is, there must be at least one negative Lyapunov exponent within the spectrum. In order to have a state of chaos, there must be at least one positive Lyapunov exponent. In a three-dimensional continuous dissipative dynamical system, the signs of the exponents within the spectrum dictate the system dynamics.

For example, the following spectrum elicits the accompanying system dynamics:

$(+, 0, -) \rightarrow$ strange attractor (i.e., chaos)
$(0, 0, -) \rightarrow$ two torus
$(0, -, -) \rightarrow$ limit cycle
$(-, -, -) \rightarrow$ fixed point

Lyapunov exponents are defined as the average exponential rate of divergence or convergence of nearby trajectories in state space. The states of nearby trajectories are closely related and therefore predictions are possible, while the states of exponential divergent trajectories are uncorrelated and predictions are impossible. The ability to quantify the separation of trajectories makes the Lyapunov exponent to also function as a measure of the average predictability of a system that exhibits nonlinear dynamics.

It is common to focus only on the largest Lyapunov exponent (Dingwell and Cusumano 2000; Dingwell et al. 2000, 2001; Harbourne and Stergiou 2003; Stergiou et al. 2004; Desalvo et al. 2006; Kikuchi et al. 2006; England and Granata 2007; Lockhart and Liu 2008; Smith et al. 2010; Decker et al. 2011). As discussed previously, a qualitative picture of the system's dynamics is provided by the signs of the Lyapunov exponents. As time evolves, eventually it is the largest positive Lyapunov exponent that determines the diameter of the ellipsoid, and therefore, the predictability of a system that exhibits nonlinear dynamics. Directions of local instabilities are determined by positive Lyapunov exponents. Chaotic systems must have at least one positive Lyapunov exponent. Therefore, the calculation of a positive largest Lyapunov exponent is sufficient to indicate the presence of chaos in the system and represents local instability in a particular direction. This, however, is only true for systems that do not contain uncorrelated noise. As a result, it is not sufficient in the calculation of experimental time series that will always contain some amount of uncorrelated noise. Lyapunov exponents are ultimately a measure of predictability and thus quantify the rate at which a system is processing information. Therefore, Lyapunov exponents should appropriately be expressed in a unit of bits of information/s or bits/orbit.

When calculated in units of bits/s, it is possible to calculate the time horizon. When a system has a positive Lyapunov exponent, there is a time horizon beyond which prediction of the system's behavior breaks down. Let $|\delta_0|$ be the error between our estimate and the true initial state of the system. After time t,

$$|\delta_t| \approx |\delta_0| e^{\lambda t} \tag{4.7}$$

Now, let a be a measure of our tolerance; hence, prediction becomes intolerable when $|\delta_t| \geq a$. This occurs at a time,

$$t_{\text{Horizon}} \approx \frac{1}{\lambda} \ln \frac{a}{|\delta_0|} \tag{4.8}$$

For example, if we have a tolerance of $a = 10^{-3}$ and estimate the initial state's uncertainty to within $|\delta_0| = 10^{-7}$, then we can predict the state of the system while remaining within the tolerance for a time of $4\ln 10/\lambda$. Or, a more obvious example with regard to maintaining units of bits/s, if we can specify an initial point with an accuracy of 20 bits, for a system with $\lambda_1 = 2.16$ bits/s, we can predict the behavior of the system as far out as 9.26 s.

DIFFERENT ALGORITHMS TO COMPUTE LYAPUNOV EXPONENTS

Several different algorithms have been proposed to compute the Lyapunov exponents. They can be classified largely into two main groups: (1) algorithms based on differential equations (Shimada and Nagashima 1979; Benettin et al. 1980; Eckmann and Ruelle 1985; Geist et al. 1990) and (2) algorithms based on a trajectory method (Sano and Sawada 1985; Wolf et al. 1985; Farmer and Sidorowich 1987; Sato et al. 1987; Casdagli 1989; Abarbanel et al. 1990; Bauer et al. 1991; Ellner et al. 1991; Wales 1991; Rosenstein et al. 1993; Kantz 1994; Darbyshire and Broomhead 1996; Wurdeman and Stergiou 2013; Wurdeman et al. 2013, 2014). The first group of algorithms is applied when equations for the system are available. In experimental data the equations that govern the system are not known, and only a measured scalar time series is available for the computation of the Lyapunov exponent. Therefore, in the following sections, we will discuss the two most widely used algorithms to compute the largest Lyapunov exponent, which belong to the second group of algorithms. Both of these algorithms require reconstruction of the state space (refer to Chapter 3 regarding the reconstruction of the state space).

WOLF ET AL. ALGORITHM

The first algorithm to compute Lyapunov exponents from experimental data was introduced by Wolf et al. (1985). This algorithm has been used extensively in the human movement literature (Harbourne and Stergiou 2003; Kurz and Stergiou 2007; Smith et al. 2010; Wurdeman and Stergiou 2013; Wurdeman et al. 2013, 2014; and many others), and the corresponding software is available at the book editor's website and all software used in this book. Several implementation notes are also given below to assist the potential user. Wolf et al.'s algorithm is based on monitoring the average divergence of nearby trajectories from a single reference trajectory to estimate the largest Lyapunov exponent. Note that this has mistakenly been understood in the past to mean a single orbit of the attractor; however, because the time series is continuous, then in actuality, the reference trajectory is the entire time series and not a single orbit. In theory, this method can also be used to compute the whole spectrum of Lyapunov exponents. However, Wolf et al. mention that the computation of negative Lyapunov exponents can be numerically unstable for experimental data, and it is limited for practical applications. Therefore, our discussion will be focused on the computation of the largest Lyapunov exponent.

PROCEDURE

1. Let $x(t)$ be a scalar time series with length N, where $t = 1, 2,..., N$. Select the embedding dimension (m) and time lag (τ) for state-space reconstruction.
2. Randomly select an embedded point as an initial condition. This embedded point is a delay vector which has m elements, $x(t)$, $x(t + \tau),..., x(t + (m - 1)\tau)$; also, this vector generates the reference trajectory. Because any point within the attractor has an equal probability of being selected as the random point with which to begin, for algorithm implementation purposes, the first point on the time series is chosen.
3. Select its nearest neighboring point, represented by delay embedded vector, $x(t_0)$, $x(t_0 + \tau),..., x(t_0 + (m - 1)\tau)$ on another trajectory. This nearest neighboring point is found by calculating the Euclidean distance to all points in the attractor and then identifying the point that is the small distance of separation. This distance between points (L) is easily calculated using dot product:

$$L = x(t), x(t + \tau),..., x(t + (m - 1)\tau)) \cdot x(t_0), x(t_0 + \tau),..., x(t_0 + (m - 1)\tau) \quad (4.9)$$

4. Let the initial distance between these two vectors be $L(t_0)$, and then $L'(t_1)$ after a time evolution of t_1.
5. Calculate the exponential growth in separation between these trajectories as the log base 2 of the distance after time evolution $(L'(t_1))$ is divided by the initial distance $(L(t_0))$ (Figure 4.7). This must then be normalized to the time evolution by dividing the calculated exponential divergence by the time the points were allowed to propagate through their respective trajectories, t_1. In practice, t_1 is equal to dt multiplied by n, where dt is equal to the time between data samples or the inverse of the sampling frequency, and n is the number of time steps or points that the point on the reference

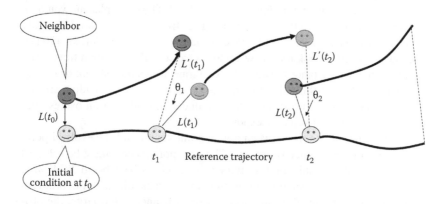

FIGURE 4.7 Wolf et al. algorithm: the evolution of trajectories and replacement procedure for the calculation of the largest Lyapunov exponent.

trajectory and the neighboring point are allowed to move through on their respective trajectories before distance calculation occurs. This can be calculated as follows:

$$Z_1 = \frac{(\log_2(L'(t_1)/L(t_0)))}{(dt \times n)} \qquad (4.10)$$

Implementation notes: The time evolution, t_1, is set *a priori* to running the algorithm. This is done by determining an appropriate n value, or number of samples through which the two-point vectors are followed along their respective trajectories. If n is chosen to be too small, then not enough of the attractor is probed and limitations have been placed on the time for the neighboring points to diverge. On the other hand, if n is chosen to be too large, then the neighboring points are followed beyond the initial period of rapid divergence, which is the point dominated by the largest Lyapunov exponent, and thus, the period is desired to be measured. In order to determine an appropriate n value, one should examine pilot data. Specifically, one can start by calculating the largest Lyapunov exponent for $n = 1, 2,...,$ ($f/2$), where f is the sampling frequency (although calculating to a max of $n = 20$ is often sufficient). Then, a plot of n versus the largest Lyapunov exponent is constructed, with n on the abscissa (Figure 4.8). Within this plot, there will be a region with a plateau. As the largest Lyapunov exponent represents a rate of divergence, the plateau region represents where a constant rate occurs. The proper n value should be one which is within this plateau region. If the pilot data are for multiple conditions or pathologies, then an n value that is able to be contained approximately within the plateaus for all is necessary. Note the width of this plateau will be partially dependent upon the sampling rate and also the system itself. If the sampling rate is very low, then the time between the point vectors is increased. In other words, the time between the point vectors for $n = 3$ at 60 Hz is equal to the time between the point vectors for $n = 6$ at 120 Hz. Thus, the plateau would be shorter for 60 Hz as a time evolution change from n of 3 to 6 would roughly approximate from n of 6 to 12 (twice as many points on the plot) for 120 Hz.

6. Now, we need to look for a new vector because if the evolution time is too large, then the distance between the two trajectories may shrink or rapidly expand if they go through a folding region of the attractor yielding erroneous results. This can result in either an underestimation or an overestimation of the largest Lyapunov exponent.

7. Let $L(t_1)$ be the length between a new point vector and the evolved point vector on the reference trajectory. The new point vector must be selected so that $L(t_1)$ is small, or less than a distance to be labeled *SCALMX*. *SCALMX* is the variable that represents the largest distance the program will search for a neighboring point. If this distance is too large, the program has potential for selecting a point vector that lies on a different trajectory. This distance is set *a priori* in the computer program prior

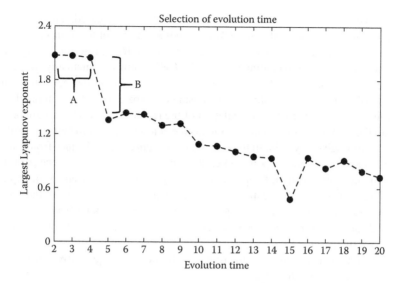

FIGURE 4.8 Plotting a range of time evolutions (*n*) against their calculated largest Lyapunov exponent can help with the selection of a proper time evolution. From this example, data of an individual walking on a treadmill, we can see an initial plateau region (A). Following this initial plateau, there is dramatic drop in the Lyapunov exponent (B). In order to capture the dynamics reflected by the largest Lyapunov exponent, a time evolution within this plateau (A) should be chosen. This region is analogous to the initial period of rapid exponential divergence selected in the Rosenstein algorithm. For multiple conditions, a time evolution should be chosen that captures this plateau region for all conditions.

to running the algorithm. It needs to be set small so that a neighbor is selected nearby in the attractor. Nearby points in an attractor are being described under similar states within the state space. This is critical for these points to have similar initial conditions (remember sensitive dependence on initial conditions from earlier in the chapter). The point vectors will also need to be separated by a minimum distance of *SCALMN*, which is theoretically the point at which noise dominates the signal. In implementation, *SCALMN* is a value greater than 0, which assures when searching for a replacement neighbor that the reference trajectory is not chosen as it would have separation calculated to be 0.

8. Furthermore, the angular separation, θ_1 between the new point vector and the evolved point vector on the reference trajectory, must be small. This is recommended by Wolf et al. to be either 0.3 or 0.2 radians.

   Implementation notes: Now, it is critical to understand that *SCALMX* and θ_1 are actually dynamic values and change throughout computation of the largest Lyapunov exponent. Specifically, replacement nearest neighbors are first sought. If the distance to the potential replacement point is less than *SCALMX*, then it is checked to ensure that it is at an angle less than θ_1. If the point does not meet these criteria, then a new point less than *SCALMX* is checked against angular separation. If points continue to fail meeting both criteria such that no points exist, then *SCALMX* is increased. This process continues until eventually *SCALMX* reaches a multiple of five times its original value, at which point θ_1 is doubled and *SCALMX* is reset to its original value and the search continues with *SCALMX* again systematically increasing as necessary. *SCALMN* is typically set very low, on the magnitude of 0.0001. While theoretically this is considered to be a noise floor, in practice this value ensures that the calculation of the replacement nearest neighbor is not the actual reference point vector. As the computer program systematically goes through every point in the time series and checks the distance from each point and the reference point, when the for-loop gets to the reference point it will calculate a distance separation of 0. Without the requirement of separation greater than *SCALMN*, the computer program will try to initiate the calculation of exponential divergence with the reference point from itself.

9. If these conditions are not met and a new vector cannot be found, then retain the point.
10. Repeat this procedure until the reference trajectory has gone over the entire data samples (Figure 4.9).
11. The largest Lyapunov exponent is calculated then as the average of the local expansion/contraction rates (Z) using the following equation:

$$\lambda_1 = \frac{(Z_1 + Z_2 + \cdots + Z_M)}{M} \tag{4.11}$$

where M is the total number of replacement steps. Or the entire calculation can be represented by a single equation as presented by Wolf et al.:

$$\lambda_1 = \frac{1}{t_M - t_0} \sum_{k=1}^{M} \log_2 \frac{L'(t_k)}{L(t_{k-1})} \tag{4.12}$$

where M is the total number of replacement steps.

For Wolf et al.'s algorithm, there are a few other considerations (and misconceptions). First, with regard to data requirements, it is believed that there needs to be a large number of data points. Wolf et al. stated that the minimum data length depends on three factors:

1. The number of points necessary to provide an adequate number of replacement points
2. The number of orbits of data necessary to probe stretching of the attractor
3. The number of data points per orbit that allow for proper attractor reconstruction with delay coordinates

From these three points, Wolf et al. go on to give a specific range of necessary data points as 10^m–30^m, where m is the attractor-embedded dimension. However, capturing 100,000–24,300,000 data points for a system is difficult if that system is a person

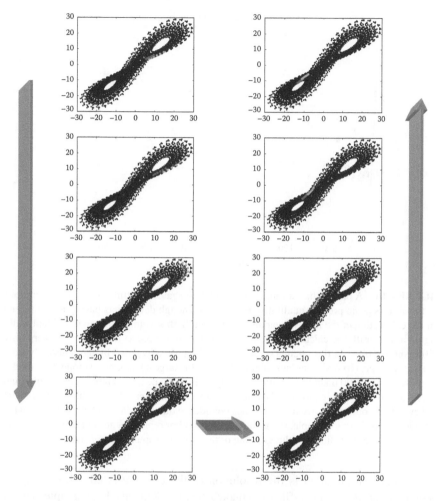

FIGURE 4.9 Wolf et al. algorithm: the reference and replacement trajectories. The reference trajectory is followed along the entire embedded data points on the attractor.

performing some task such as walking and sampling rates are anywhere from 60 to 120 Hz (at 120 Hz, it would take nearly 14 min to get 100,000 data points). This difficulty is compounded when examining pathological motion. Hence, it is important to focus on the three points given by Wolf et al. noting that the estimated number of data points provided was not based on human movement science, and in reality, the number of data points needed remains a question. From Wolf et al. however, we are given a means to examine qualitatively if we have enough data to have confidence in our estimated largest Lyapunov exponent. If the running average is plotted against the iteration within the calculation, there becomes a point where we can see the average reaches a steady state (Figure 4.10). If there is not enough data, there will not be such a steady state and there is less confidence in the estimated largest Lyapunov exponent.

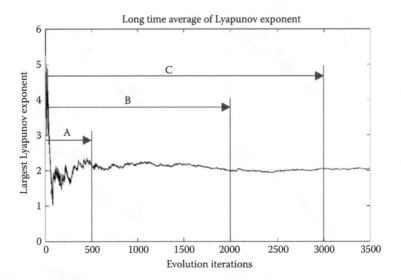

FIGURE 4.10   A plot of the running average, plotted against the time evolution or iterations on the abscissa, can provide qualitative evidence of enough data points having been utilized for the calculation of the largest Lyapunov exponent. In this example, for an individual walking on a treadmill, the calculation was performed with $n = 3$. (A) If the data set were only 1500 points (500 × 3), the calculation would still be unsteady, noted by the nonsteady state running average. (B) A similar lack of confidence in the largest Lyapunov exponent is noted if there were only 2000 potential iterations through which the nearest neighbors can evolve and be replaced by a new neighbor. (C) The steady state reached when 3000 neighbor replacement and evolution points have occurred provides confidence that enough data have been available for calculation. In this example, there were 3500 neighbor replacements and evolution points utilized, so we are confident in the estimate of the largest Lyapunov exponent in this case.

Another consideration is the resolution of the data collected. This is highly system-dependent so it is difficult to make general statements. For example, a good estimate can be made with 5 bits resolution for the Lorenz and Rossler attractors. As a conservative guidance, capturing 8 bits resolutions is a good minimum guideline.

ROSENSTEIN ET AL. ALGORITHM

Rosenstein et al. (1993) introduced another algorithm to compute the largest Lyapunov exponent. This algorithm has also been used extensively in the human movement literature (Dingwell and Cusumano 2000; Dingwell et al. 2000, 2001; England and Granata 2007; and many others) and the corresponding software is widely available from a variety of sources. Rosenstein et al. introduced this algorithm as a remedy to the existing methods, stating that those methods suffer from at least one of the following drawbacks: (1) unreliable for small data sets; (2) computationally intensive; and (3) relatively difficult to implement. Rosenstein et al.'s algorithm is based on the idea that any two randomly chosen initial conditions will have exponential divergence at a rate given by the largest Lyapunov exponent. The average divergence at time t is defined as $D(t) = C \times e^{\lambda_1 t}$, where C is a constant that normalizes the initial separation and λ_1 is the largest Lyapunov exponent.

PROCEDURE

1. Let $x(t)$ be a scalar time series with length N, where $t = 1, 2,..., N$. Select the embedding dimension (m) and time lag (τ) for time delay embedding reconstruction.

2. Randomly select an embedded point as an initial condition. This embedded point is a delay vector that has m elements, $x(t), x(t + \tau),..., x(t + (m - 1) \times \tau)$, and lies upon its own specific trajectory.

3. Select its nearest neighboring embedded point that similarly has m elements, $x(t_0), x(t_0 + \tau),..., x(t_0 + (m - 1) \times \tau)$. When selecting a nearest neighbor, it is stipulated that the neighboring point must have a temporal separation greater than the mean period of the time series. This is easily implemented as the reciprocal of the mean frequency of the power spectrum or the median frequency of the magnitude spectrum. This stipulation prevents the selection of a neighboring point that lies on the same trajectory.

4. Compute the distance between these two vectors on the trajectories at each step (Figure 4.11). This will yield a time series: $d(1), d(2),..., d(K)$, where K is the last embedded point in the attractor. Then calculate the natural logarithm of these distances. This now creates a time series: $\ln(d(1)), \ln(d(2)), \ln(d(3)),..., \ln(d(K))$, where K is the final embedded point of the attractor.

5. There are $M = N - (m - 1)\tau$ embedded points (delay vectors) on the attractor. Repeat the earlier procedure for all these delay vectors.

6. Now, we should have M time series of $d(1), d(2),..., d(K)$. Importantly, each time series will be of a different length based on the location within the attractor of the original two neighboring points. Specifically, if one of the original neighboring points selected was the third from the last point in the original data time series, then its trajectory will only have two more embedded points and the time series of distances would only be $d(1), d(2), d(3)$. For this reason, in the implementation of this algorithm, it may be stipulated that embedded points located within a certain number of points from the end of the attractor should be excluded from selection as original neighboring points. This will speed up processing time as these shorter time series of distances will not be desired in future steps.

7. Now average the distances located at similar points in their time series (i.e., average all $d(1)$ values, then all $d(2)$ values, etc.). This will provide a new time series of average distances: $X = \langle d(1) \rangle, \langle d(2) \rangle,..., \langle d(i) \rangle$, where i is the number of embedded points on the shortest time series of distances.

8. Next, calculate the natural log of each of the average distances, yielding a new time series of $\ln\langle d(i) \rangle$, where i is $1, 2,...,$ up to the number of average distance measures within the time series X.

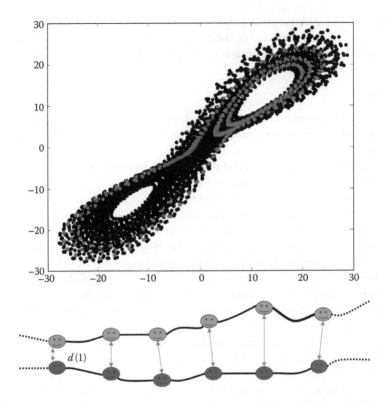

FIGURE 4.11 Top: The trajectories generated by two nearby vectors. Bottom: The distance between these two vectors are calculated at each iteration. There is no replacing of trajectories.

9. Now plot $\ln\langle d(i)\rangle$ versus time (Figure 4.12).
10. The largest Lyapunov exponent is finally extracted by using a least-square fit to the initial linear region in the plot of greatest slope, representing the initial rate of rapid divergence (Figure 4.13).

   Implementation notes: When plotting $\ln\langle d(i)\rangle$ versus time, time can be maintained within the domain of samples or more properly converted from samples to actual time through multiplying by the inverse of the sampling frequency. If time is kept in the domain of samples, then the subsequent units for the largest Lyapunov exponent is divergence/sample, which is difficult to comprehend and loses translation across studies if sampling is done under different rates. If time is converted to seconds, then the unit for the largest Lyapunov exponent is divergence/second. Note that the natural logarithm base with which Rosenstein et al. initially implemented their algorithm prevents the expression of bits of

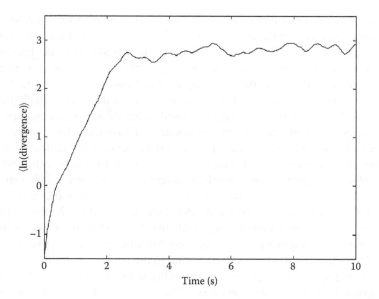

FIGURE 4.12 Plot of $\ln\langle d(i)\rangle$ versus time.

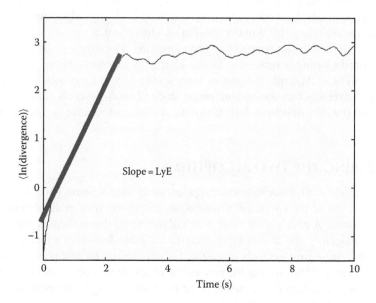

FIGURE 4.13 The largest Lyapunov exponent is the slope of the initial region of rapid exponential expansion, noted as an early period on the graph of $\ln\langle d(i)\rangle$ versus time with increased slope.

information with bits being binary. In addition, we are aware of research work being generated specific to gait which has converted time to strides by multiplying time and average cadence. In this situation, the resultant units are expressed as divergence/stride. This method, however, is not recommended as it makes a strong untested assumption with regard to information processing. Conversion into units of divergence/stride indicates that information is processed based on the stride cycle. This is problematic as the person who moves slower will have more time to process information than the person who is moving quicker. For example, if both individuals' movement trajectories have a largest Lyapunov exponent of 2 bits/stride and were necessarily needing to process 2 bits of information to maintain locomotion, then this will correctly occur in one stride for each individual. However, the quicker individual is actually able to process information at a much quicker rate in terms of seconds. Thus, we may begin to see implications for motor control whereby the processing time of the slower individual is contributing to the person's naturally selected walking speed or compromising his ability to successfully recover from a potential fall due to slow processing time. As a result, it is recommended that the time domain of seconds is still used as originally put forward by Rosenstein et al. and Wolf et al. Another interesting note is that when calculating the slope of the linear region in the plot of $\ln\langle d(i)\rangle$ versus time, the investigator is essentially determining the average of the derivative of this region. If the reader remembers the Wolf et al. algorithm implementation notes (see point 5 under Wolf et al. algorithm), a method is outlined for determining an appropriate time evolution. The investigator is guided toward plotting n versus the largest Lyapunov exponent. If the investigator were to integrate the plot of n versus the largest Lyapunov exponent, or conversely plot the instantaneous slope of $\ln\langle d(i)\rangle$ versus time against time (i.e., the first time derivative), the resulting plots have similar shape.

COMPARING THE TWO ALGORITHMS

The Rosenstein et al. algorithm was proposed as an improvement for existing algorithms to compute the Lyapunov exponent, including the Wolf et al. algorithm, for several reasons. A concern for Wolf et al.'s algorithm is that it focuses only on one reference trajectory and does not utilize all the available data. This is incorrect, however, as the entire time series is propagated with potential for any point to serve as a replacement neighbor during the new neighbor selection process. All other points that may not get selected as a neighboring point still serve the purpose as a space holder during the time propagation.

Another interesting point that is often mentioned as a weakness of the Wolf et al. algorithm is its assumption of the presence of exponential divergence without verification, not being able to distinguish chaos from noise. On the other hand, Rosenstein et al.'s algorithm seems to be able to make this distinction by inspecting a plot of $\ln\langle d(i)\rangle$ versus time (s) with increasing embedding dimensions. For a system with finite

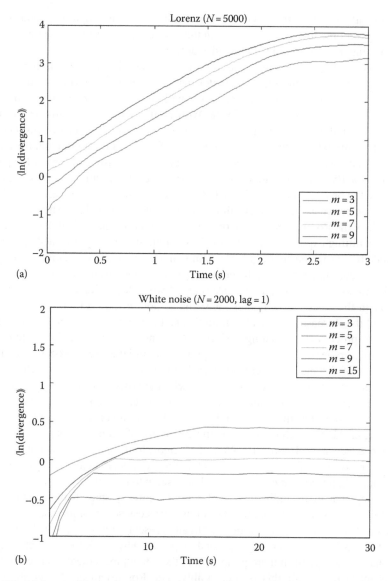

FIGURE 4.14 (a) Effects of embedding dimension for the computation of the largest Lyapunov exponent using the Lorenz attractor ($N = 5000$); with $m = 3$ (bottom), $m = 5$ (next up), $m = 7$ (next up), $m = 9$ (top). (b) Effects of embedding dimension for the computation of the largest Lyapunov exponent using White noise ($N = 2000$; lag = 1); with $m = 3$ (bottom); $m = 5$ (next up); $m = 7$ (next up); $m = 9$ (next up); and $m = 15$ (top).

dimension, when the embedding dimension is large enough to unfold the attractor, the scaling regions with different embedding dimensions converge (Figure 4.14a), whereas the scaling region of a stochastic system flattens (Figure 4.14b). Rosenstein et al.'s algorithm, however, does require the selection of a "long linear region" with which to extract the largest Lyapunov exponent. This region is not well defined and can influence the final outcome specifically when investigating experimental data. To overcome this, and especially in the gait-related literature, researchers have started using a set region of 0–0.5 strides or 0–1 stride.

Rosenstein et al.'s algorithm has traditionally been believed to be robust with short and noisy data, and therefore better than Wolf et al.'s algorithm. However, as Rosenstein et al. mention in their paper, a "small data set" is comparative to the data requirement previously discussed in the Wolf et al. paper. The requirement of data is still suggested by Rosenstein et al. to be $N > 10^D$, where D is the dimension of an attractor, comparable to the 10^D reported by Wolf et al. As for noisy data, the results of their study indicated as great as 55.4% error in their estimated largest Lyapunov exponent for the Rossler system, when the signal-to-noise ratio was 100, which is considered to be moderate noise level. Cignetti et al. (2012) provided results for direct comparison between the two algorithms when examining gait data. Their results did in fact show the Rosenstein et al. algorithm to be better for theoretical data. However, when examining experimental data, the Wolf et al. algorithm performed superiorly. Specifically, the Rosenstein et al. algorithm showed increased dynamic stability in elderly gait compared to young, healthy individuals, which would seem to be counter-intuitive to common sense and the vast body of work displaying decreased dynamic stability in the elderly gait. Interestingly, the authors began to highlight one of the pitfalls of the Rosenstein et al. algorithm that had not previously been drawn to light. Within the process of calculating the largest Lyapunov exponent, the Rosenstein et al. algorithm averages data at two separate points; the initial averaging occurs when the time series of distances is averaged at each point (see step 7 above for Rosenstein et al. algorithm). Next, the averaging occurs with the process of applying a regression line to a specific region. The longer the regression line, the more rates that are being averaged together. On the other hand, the Wolf et al. algorithm performs a single averaging of the data, which occurs with the average of each calculated local rate of divergence (see step 11 above for Wolf et al. algorithm). Just as oversmoothing data can lose important information, it seems that the Rosenstein et al. algorithm may be losing important information. This would only seem to be further compounded when considering that many individuals will actually initially smooth their data with a digital filter before applying either algorithm (a process not recommended due to the above mentioned presence of averaging already present within the algorithm).

At this point, the reader may be wondering then why the Rosenstein et al. algorithm has seemingly been more prominent in the human movement science research. The primary reason for this is accessibility. The Rosenstein et al. algorithm was made freely available online in a software package that is readily downloadable. Only recently (2014), through this book and correspondence with Dr. Wolf, has the Wolf et al. algorithm been made available in a software program downloadable for MATLAB®. It should be noted, however, that the use of the Wolf et al. algorithm within all arenas of science has been historically and still is used far more than the Rosenstein et al. algorithm.

There has been further confusion in the literature stemming from the introduction of a short-term and long-term Lyapunov exponent (Dingwell et al. 2000, 2001; Dingwell and Marin 2006). The short-term and long-term exponents, or short-term and long-term divergence exponents, represent slopes on two different regions of the divergence plot constructed in step 9 above for Rosenstein's algorithm. Referring back to Figure 4.13, under these alternative conventions, the slope of initial rapid exponential divergence is labeled the short-term divergence exponent. This is based on the short amount of time over which the average slope is calculated (e.g., 0–1 stride), which is consistent with the theoretical definition of largest Lyapunov exponent. A calculation of the average slope of the plot on right side of the figure, where there is a distinctly different and much flatter slope, is labeled the long-term divergence exponent. The label "long-term" is the result of the calculation occurring over a longer period of time and occurring further out, typically calculated over a range of 4–10 strides when curves are normalized to stride time. However, recent work has found the long-term divergence exponent to be merely an artifact of the shape of the attractor, representing a point within the attractor when nearest neighbors are no longer able to diverge due to the bounded shape of the attractor. Bruijn et al. (2012) concluded in their modeling study, "Our findings support the use of [short-term divergence exponents], but not [long-term divergence exponents], as a measure of human gait stability." The research group that had originally introduced the long-term divergence exponent also appears to have realized the triviality of the flatter region in the divergence curve as they have stopped reporting this variable (Buerskens et al. 2014a,b; Kao et al. 2014).

SUMMARY

In this chapter, first we discussed properties of a chaotic system, then we discussed Lyapunov exponents that can be used as a dynamic diagnostic method for chaotic systems. There are as many Lyapunov exponents as the number of dimensions of state space. However, the largest Lyapunov exponent is considered the most important. It quantifies the average exponential rates of divergence or convergence of nearby trajectories in state space. As nearby trajectories separate rapidly, it produces instability, and the largest Lyapunov exponent estimates this instability.

There are various algorithms to compute Lyapunov exponents, and we have looked at two prominent ones: the Wolf et al. and Rosenstein et al. algorithms. The Rosenstein et al. algorithm was proposed as a remedy to previous algorithms, including the Wolf et al. algorithm. However, the Rosenstein et al. algorithm also has significant drawbacks. Therefore, as with the Wolf et al. algorithm, we need to be aware of these limitations when we use the algorithm with biological data.

EXERCISES

1. Is there a universally accepted definition of chaos? State some properties that a chaotic system should have.
2. State the weaknesses of the Wolf et al. algorithm.
3. State the weaknesses of the Rosenstein et al. algorithm.
4. State the differences between the Wolf et al. and the Rosenstein et al. algorithms.
5. The algorithms mentioned in this chapter cannot distinguish between chaotic and stochastic systems. Is there any method we can apply to remedy this problem (the answer may not be in this chapter).

REFERENCES

Abarbanel, H.D.I., R. Brown, and J.B. Kadtke. (1990). Nonlinear prediction for time series with broadband fourier spectra. *Physical Review A*, 41(4):1782–1807.

Aguirre, L.A. and A. Aguirre. (1997). A tutorial introduction to nonlinear dynamics in economics. *Nova Economia*, 7(2):9–48.

Bauer, H.U., J. Deppisch, and T. Geisel. (1991). Hierarchical training of neural networks and prediction of chaotic time series. *Physics Letters A*, 158:57–62.

Benettin, G., L. Galgani, A. Giorgilli, and J.M. Strelcyn. (1980). Lyapunov characteristic exponents for smooth dynamical systems and for Hamiltonian systems:A method for computing all of them. Part 2: Numerical application. *Meccanica*, 15(1):21–30.

Brandstater, A., J. Swift, H.L. Swinney, A. Wolf, J.D. Farmer, E. Jen, and J.P. Crutchfield. (1983). Low dimensional chaos in a hydrodynamic system. *Physical Review Letters*, 51(16):1442–1445.

Bruijn, S.M., D.J. Bregman, O.G. Meijer, P.J. Beek, and J.H. van Dieen. (2012). Maximum Lyapunov exponents as predictors of global gait stability: A modelling approach. *Medical Engineering and Physics*, 34(4):428–436.

Buerskens, R., J.M. Wilken, and J.B. Dingwell. (2014a). Dynamic stability of superior vs. inferior body segments in individuals with transtibial amputation walking in destabilizing environments. *Journal of Biomechanics*, 47(12):3072–3079.

Buerskens, R., J.M. Wilken, and J.B. Dingwell. (2014b). Dynamic stability of individuals with transtibial amputation walking in destabilizing environments. *Journal of Biomechanics*, 47(7):1675–1681.

Buzzi, U.H., N. Stergiou, M.J. Kurz, P.A. Hageman, and J. Heidel. (2003). Nonlinear dynamics indicates aging affects variability during gait. *Clinical Biomechanics*, 18(5):435–443.

Casdagli, M. (1989). Nonlinear prediction of chaotic time series. *Physica D*, 35:335–356.

Cignetti, F., L.M. Decker, and N. Stergiou. (2012). Sensitivity of the Wolf's and Rosenstein's algorithms to evaluate local dynamic stability from small gait data sets. *Annals in Biomedical Engineering*, 40(5):1122–1130.

Darbyshire, A.G. and D.S. Broomhead. (1996). Robust estimation of tangent maps and Lyapunov spectra. *Physica D*, 89(3):287–305.

Decker, L.M., C. Moraiti, N. Stergiou, and A.D. Georgoulis. (2011). New insights into anterior cruciate ligament deficiency and reconstruction through the assessment of knee kinematic variability in terms of nonlinear dynamics. *Knee Surgery, Sports Traumatology, Arthroscopy*, 19(10):1620–1633.

Desalvo, A., S. Giannerini, and R. Rosa. (2006). Chaos, chaotic phenomena of charged particles in crystal lattices. *Chaos*, 16(2):023114-1–023114-12

Dingwell, J.B. and J.P. Cusumano. (2000). Nonlinear time series analysis of normal and pathological human walking. *Chaos*, 10(4):848–863.

Dingwell, J.B., J.P. Cusumano, P.R. Cavanagh, and D. Sternad. (2000). Slower speeds in patients with diabetic neuropathy lead to improved local dynamic stability of continuous overground walking. *Journal of Biomechanics*, 33(10):1269–1277.

Dingwell, J.B., J.P. Cusumano, P.R. Cavanagh, and D. Sternad. (2001). Local dynamic stability versus kinematic variability of continuous overground and treadmill walking. *Journal of Biomechanical Engineering*, 123(1):27–32.

Dingwell, J.B. and L.C. Marin. (2006). Kinematic variability and local dynamic stability of upper body motions when walking at different speeds. *Journal of Biomechanics*, 39(3):444–452.

Donker, S.F., M. Roerdink, A.J. Greven, and P.J. Beek. (2007). Regularity of center-of-pressure trajectories depends on the amount of attention invested in postural control. *Experimental Brain Research*, 181(1):1–11.

Eckmann, J.P. and D. Ruelle. (1985). Ergodic theory of chaos and strange attractors. *Reviews of Modern Physics*, 57(3):617–656.

Ellner, S., A.R. Gallant, D.F. McGaffrey, and D. Nychka. (1991). Convergence rates and data requirements for the Jacobian-based estimates of Lyapunov exponents from data. *Physics Letters A*, 153:357–363.

England, S.A. and K.P. Granata. (2007). The influence of gait speed on local dynamic stability of walking. *Gait Posture*, 25(2):172–178.

Farmer, J.D. and J.J. Sidorowich. (1987). Predicting chaotic time series. *Physical Review Letters*, 59(8):845–848.

Geist, K., U. Parlitz, and W. Lauterborn. (1990). Comparison of different methods for computing Lyapunov exponents. *Progress of Theoretical Physics*, 83(5):875–893.

Gleick, J. (1987). *Chaos: Making a New Science*. Viking Penguin, New York.

Goldberger, A.L., D.R. Rigney, and B.J. West. (1990). Chaos and fractals in human physiology. *Scientific American*, 262(2):42–49.

Gollub, J.P., E.J. Romer, and J.E. Socolar. (1980). Trajectory divergence for coupled relaxation oscillators: Measurements and models. *Journal of Statistical Physics*, 23(3):321–333.

Guckenheimer, J. and G. Buzyna. (1983). Dimension measurements for geostrophic turbulence. *Physical Review Letters*, 51:1438–1441.

Harbourne, R.T. and N. Stergiou. (2003). Nonlinear analysis of the development of sitting postural control. *Developmental Psychobiology*, 42(4):368–377.

Hassell, M.P., H.N. Comins, and R.M. May. (1991). Spatial structure and chaos in insect population dynamics. *Nature*, 353:255–258.

Kantz, H. (1994). A robust method to estimate the maximal Lyapunov exponent of a time series. *Physics Letters A*, 185(1):77–87.

Kao, P.C., J.B. Dingwell, J.S. Higginson, and S. Binder-Macleod. (2014). Dynamic instability during post-stroke hemiparetic walking. *Gait Posture*, 40(3):457–463.

Kikuchi, A., T. Shimizu, A. Hayashi, T. Horikoshi, N. Unno, S. Kozuma, and Y. Taketani. (2006). Nonlinear analyses of heart rate variability in normal and growth-restricted fetuses. *Early Human Development*, 82(4):217–226.

Kurz, M.J. and N. Stergiou. (2007). Do horizontal propulsive forces influence the nonlinear structure of locomotion? *Journal of Neuroengineering Rehabilitation*, 15(4):30.

Kyvelidou, A., R.T. Harbourne, V.K. Shostrom, and N. Stergiou. (2010). Reliability of center of pressure measures for assessing the development of sitting postural control in infants with or at risk of cerebral palsy. *Archives of Physical Medicine and Rehabilitation*, 91(10):1593–1601.

Lamoth, C.J. and M.J. van Heuvelen. (2012). Sports activities are reflected in the local stability and regularity of body sway: older ice-skaters have better postural control than inactive elderly. *Gait Posture*, 35(3):489–493.

Lamoth, C.J., R.C. van Lummel, and P.J. Beek. (2009). Athletic skill level is reflected in body sway: a test case for accelerometry in combination with stochastic dynamics. *Gait Posture*, 29(4):546–551.

Lockhart, T.E. and J. Liu. (2008). Differentiating fall-prone and healthy adults using local dynamic stability. *Ergonomics*, 51(12):1860–1872.

Longstaff, M.G. and R.A. Heath. (1999). A nonlinear analysis of the temporal characteristics of handwriting. *Human Movement Science*, 18(4):485–524.

Lorenz, E.N. (1963). Deterministic nonperiodic flow. *Journal of Atmospheric Sciences*, 20:130–141.

Malraison, B., P. Attens, P. Berge, and M. DuBois. (1983). Dimensions of strange attractors: An experimental determination for the chaotic regime of two convective systems. *Journal de Physique Lettres*, 44:L897–L902.

Mees, A.I. and C. Sparrow. (1987). Some tools for analyzing chaos. *Proceedings of the IEEE*, 75(8):1058–1070.

Peel, D.A. and A.E.H. Speight. (1994). Hysteresis and cyclical variability in real wages, output and unemployment: empirical evidence from nonlinear methods for the United States. *International Journal Systems Science*, 25(5):943–965.

Piccoli, H.C. and H.I. Weber. (1998). Experimental observation of chaotic motion in a rotor with rubbing. *Nonlinear Dynamics*, 16:55–70.

Rosenstein, M.T., J.J. Collins, and C.J. De Luca. (1993). A practical method for calculating largest Lyapunov exponents from small data sets. *Physica D*, 65:117–134.

Sano, M. and Y. Sawada. (1985). Measurement of the Lyapunov spectrum from a chaotic time series. *Physical Review Letters*, 55(10):1082–1085.

Sato, S., M. Sano, and Y. Sawada. (1987). Practical methods of measuring the generalized dimension and the largest Lyapunov exponent in high dimensional chaotic systems. *Progress in Theoretical Physics*, 77:1–5.

Schaffer, W.M. (1985). Order and chaos in ecological systems. *Ecology*, 66:93–106.

Shimada, I. and T. Nagashima. (1979). A numerical approach to ergodic problem of dissipative dynamical systems. *Progress of Theoretical Physics*, 61(6):1605–1616.

Smith, B.A., N. Stergiou, and B.D. Ulrich. (2010). Lyapunov exponent and surrogation analysis of patterns of variability: Profiles in new walkers with and without Down syndrome. *Motor Control*, 14(1):126–142.

Stergiou, N., C. Moraiti, G. Giakas, S. Ristanis and A.D. Georgoulis. (2004). The effect of the walking speed on the stability of the anterior cruciate ligament deficient knee. *Clinical Biomechanics*, 19(9):957–963.

Swinney, H.L. (1983). Observations of order and chaos in nonlinear systems. *Physica D*, 7: 3–15.

Timmer, J., S. Haussler, M. Lauk and C.H. Lucking. (2000). Pathological tremors: Deterministic chaos or nonlinear stochastic oscillators? *Chaos*, 10(1):278–288.

Wales, D.J. (1991). Calculating the rate of loss of information from chaotic time series by forecasting. *Nature*, 350:485–488.

Wolf, A., J.B. Swift, H.L. Swinney and J.A. Vastano. (1985). Determining Lyapunov exponents from a time series. *Physica D*, 16:285–317.

Wurdeman, S.R., S.A. Myers, A.L. Jacobsen, and N. Stergiou. (2013). Prosthesis preference is related to stride-to-stride fluctuations at the prosthetic ankle. *Journal of Rehabilitation Research and Development*, 50(5):671–686.

Wurdeman, S.R., S.A. Myers, A.L. Jacobsen, and N. Stergiou. (2014). Adaptation and prosthesis effects on stride-to-stride fluctuations in amputee gait. *PLoS One*, 9(6):e100125.

Wurdeman, S.R., S.A. Myers, and N. Stergiou. (2013). Transtibial amputee joint motion has increased attractor divergence during walking compared to non-amputee gait. *Annals in Biomedical Engineering*, 41(4):806–813.

Wurdeman, S.R., S.A. Myers, and N. Stergiou. (2014). Amputation effects on the underlying complexity within transtibial amputee ankle motion. *Chaos*, 24(1):013140.

Wurdeman, S.R. and N. Stergiou. (2013). Temporal structure of variability reveals similar control mechanisms during lateral stepping and forward walking. *Gait Posture*, 38(1): 73–78.

Yoshino, K., T. Motoshige, T. Araki, and K. Matsuoka. (2004). Effect of prolonged free-walking fatigue on gait and physiological rhythm. *Journal of Biomechanics*, 37(8):1271–1280.

5 Surrogation

Sara A. Myers

CONTENTS

Introduction 111
Nonlinearity 112
General Principles of Surrogation 113
Hypothesis Testing (Discriminating Criterion) 119
Linear Surrogate Methods 124
    Algorithm 0 124
    Algorithm 1 (Fourier Transform) 126
    Algorithm 2 134
    Iterated Amplitude-Adjusted Fourier Transform 136
Rejection of Null Hypothesis 146
Pseudoperiodic Surrogate Method 147
Discriminating Statistics for PPS 154
Summary 156
Exercises 156
Appendix 5.A: Knee Joint Flexion/Extension Angle (Degrees) 157
    Original Series 157
    PPS Surrogate Series 162
References 168

> Progress is impossible without change, and those who cannot change their minds cannot change anything.
>
> **George Bernard Shaw (1856–1950)**

INTRODUCTION

One of the goals of time series analysis is to understand the underlying mechanisms that generate different dynamics for different time series. If a time series is not a product of random process, then we can assume that some kind of dynamics govern the time series. The question is what kinds of dynamics are controlling the time series. For nonlinear time series analysis, our focus is on nonlinear dynamics, and one of the goals is to characterize those dynamics by applying nonlinear tools. However, it is important to establish evidence of nonlinearity in a time series first in order to avoid obtaining possible spurious results by applying nonlinear tools to the system that does not contain nonlinearity. Second, nonlinearity is considered as one of the key features of time series that exhibit chaos, which has been shown to have a potential link with overall health of the biological system (Amato 1992; Buchman et al. 2001; Cavanaugh et al. 2010; Garfinkel et al. 1992; Goldstein et al. 1998; Orsucci 2006; Slutzky et al. 2001; Toweill and Goldstein 1998; Wagner et al. 1996). Therefore, in terms of detecting chaos in a time series, identifying the presence of nonlinearity in the system is essential.

NONLINEARITY

Nonlinear analysis characterizes the nonlinear properties of time series data. For these analysis tools to provide meaningful results, they must be applied to time series that contain nonlinear structures. When nonlinear tools are used on data without nonlinear structures, false results are obtained due to practical limitations of nonlinear measures. Therefore, it is important to establish the evidence of nonlinearity in a time series prior to applying nonlinear tools.

Before getting into a discussion of methods to identify possible nonlinearity in data, let us first define a nonlinear system. A nonlinear system is defined as a system that does not have a linear origin. This includes a system that may contain nonlinearity, but the underlying dynamics are linear. In this case, the presence of nonlinearity is caused by some measurement distortion, but it is originally generated by a linear stochastic process. We will look at such a case in detail later in this chapter. Furthermore, discussion in this chapter will be limited only to a stationary time series and will not include nonstationary stochastic processes. A time series is considered nonstationary if its distribution changes across time. In other words, the mean and variance of the time series change over different time intervals. Applying surrogate methods to nonstationary time series can lead to problems regarding the proper interpretation of results (Breakspear and Terry 2002; Palus 1996). For example, when the null hypothesis is rejected in a surrogate analysis, there is no way of knowing whether nonlinearity exists in the data or whether the data were generated by a nonstationary stochastic process. This problem was noted by Breakspear and Terry (2002) in their study of electroencephalographic (EEG) data (Breakspear and Terry 2002). The problem of nonstationarity was also highlighted by Peng et al. (1995) in the analysis of heart rate variability. Specifically, nonstationarity makes it difficult to determine whether the structure of the time series is the result of the dynamics of the system or from changes in the external environment. Therefore, we will restrict our discussion to time series that are stationary.

There are two major approaches to identify the evidence of nonlinearity in a time series in general. The first approach involves the direct application of nonlinear measures (Kaplan and Glass 1995; Mitra et al. 1997), while the second approach involves the application of surrogate methods (Breakspear and Terry 2002; Dingwell and Cusumano 2000; Palus 1996; Stergiou et al. 2004). Methods commonly used for the first approach include the application of the correlation dimension or the largest Lyapunov exponent. The correlation dimension is a measure of self-similarity of a time series, while the largest Lyapunov exponent quantifies the exponential rate of divergence of nearby trajectories in the state space (see Chapters 3, 4, and 8). Both of these measures are applied to attractors reconstructed from an original time series in the state space. Attractors are often associated with nonlinearity and possibly chaotic dynamics. However, the use of these two popular nonlinear measures with experimental data can give spurious results. It has been reported that the correlation dimension of a time series with linear correlations can mimic low-dimensional behavior of the system by giving finite noninteger values (Osborne and Provencale 1989). Noise in a time series can cause the largest Lyapunov exponent to be positive, indicating the presence of chaos where there is none (Rapp et al. 1993). The use of other nonlinear measures besides correlation dimension and the largest Lyapunov exponent are also limited in terms of detecting nonlinearity in a time series since the probability distributions of those measures on time series with finite data length are unknown (Palus 1995; Pompe 1993; Prichard and Theiler 1995). Thus, applications of these nonlinear measures alone in detecting nonlinearity, possibly chaotic behavior in the system have been shown to be difficult (Miller et al. 2006; Schreiber and Schmitz 2000; Theiler and Rapp 1996). Moreover, applications of these nonlinear measures often involve subjective judgment of a researcher such as finding an appropriate scaling region or threshold value and lack in certainty. We particularly observe such procedures with methods like detrended fluctuation analyses and recurrence quantification analyses. To compensate for these weaknesses of the first approach of direct applications of nonlinear measures, the second approach of applying surrogate methods is often used. The second approach can be considered as an indirect approach in a sense that attempts to identify the evidence of nonlinearity by excluding that a time series has a linear origin through statistical hypothesis testing.

GENERAL PRINCIPLES OF SURROGATION

Surrogate methods were originally developed to prevent misdiagnoses of random stochastic processes from being characterized as chaotic dynamical processes or vice versa (Stergiou et al. 2004; Theiler et al. 1992; Theiler and Rapp 1996). They take a form of hypothesis testing to determine whether a given time series is consistent with a specific null hypothesis. The general procedure of a surrogate method is as follows (Figure 5.1). First, a null hypothesis is specified, and from the original time series an ensemble of surrogate time series is generated that are consistent with this null hypothesis. The null hypothesis is typically what researchers want to show that is not true. An example of null hypothesis would be that the time series was generated by a linear stochastic process. If the data are nonlinear, the test statistic results will be the difference between the original and surrogate time series and the null hypothesis will be proven false. If the results are the same, the null hypothesis fails to be proven false, and the original time series is a linear stochastic process. These surrogate time series must preserve some properties (mean, variance, and/or power spectra), which correspond to the underlying null hypothesis. Then, discriminating statistics such as the correlation dimension are computed for both the original and the ensemble of surrogate time series. The values of the discriminating statistics between the original time series and the distribution of values of discriminating statistics obtained from the surrogate time series are compared. If the value of the discriminating statistics from the original time series does not fall within the distribution of the discriminating statistics of the surrogates, the null hypothesis should be rejected. As it is stated differently, if the results between original and surrogate are different, the null is rejected, and if

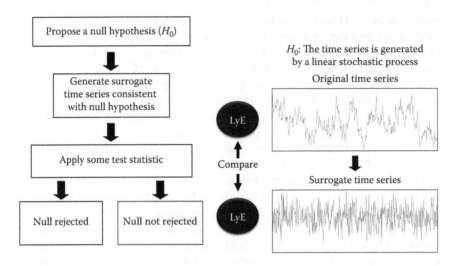

FIGURE 5.1 The general procedure of surrogate methods. These steps can be applied with one of the surrogate algorithms presented in this chapter. If the discriminant statistics are significantly different between the original time series and the surrogate time series, the null is rejected.

the discriminating statistic is the same between original and surrogate, the null is accepted. The following tools are examples of discriminating statistics that have been used before for this purpose: the correlation dimension (Diks 1996; Grassberger and Procaccia 1983; Small 2005; Small and Judd 1998; Small and Tse 2002; Yu et al. 2000), the largest Lyapunov exponent (Kantz and Schreiber 1997; Wolf et al. 1985), approximate entropy (Miller et al. 2006; Pincus 1991), sample entropy (Lamoth et al. 2010, 2011; Rathleff et al. 2011), higher and cross moments (Keenan 1985; Tsay 1986), a simple skewed difference statistic (Theiler et al. 1992), Volterra polynomials (POL) (Barahona and Poon 1996; Kugiumtzis 1999), and the local average mapping (LAM) (Schreiber and Schmitz 1997).

This approach to use surrogate methods for determining whether a given time series is consistent with a specific null hypothesis has been applied to identify the evidence of nonlinearity in many biological systems such as postural control, ECG, EEG, gait mechanics, and so forth (Acharya et al. 2005; Breakspear and Terry 2002; Buzzi et al. 2003; Chang et al. 1994; Cignetti et al. 2009; Collins and De Luca 1995; Costa et al. 2014; Ehlers et al. 1998; Govindan et al. 1998; Hausdorff et al. 1995; Ivanov et al. 1996; Janjarasjitt et al. 2008; Kugiumtzis 2001; Kunhimangalam et al. 2008; Kurz et al. 2008; Ladislao and Fioretti 2007; Little et al. 2006; Martinerie et al. 1998; Miller et al. 2006; Myers et al. 2013; Nurujjaman et al. 2009; Palus 1996; Porta et al. 2007; Preatoni et al. 2010; Rieke et al. 2003; Rombouts et al. 1995; Stam et al. 1997; Stergiou et al. 2004; Zhang et al. 2007; Zhao et al. 2008; Wurdeman et al. 2014). Table 5.1 details the surrogate methodology and whether determinism was found in these studies. Throughout the various methods and biological time series utilized in these studies, a common theme was the presence of nonlinear patterns and consistence of rejecting the null hypothesis in biological time series.

TABLE 5.1

A Selection of Studies in the Literature That Have Implemented Surrogate Methods in Biological Signals

Article	Measured Behavior	Surrogate Procedure	Discriminating Criterion	Rejecting the Null, Results
Collins and De Luca (1995)	Posture	Algorithm 0	Scaling exponent	**Yes**, correlations in the time series are due to underlying dynamic processes.
Stergiou et al. (2004)	Gait	Algorithm 1	Lyapunov exponent (LyE)	**Yes**, gait variability is deterministic in patients with Parkinson's even without medication.
Stam et al. (1997)	EEG	Algorithm 1	Correlation coefficients	**Yes**, it may be deterministic; however, the test is not definitive.
Ehlers et al. (1998)	EEG	Algorithm 1	Slope asymmetry, correlation dimension, one percent radius, redundancy, Kaplan's δ/ε.	**Yes**, EEG is not modeled effectively as linearly filtered Gaussian noise.
Ivanov et al. (1996)	EEG	Algorithm 1	Correlation dimension, correlation parameter (P_a)	**Yes**, data differed significantly from linear stochastic time series.
Martinerie et al. (1998)	Intracranial recordings	Algorithm 1	Correlation density	**Yes**, data differed significantly from stochastic fluctuations.
Breakspear and Terry (2002)	EEG	Algorithm 1	Phase synchrony	**Yes**, phase coherence cannot be described by purely linear methods for a small number of EEG epochs.
Govindan et al. (1998)	ECG	Algorithm 1	Correlation dimension	**Yes**, the results indicate the presence of nonlinear structure in the time series.
Rombouts et al. (1995)	EEG	Algorithm 2	Correlation dimension	**Yes**, evidence for nonlinearity is found yet EEG dynamics are low dimensional.
Chang et al. (1994)	Spinal cord monosynaptic reflex	Algorithm 1	Local flow, local dispersion, and nonlinear prediction	**Yes**, deterministic structure was found in 2/4 of the time series for the decerebrate state.
Palus (1996)	EEG	Algorithm 1	Slopes of redundancy	**Yes**, the hypothesis of a linear stochastic process is rejected.

(Continued)

TABLE 5.1 (Continued)
A Selection of Studies in the Literature That Have Implemented Surrogate Methods in Biological Signals

Article	Measured Behavior	Surrogate Procedure	Discriminating Criterion	Rejecting the Null, Results
Miller et al. (2006)	Gait	Algorithm 1, PPS	LyE, approximate entropy (ApEn)	**Yes**, significant differences were found for both LyE and ApEn values.
Hausdorff et al. (1995)	Gait	Algorithm 0	Scaling exponent a from DFA	**Yes**, fluctuations in the stride intervals were unlike those obtained from an uncorrelated random walk.
Buzzi et al. (2003)	Gait	Algorithm 1	LyE	**Yes**, LyE were found to be significantly different indicating that the time series may reflect nonlinear processes.
Zhang et al. (2007)	ECG, speech	PPS	Correlation coefficient, average cycle divergence rate (ACDR, analogous to LyE), and clustering coefficient	**Yes**, differences were observed in all measures.
Rieke et al. (2003)	EEG from epilepsy patients	IAAFT	Coarse-grained flow average (Kaplan and Glass 1995)	**Yes**, nonlinearity is evident in the EEG.
Kugiumtzis (2001)	Simulations, EEG, exchange rate data	Algorithm 2, IAAFT	Volterra polynomials, local average mapping, mutual information, LyE, correlation dimension, simple nonlinear averages	**Yes**, but results depend on the parameter examined suggesting surrogate testing should be performed using multiple methods and parameters.
Kurz et al. (2008)	Robot gait	PPS	LyE	**Yes**, support the notion that the deterministic variations present in gait may be partly governed by the intrinsic mechanical dynamics of the locomotive system.
Kunhimangalam et al. (2008)	EEG	Algorithm 1	Correlation dimension, LyE	**Yes**, in case of LyE of EEG data, the change due to surrogating is small suggesting that it is not representing the system complexity properly but there is a marked change in the case of correlation dimension value due to surrogating.

(Continued)

TABLE 5.1 (*Continued*)
A Selection of Studies in the Literature That Have Implemented Surrogate Methods in Biological Signals

Article	Measured Behavior	Surrogate Procedure	Discriminating Criterion	Rejecting the Null, Results
Janjarasjitt et al. (2008)	Neonatal EEG	Algorithm 1	Correlation dimension	**Yes**, dimensional complexity cannot be rejected for active sleep but can be for other sleep states.
Acharya et al. (2005)	EEG during sleep	Algorithm 1	Correlation dimension, fractal dimension, LyE, ApEn, Hurst exponent, phase space plot, recurrence plots	**Yes**, correlation dimension and ApEn show that the original data contain nonlinear features.
Nurujjaman et al. (2009)	EEG	Algorithm 0	Probability distribution function, Hurst exponent	**Yes**, the activity of an epileptic brain is non-Gaussian in nature, but not normal brain activity.
Little et al. (2006)	Speech	IAAFT	Time-delayed mutual information	**Yes**, the assumption of dynamical nonlinearity and/or non-Gaussianity is supported but linear Gaussian theory is also a weak approximation.
Porta et al. (2007)	Short-term heart beat intervals	Algorithm 0, Algorithm 1, Algorithm 2, IAAFT	Porta's (P) method, modified Kantz and Schreiber's (MKS) method, Sugihara and May's (SM) method	**No**, short-term heart period variability at rest was mostly linear.
Ladislao and Fioretti (2007)	Posture	IAAFT	LyE	**Yes**, postural sway derives from a process exhibiting weakly chaotic dynamics.
Cignetti et al. (2009)	Cross country skiing joint angles	Algorithm 1	LyE, correlation dimension	**Yes**, temporal variations in the data had a deterministic origin.
Zhao et al. (2008)	Human cardiac data	PPS	Complexity, correlation dimension	**Yes**, bounded aperiodic determinism exists in ECG and pulse time series but dynamic noise means that it is not possible to conclude the underlying system is chaotic.

(Continued)

TABLE 5.1 (Continued)
A Selection of Studies in the Literature That Have Implemented Surrogate Methods in Biological Signals

Article	Measured Behavior	Surrogate Procedure	Discriminating Criterion	Rejecting the Null, Results
Preatoni et al. (2010)	Race walking joint angles and ground reaction forces	PPS	Sample entropy (SampEn)	**Yes,** SampEn was significantly lower for all measures than the surrogates.
Myers et al. (2013)	Gait (lower limb joint angles)	PPS	LyE	**Yes,** significant differences were found for the ankle and knee joint angle time series at baseline and ankle postvascular occlusion.
Costa et al. (2014)	Glucose levels	Algorithm 0	SampEn	**Yes,** the 100 shuffled surrogate time series were consistently more entropic than the original first difference time series.
Wurdeman et al. (2014)	Gait (ankle motion)	PPS	LyE	**Yes,** results revealed the presence of underlying deterministic structure.

Since surrogate methods take the form of a null hypothesis testing, considerations must be given to the selection of discriminating statistics and discriminating criteria. Hypothetically, it should not matter which discriminating statistic is used. However, there are two different views on the selection of discriminating statistics. One view is that all nonlinear statistics should be able to detect the presence of nonlinearity by rejecting the null hypothesis at different significance levels. The alternative view is that the mismatch between a surrogate algorithm and discriminating statistics can lead to a spurious result. There are many different surrogate algorithms, which will determine which discriminating statistic is appropriate, based on the origination of the time series data. In general, a discriminating statistic must give consistent results for both surrogates and original time series if the null hypothesis is true. If the null hypothesis is not true, the discriminating statistic of the original time series should be different from the distribution of the discriminating statistics for its surrogates. The use of multiple discriminating statistics is encouraged in order to establish the evidence of nonlinearity in a time series since there may be cases where one discriminating statistic is not sufficient (Kugiumtzis 2001). For example, using parameters such as the largest Lyapunov exponent, correlation dimension, global false nearest neighbors, average mutual information and others on both simulated and actual EEG data, Kugiumtzis (2001) argued that different nonlinear methods characterize different aspects of data. However, if there is nonlinearity in the data, those different nonlinear methods should be able to detect the presence of nonlinearity by rejecting the null hypothesis at different significance levels respectively. On the other hand, it has been pointed out that the mismatch between surrogate algorithm and discriminating statistics can occur and can lead to a spurious result (Small et al. 2001, 188101). Therefore, considerations should be given to the right match between a specific surrogate algorithm and discriminating statistics (Zhang et al. 2007). We will show some examples of mismatch between a discriminating statistics and surrogate algorithm later in this chapter.

HYPOTHESIS TESTING (DISCRIMINATING CRITERION)

In this section, hypothesis testing will be discussed. The first question that needs to be answered after computing discriminating statistics for both original time series and its surrogates is what criteria should be used to determine whether the null hypothesis should be rejected or not. One way to conduct a hypothesis test is by using a parametric criterion. The mean (μ_H) and standard deviation (σ_H) of discriminating statistics for surrogate data are used to calculate the significance S with a unit of "sigma," which in turn is used to construct a confidence level of inference (Theiler et al. 1992):

$$S = \frac{|Q_D - \mu_H|}{\sigma_H} \tag{5.1}$$

For example, the rejection of the null hypothesis at the 95% level of confidence is indicated by significance of about two "sigmas." The assumption for this criterion is that the distribution of discriminating statistics is Gaussian. However, it has been shown that the distributions of many nonlinear measures do not follow a Gaussian distribution (Schreiber and Schmitz 2000; Theiler et al. 1992).

Therefore, another criterion, the rank-order criterion is often used in the literature since it is more robust in terms of defining significance. This criterion namely examines the ranks of discriminating statistics of an original time series and surrogates. Suppose N surrogate time series were generated from the original time series and the discriminating statistics Q were computed for each surrogate time series and the original time series. Then, there are $(N + 1)$ Q's in total. Let Q_D be the discriminating statistics value for the original time series, and $Q_1, Q_2, \ldots, Q_N$ be the discriminating statistic's values for the surrogates. Now, all these $(N + 1)$ discriminating statistic's values are ranked in an increasing order. If the original time series is generated by a process which is consistent with the null hypothesis, the probability of Q_D to be the smallest or the largest will be $1/(N + 1)$. According to the rank-order criterion, the null hypothesis is rejected when Q_D is the smallest or the largest values among $(N + 1)$ Q's. For a one-sided test, $1/(N + 1)$ is regarded as a false rejection rate while $2/(N + 1)$ for a two-sided test. Therefore, in order to conduct hypothesis testing at 95% significance level, 19 surrogates must be generated for a one-sided test and 39 surrogates for a two-sided test.

Let us look at an example of a surrogate test using sample entropy (SampEn), which is a measure of regularity as a discriminating statistics (Example Box 5.1). Nineteen surrogate time series were generated from an original time series. Twenty sample entropy (SampEn) values were computed for the original time series and the nineteen surrogates. After ranking those 20 SampEn values, we may reject the null hypothesis at 95% confidence level if the SampEn value of the original time series was the smallest value (Figure 5.2; Appendix 5.A). In this case, the probability of a false rejection is 5%.

EXAMPLE BOX 5.1   EXAMPLE OF SURROGATE TESTING

This example uses the data from Appendix 5.A to go through the steps of surrogate testing. For space purposes, only the original and one surrogate time series are included. For this example, sample entropy (SampEn) will be used as the discriminant, which is a measure of regularity. The data are a continuous knee flexion/extension time series from walking.

1. *Plot the data and identify the null hypothesis.* It is important to plot the data to quickly inspect that the data are as expected (no missing points, proper length, etc.). Identifying the null hypothesis will determine which surrogate algorithm should be implemented. In our example, a knee flexion/extension time series is used that has inherent periodicity due to the repetition of gait cycles. The repeating cycles of the time series are evident in the graph in the following. Therefore, an appropriate null hypothesis would be that our time series is consistent with a periodic orbit perturbed by uncorrelated noise. To test this hypothesis, we will need to use the pseudoperiodic surrogate (PPS) method.

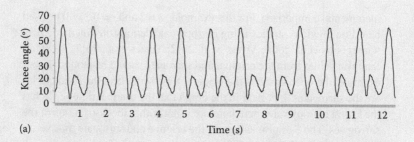

(a)

2. *Calculate and choose parameters for surrogate method.* As mentioned
   earlier, the PPS algorithm is appropriate for this data. To implement
   the PPS algorithm, the state space must be reconstructed. Thus, the
   embedding dimension and the time lag from the original series must
   be calculated to generate the surrogate time series. Another parameter
   that must be determined is the noise radius, which defines the amount
   of noise in a surrogate. The proper ρ is selected to maximize the number of short segments that are the same for the original time series and
   the surrogate. For this particular time series, the embedding dimension
   is 6, time lag is 10 and the noise radius is 0.5.
3. *Generate a series of surrogates.* Using the same parameters, a series
   of 19 surrogates should be calculated from the original time series.
   Each of these surrogates should be plotted to ensure that it was generated correctly. In the example, the dotted line is the original time
   series and the 19 surrogates are all plotted in black. The surrogates
   resemble the original time series, which is correct. Only 1.5 s of data
   is shown for clarity purposes.

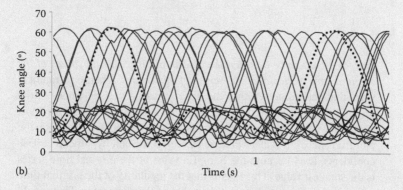

(b)

4. *Calculate the discriminating statistic.* SampEn, a measure of regularity is our chosen discriminating statistic. To calculate SampEn, some
   parameters need to be chosen first. Briefly, SampEn calculates the loga-
   rithmic probability that run patterns that are close (within tolerance r)
   for m observations remain close (with the same tolerance r) on the next

incremental comparison. For this example, $m = 2$ and $r = 0.2$ will be used based on previous studies using entropy calculations on kinematic data (Georgoulis et al. 2006; Myers et al. 2012; Yentes et al. 2013). Next, all SampEn values from the original and surrogate should be plotted. In our example, the open circle is the original time series and the solid circles are the surrogates. It is clear in the graph that the original time series has the lowest entropy value and therefore is not within the distribution of the surrogates. The SampEn values for the original and surrogate time series from Appendix 5.A are 0.373 and 0.401, respectively. Keep in mind, however, that each time a surrogate series is generated, it adds dynamics noise. So, a surrogate you generate from the example data will not match the provided surrogate series. However, you can use the example surrogate series to test whether your SampEn calculations are correct using the same parameters used in this example.

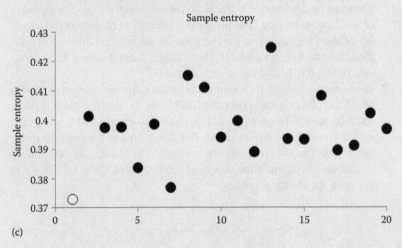

(c)

5. *Test for significance between the discriminating statistic values of the original time series and the series of surrogates.* There are multiple ways that determine whether the discriminating statistic values of the original time series are different from the surrogates. One of the most common ways as used in this example is a simple rank test. Based on the plot from step 4, it is clear that we can reject the null hypothesis at 95% confidence level because the SampEn value of the original time series is the smallest value. This means that the regularity of the original time series is significantly different than that of the surrogates. That would leave a 5% probability that our rejection of the null is false. Remember the null hypothesis was that our original knee joint flexion/extension time series is consistent with a periodic orbit perturbed by uncorrelated noise. Since we rejected the null hypothesis, we have concluded that our time series is not an orbit with noise, but contains identifiable dynamics.

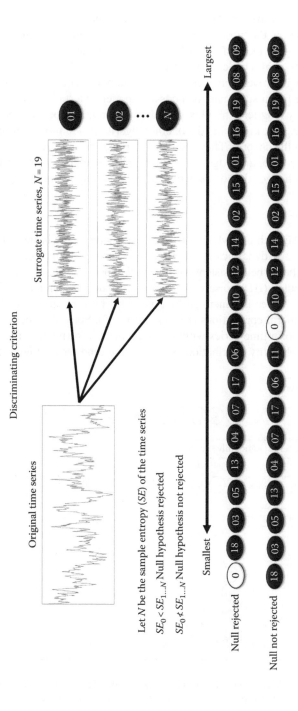

FIGURE 5.2 An example of surrogate testing with the sample entropy (SampEn) as the discriminant statistic. A total of 19 surrogates are generated and SampEn is calculated for the original and each surrogate. The process of generating 19 surrogate time series is the same, regardless of which surrogation algorithm is determined to be appropriate for the data. A rank order test is used to verify that the original time series has the lowest SampEn. The null hypothesis would be rejected if SampEn of the original series has the lowest value of all of the surrogate series values. The null would be accepted if the SampEn value for the original is not the lowest value. (Adapted from Pincus, S.M. et al., *J. Clin. Monit.*, 7(4), 335, 1991.)

LINEAR SURROGATE METHODS

As we have mentioned earlier in the chapter, there are many different surrogate algorithms. In this section, the most commonly applied surrogate algorithms, which are called linear surrogate methods, will be discussed. Linear surrogate methods were originally developed by Theiler and colleagues (Theiler et al. 1992; Theiler and Rapp 1996), and later improvements were made by Schreiber et al. (Schreiber and Schmitz 2000). These linear surrogate methods are applied to a stationary irregular time series without any long-term trend or periodicity. If trends, especially periodic trends, are present (i.e., gait kinematic data), other algorithms are more appropriate as we will see later in the chapter. They are known as Algorithm 0, Algorithm 1 or Fourier transform surrogate, and Algorithm 2 or amplitude adjusted Fourier transform (AAFT), and each algorithm deals with a different null hypothesis.

Algorithm 0

First, let us examine Algorithm 0, which is used to test whether there is any evidence that a time series has any dynamics at all. Therefore, surrogate time series generated by Algorithm 0 should be consistent with the null hypothesis of an independent and identically distributed (IID) noise with unknown (random) mean and variance. Such a surrogate time series is generated by randomly shuffling an original time series, destroying temporal correlations (Example Box 5.2). Since this method permutes temporal order of a time series without replacement, a surrogate time series preserves the same probability distribution as the original time series (Figure 5.3).

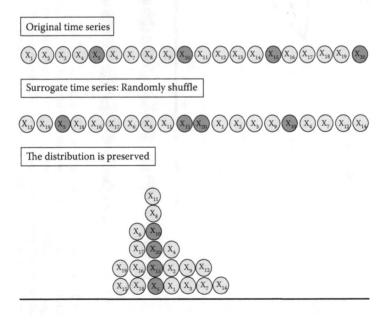

FIGURE 5.3 A graphical representation of the Theiler et al. Algorithm 0 surrogate. The original and surrogate (created using the Algorithm 0) time series have the same frequency distribution, even though they now have completely different time structure.

**EXAMPLE BOX 5.2   NUMERICAL EXAMPLE OF
THEILER ET AL. ALGORITHM 0 SURROGATE METHOD**

This example uses the following 20 data points from 20 s of standing posture
sampled at 1 Hz.
{0.76, 0.64, 0.34, 0.60, 0.55, 0.27, 0.29, −0.39, 0.04, −0.19, −0.21, −0.51, −0.93,
−0.48, 0.69, 1.63, 0.13, 1.5, 1.26, 1.5}.

1. *Plot the data and identify the null hypothesis.* The null hypothesis
   for A0 is that the data are consistent with independent and identically
   distributed noise with unknown mean and variance.

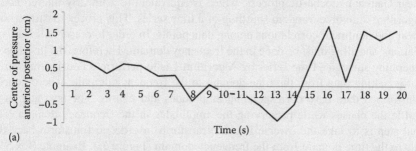

(a)

2. *Randomly shuffle the original time series.* This can be done with the
   `randn` function in MATLAB®. After shuffling, our time series is as
   follows:
   {0.60, 0.13, −0.19, −0.48, 1.5, −0.93, 0.76, 1.26, 1.63, 0.29, 0.04, 0.64,
   −0.21, 0.69, 1.5, 0.27, 0.34, −0.39, 0.55, −0.51}.

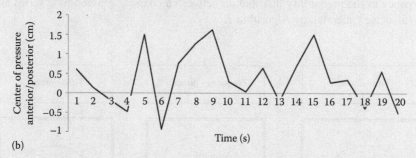

(b)

This step would be repeated so that a total of at least 19 surrogates are
generated to be able to reject the null with 95% confidence that the
original time series is not within the distribution of the surrogates.

3. *Calculate the discriminant statistic.* For this example, the discriminant is not calculated because the 20 points data series would be too
   short to provide meaningful results, but this would be the next step.

4. *Test for significance between the discriminating statistics values of
   the original time series and the series of A0 surrogates.*

Suppose, surrogate time series are generated by Algorithm 0 and some discriminating statistic is applied, and the null hypothesis of the test is rejected. What does this indicate? The rejection of the null hypothesis of IID noise implies the evidence of some structure in a time series. If the null is accepted, it means that the original time series has no determinable dynamics, that is, there are no correlations among the data points of the time series. Thus, the next step is to test whether this structure has a linear origin or not by using Algorithm 1 or Algorithm 2.

ALGORITHM 1 (FOURIER TRANSFORM)

The null hypothesis in Algorithm 1 addresses that a time series is generated from a linear Gaussian stochastic process, which is equivalent to a linearly filtered noise. Algorithm 0 involves random shuffling of a time series. This process destroys both linear and nonlinear correlations among data points. In order to preserve linear correlations, shuffling must be done in the frequency domain. Therefore, the first step of generating surrogate time series by Algorithm 1 is to perform a Fourier transform, that is, taking data from the time domain to the frequency domain, where Fourier transformed data have corresponding amplitudes and phases. The next step is to shuffle the phases while preserving the amplitudes in the frequency domain. The final step is to take the inverse Fourier transform in order to transform back the data to the time domain from the frequency domain (Figure 5.4; Example Box 5.3). A surrogate time series generated by Algorithm 1 preserves the linear correlations, which are represented by the discrete Fourier power spectrum as the original time series while any additional structure should be destroyed. However, surrogate time series does not preserve the probability distribution of the original data, which can lead to a false rejection of the null hypothesis. There is an especially obvious discrepancy in the probability distribution between a coarsely grained time series and its surrogate generated by Algorithm 1.

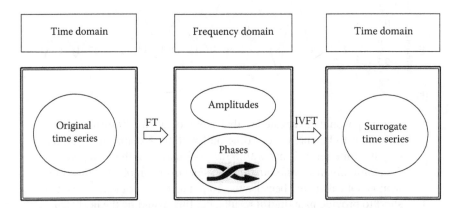

FIGURE 5.4 The original time series undergoes fast Fourier transformation to move the series from the time domain to the frequency domain. Then phase randomization is performed. Inverse Fourier transformation provides the resulting surrogate time series.

EXAMPLE BOX 5.3   NUMERICAL EXAMPLE OF THEILER ET AL. ALGORITHM 1 SURROGATE METHOD

This example will use the same 20 data point time series as Example Box 5.2, but continue through the steps for the A1 algorithm.

1. *Plot the data and identify the null hypothesis.* The appropriate null hypothesis for the A1 algorithm is that the time series is generated from a linear Gaussian stochastic process equivalent to a linearly filtered noise. The time series is: {0.76, 0.64, 0.34, 0.60, 0.55, 0.27, 0.29, −0.39, 0.04, −0.19, −0.21, −0.51, −0.93, −0.48, 0.69, 1.63, 0.13, 1.5, 1.26, 1.50}.

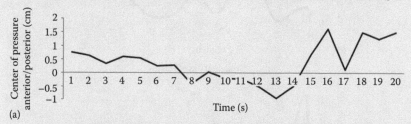

(a)

2. *Perform a Fourier transform.* Since randomly shuffling the time series removes linear and nonlinear correlations among data points, shuffling must be done in the frequency domain. This can be done with the `fft` function in MATLAB®. After the transform, the series is "moved" from the time domain to the frequency domain. The result is a list of coefficients representing real and imaginary parts. The coefficients represent the amount that each frequency contributes to the overall signal. Plots of the real and imaginary parts of each Fourier coefficient are as follows:

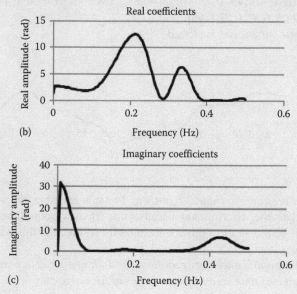

(b)

(c)

3. *Shuffle the phases while preserving the amplitudes.* The graphs in the following are the real and imaginary amplitudes of the Fourier coefficients after the phases have been shuffled. It is clear that the frequency contributions are different from the original.

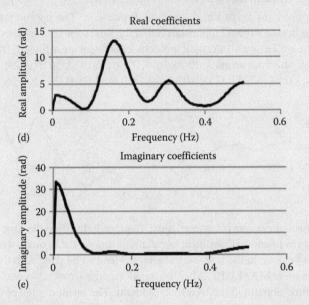

(d)

(e)

4. *Take the inverse Fourier transform.* This step takes the data back into the time domain. The surrogate time series is {1.00, 1.10, 1.09, 0.72, 0.65, 0.64, −0.14, −0.42, −0.52, −0.63, −0.83, −0.16, 0.06, 0.44, 0.44, 1.11, 1.05, 0.37, 0.57, 0.98}.
The new time series is plotted:

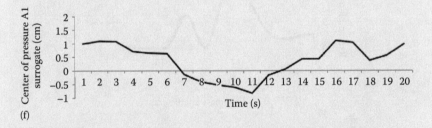

(f)

5. *Calculate the discriminant statistic.* For this example, we will not calculate the discriminant because the 20 data point time series would be too short to provide meaningful results, but this would be the next step.
6. *Test for significance between the discriminating statistics values of the original time series and the series of A1 surrogates.*

Let us look at an example. An autoregressive time series with length $N = 2000$ called AR is generated by the following Equation 5.2:

$$X_{t+1} = 0.9X_t + \delta \qquad (5.2)$$

where δ is an error term.

AR is generated by the linear Gaussian stochastic process. Thus, the null hypothesis of Algorithm 1 should not be rejected. Another time series called AR2 is created by making AR coarse (removing the precisions). Even though little difference is visually observed between the plots of the two time series, the number of unique values each time series has is quite different (Figure 5.5a). The number of unique values of AR is the same as its data length (2000) while AR2 only has 71 unique values, even though it is still 2000 data points long. Nineteen surrogate time series are generated from AR and AR2, respectively, but again it is hard to differentiate between the surrogate time series of each time series by a visual inspection (Figure 5.5b). However, the results of the null hypothesis testing using the SampEn as discriminating statistics are different between AR and AR2 (Figure 5.5c). For AR, the SampEn value of the original time series falls within the distribution of the SampEn values of the surrogates, and this is what we have expected, that is, not rejecting the null hypothesis. However, the SampEn value of AR2 is the smallest SampEn values among the SampEn value of its surrogate time series. As a result, we may reject the null hypothesis at 95% confidence level. The discrepancy in the results between AR and AR2 hypothesis testing seems to be due to an increase in the number of values in surrogate time series generated from AR2. The SampEn value of AR2 is much lower than the SampEn value of AR since AR2 has fewer numbers of unique values than that of the AR2. However, the process of generating surrogate time series using the Fourier transform preserves the frequency distribution (Figure 5.6), but not the probability distribution (Figure 5.7). Thus, Algorithm 1 increases the number of unique values in surrogate time series generated from AR2: they all have 2000 unique values. This jump in the increase in the number of values in the surrogate time series is reflected in the value of SampEn of surrogates generated from AR2. It created discrepancies in the SampEn values between AR2 and its surrogates, causing the false rejection of the null hypothesis. In order to avoid statistical bias, it is better that the probability distribution of an original time series and surrogate are the same. Therefore, for a coarsely grained time series, Algorithm 1 may not be an appropriate surrogate method to apply.

Again, let us suppose surrogate time series are generated by Algorithm 1 and some discriminating statistics are applied, and the null hypothesis is rejected. What does the rejection of the null hypothesis of a linearly filtered noise imply? It may be indicating evidence of a more complex structure in a time series such as nonlinearity. However, even though a time series contains nonlinearity, it may be due to some distortion caused by a measurement procedure, and the origin of underlying dynamics may be linear stochastic. To test such a case, Algorithm 2 can be used.

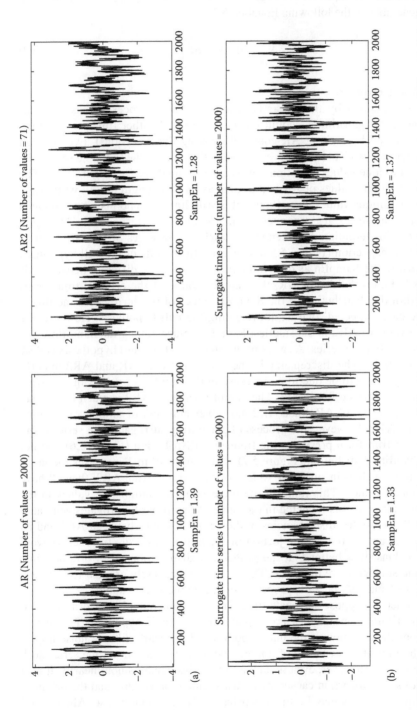

FIGURE 5.5 (a) Plots of a linear Gaussian stochastic process (AR) and a course AR (AR2), in which the precisions were removed. There is little visual difference, but the number of unique values in AR is 2000, while AR2 only has 71. (b) The surrogate time series of AR and AR2 are also visually similar. However, Algorithm 1 increases the number of unique values in AR2 to 2000.

(Continued)

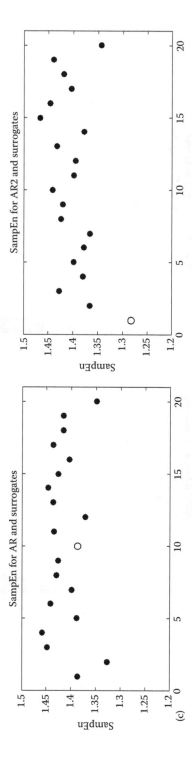

FIGURE 5.5 (Continued) (c) The open circle represents the SampEn of the original time series and the solid circles are the surrogate SampEn values on each graph. Results of testing the null hypothesis using SampEn as a discriminant statistic are different when using AR and AR2. This difference occurs because the Fourier transform increases the number of unique values in the surrogate time series generated from AR2. This increase resulted in discrepancies in the SampEn values between AR2 and its surrogates, leading to a false rejection of the null hypothesis.

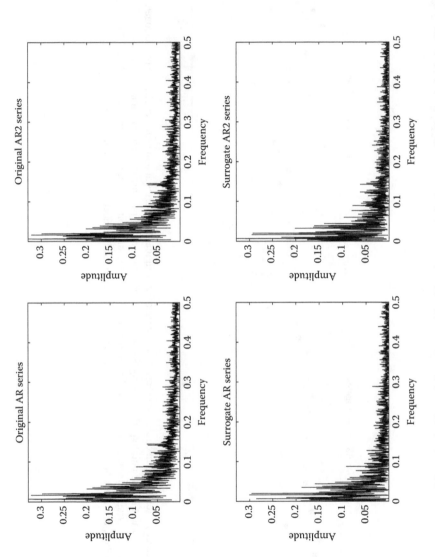

FIGURE 5.6   The power spectra of the series in Figure 5.5 are shown. Algorithm 1 preserves the frequency distribution in both the AR and AR2 time series.

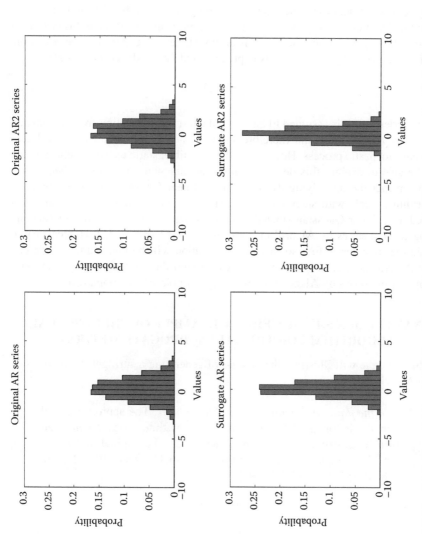

FIGURE 5.7 The probability distribution of AR and AR2 from Figure 5.5. Algorithm 1 does not preserve this distribution, which can lead to a false rejection of the null hypothesis.

ALGORITHM 2

Algorithm 2 deals with the null hypothesis of a static and monotonic nonlinear filter. Here, a measurement procedure is regarded as a nonlinear filter and enhances fluctuations in a system with linear dynamics as this linear stochastic system passes through the filter. Therefore, the time series contains nonlinearity, which enhances the system with linear dynamics as it goes through the filter, but this nonlinearity is not in the dynamics. This process is known as nonlinear distortion and is described by the following equation where $h\,(\cdot)$ is an invertible, static measurement function, $\{x_n\}$ is the underlying linear stochastic process, and $\{y_n\}$ is the observed data:

$$y_n = h(x_n) \tag{5.3}$$

A time series in test is assumed to have failed a test for originating from a Gaussian process by Algorithm 1 and therefore shown that it is not generated by a linear Gaussian stochastic process. However, if the invertible, static measurement function may be able to explain this deviation from the Gaussian distribution, then it may be shown that the underlying dynamics are a linear Gaussian stochastic process. Algorithm 2 deals with such a scenario. Since the underlying dynamics are considered as a linear Gaussian stochastic process, part of the procedure to generate surrogate time series by Algorithm 2 also involves Algorithm 1. It is necessary to rescale the time series first so that the distribution will be Gaussian, and we can apply Algorithm 1. Example Box 5.4 goes through the procedure of generating a surrogate time series by Algorithm 2 by using a simple 10 data point time series.

EXAMPLE BOX 5.4   NUMERICAL EXAMPLE OF THEILER ET AL. ALGORITHM 2 OR THE AAFT SURROGATE METHOD

This example will illustrate the process of generating a surrogate time series by Algorithm 2.

1. *Plot the data and identify the null hypothesis.* The appropriate null hypothesis for the A2 algorithm is that the time series is generated from a static and monotonic nonlinear filter. The original time series for this example is: $\{x_n\} = \{125.00, 67.37, 46.33, 49.64, 49.83, 172.36, 188.22, 157.40, 138.77, 276.97\}$.

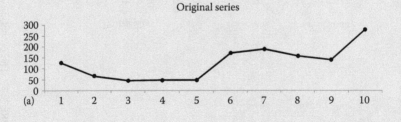

2. *Rank order $\{x_n\}$ and make a time series of rank.* If we rank order the time series, it would be: {46.33, 49.64, 49.83, 67.37, 125.00, 138.77, 157.40, 172.36, 188.22, 276.97}. So, the rank order time series would take the position of these numbers as 1–10, in the order of the original series. The time series of the ranks would be: Rank_original = {5, 4, 1, 2, 3, 8, 9, 7, 6, 10}.

3. *Generate a random time series which has the same length as $\{x_n\}$ and has a Gaussian distribution.* We call this random time series $\{y_n\}$ ={1.50, −0.28, 0.50, 1.034, −1.51, −2.34, 0.26, −0.52, 0.23, 0.32}.

4. *Sort $\{y_n\}$ in an ascending order, which is called Sorted_$\{y_n\}$.* Sorted_$\{y_n\}$ = {−2.34, −1.50, −0.52, −0.28, 0.23, 0.26, 0.32, 0.50, 1.03, 1.50}

5. *Reorder Sorted_$\{y_n\}$ according to Rank_original and let it be called Reordered_$\{y_n\}$.* Reordered_$\{y_n\}$ = {0.23, −0.28, −2.34, −1.51, −0.52, 0.50, 1.03, 0.32, 0.26, 1.50}. Reordered_$\{y_n\}$ has the same time evolution as the $\{x_n\}$, but the distribution is Gaussian.

6. *Apply Algorithm 1 on Reordered_$\{y_n\}$.* That is taking the Fourier transform and shuffling phases while keeping the amplitudes and then applying the inverse Fourier transform. This series is called Surrogate_$\{y_n\}$ = {1.07, 1.19, −0.55, −1.06, −1.48, −0.06, 0.17, −0.12, −0.28, 0.30}.

7. *Rank order Surrogate_$\{y_n\}$.* This results in Rank_Surrogate $\{y_n\}$ = {5, 4, 3, 9, 8, 6, 7, 10, 1, 2}.

8. *Reorder Rank_Surrogate $\{y_n\}$.* This sequence is called Final_reorder = {9, 10, 3, 2, 1, 6, 7, 5, 4, 8}.

9. *Arrange $\{x_n\}$ according to the Final_reorder.* Now, a surrogate has been generated as Surrogate = {188.22, 276.97, 49.83, 49.64, 46.33, 138.77, 157.40, 125.00, 67.37, 172.36}. By plotting the series in the following, it is clear that the surrogate contains the same values as the original, but in a different order.

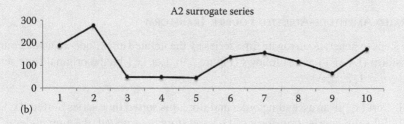

(b)

The chart following further illustrates how the surrogate series has changed from the original series. Two highlighted values show 46.33 moving from position 3 in the original series to position 5 in the surrogate series and 188.22 moving from position 7 to position 1.

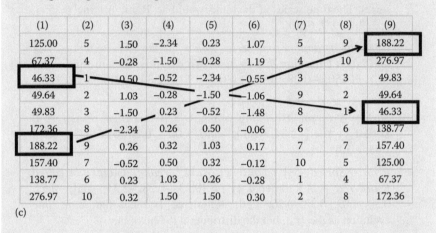

(1)	(2)	(3)	(4)	(5)	(6)	(7)	(8)	(9)
125.00	5	1.50	−2.34	0.23	1.07	5	9	188.22
67.37	4	−0.28	−1.50	−0.28	1.19	4	10	276.97
46.33	1	0.50	−0.52	−2.34	−0.55	3	3	49.83
49.64	2	1.03	−0.28	−1.50	−1.06	9	2	49.64
49.83	3	−1.50	0.23	−0.52	−1.48	8	1	46.33
172.36	8	−2.34	0.26	0.50	−0.06	6	6	138.77
188.22	9	0.26	0.32	1.03	0.17	7	7	157.40
157.40	7	−0.52	0.50	0.32	−0.12	10	5	125.00
138.77	6	0.23	1.03	0.26	−0.28	1	4	67.37
276.97	10	0.32	1.50	1.50	0.30	2	8	172.36

(c)

A surrogate time series generated by Algorithm 2 preserves the amplitude distribution of the original time series and linear correlations among data points or power spectrum of the original time series. Algorithm 2 deals with more realistic situations than Algorithm 1. However, limitations with Algorithm 2 have also been reported (Kugiumtzis 2001; Schreiber and Schmitz 1997). When a time series is short and strongly correlated, rescaling of the inverse Fourier transformed data can change the linear correlations of the time series, causing a discrepancy between the power spectrum of the original time series and the surrogate time series (Figure 5.8). This discrepancy can lead to a false rejection of the null hypothesis, especially with a discriminating statistic which is sensitive to correlations among data points such as polynomial and local average fit, mutual information, and largest Lyapunov exponent (Kugiumtzis 2001). To deal with this problem, Schreiber et al. (1996) proposed an improved method known as the iterated amplitude-adjusted Fourier transform (IAAFT), and this has been widely used (Lehnertz et al. 2001; Poggi et al. 2004; Rieke et al. 2003).

ITERATED AMPLITUDE-ADJUSTED FOURIER TRANSFORM

The steps to generate surrogate time series by the iterated amplitude-adjusted Fourier transform (IAAFT) are as follows (Figure 5.9). Let $\{x_n\}$ be the original time series where $n = 1, 2,..., N$:

1. Sort $\{x_n\}$ in an ascending order and store this sorted time series Sorted_$\{x_n\}$.
2. Take the Fourier transform of $\{x_n\}$ and store the squared, the amplitudes of the Fourier transform of $\{x_n\}$, $X_k^2 = \left|\Sigma x_n e^{2\pi k n/N}\right|^2$

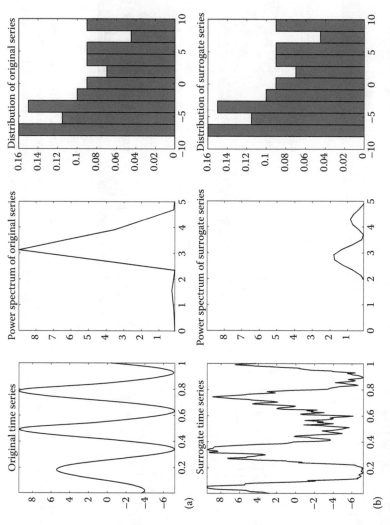

FIGURE 5.8 Theiler et al. Algorithm 2 preserves the amplitude distribution and the power spectrum of the original time series. However, when the time series is short and strongly correlated, the linear correlations of the data can change during the inverse Fourier process. When comparing the (a) original time series, power spectrum, and amplitude spectrum to the (b) surrogate time series, power spectrum, and amplitude, it is clear that the amplitude is preserved with algorithm 2, but not the power spectrum.

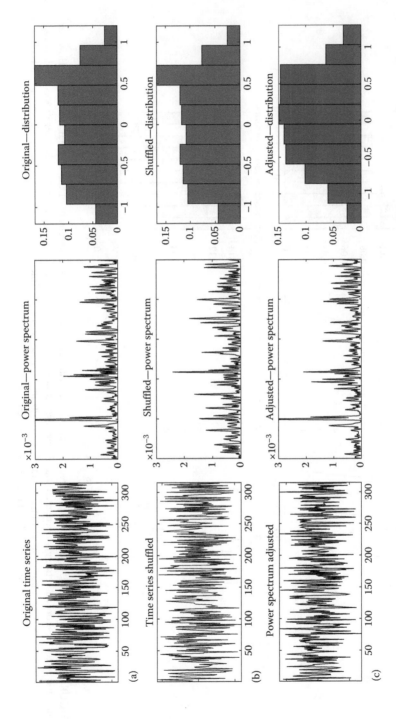

FIGURE 5.9 The IAAFT algorithm is the best to preserve the power spectrum of the original time series. (a) The original time series, power spectra, and distribution are shown. (b) The shuffled time series results in a different power spectrum, but the distribution is the same. (c) The power spectrum is adjusted by replacing the squared amplitudes of the Fourier transform of the shuffled time series with the squared amplitudes of the Fourier transform of the original time series. This brings the power spectrum closer to the original time series but results in changes to the amplitude distribution.   *(Continued)*

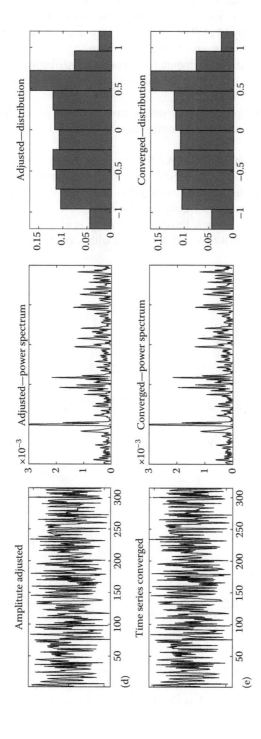

FIGURE 5.9 (*Continued*) (d) The amplitudes are then adjusted by ranking the values of the time series in (c) and replacing them with the ranked values of the time series in (b). (e). This procedure can alter the power spectrum again, so the process of adjusting the power spectrum and the amplitude distribution are repeated until convergence is achieved with both measures.

3. Shuffle $\{x_n\}$ and take the Fourier transform and call it FTRandomized$\{x_n\}$.
4. To adjust the power spectrum, replace the squared amplitudes of FTRandomized$\{x_n\}$ by $\{X_k^2\}$. The phases are kept unchanged. Then transform back by taking the inverse Fourier transform.
5. The procedure at step 4 will change the amplitude distribution. Therefore, adjust the amplitudes by ranking the values of this time series and replacing them by the values of Sorted_$\{x_n\}$.
6. However, again the procedure at step 5 may alter the power spectrum, so step 4 and step 5 are repeated until some convergence is achieved.

A surrogate time series generated by IAAFT preserves the power spectrum of an original time series much better than the other surrogate algorithms (Figure 5.10). For a numerical example, please see Example Box 5.5. This algorithm is trying to maintain the underlying linear correlations. However, there is no guarantee that iterations will eventually converge. Furthermore, there is also a concern that surrogate time series generated by IAAFT for a data with short length may not have

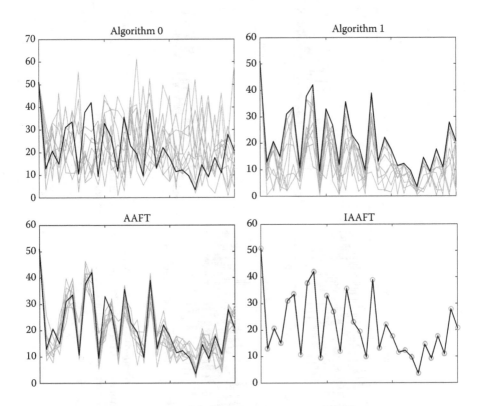

FIGURE 5.10 These plots of a portion of the power spectra of the original time series (gray) and 19 surrogate time series generated by Algorithm 0 (black), Algorithm 1 (black), AAFT (black), and IAAFT (circles). It is visually clear that the spectra are altered the least in IAAFT.

EXAMPLE BOX 5.5   NUMERICAL EXAMPLE OF THE IAAFT

This example will use the same 10 data point time series as Example Box 5.4, which is: $\{x_n\} = \{125.00, 67.37, 46.33, 49.64, 49.83, 172.36, 188.22, 157.40, 138.77, 276.97\}$.

1. *Plot the data, identify the null hypothesis, and Sort $\{x_n\}$ in an ascending order.* The appropriate null hypothesis for this algorithm is that the time series is generated from a linear Gaussian stochastic process.

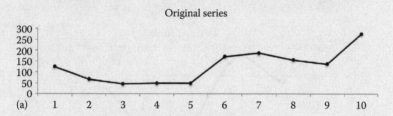

Original series

The new time series is Sorted_$\{x_n\}$ = $\{46.33, 49.64, 49.83, 67.37, 120.00, 138.77, 157.40, 172.36, 188.22, 276.97\}$.

2. *Take the Fourier transform of $\{x_n\}$ and store the squared amplitudes of the Fourier transform of $\{x_n\}$, $X_k^2 = \left|\Sigma x_n e^{2\pi kn/N}\right|^2$.*

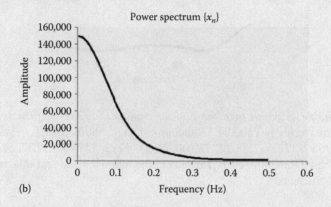

The transform moves the series from the time domain to the frequency domain. The power spectrum of $\{x_n\}$ is shown. The Fourier transform results in a list of real and imaginary coefficients in the different frequencies. The plots of the frequency components from the Fourier transform are shown in the following. The stored squared amplitudes of the Fourier transform of $\{x_n\}$ that are stored as follows: $\{X_k^2\}$ = $\{1271.89, 396.23, 170.51, 222.24, 77.16, 175.59, 77.16, 222.24, 170.51, 396.23\}$. The amplitude distribution of $\{x_n\}$ is shown on the next page.

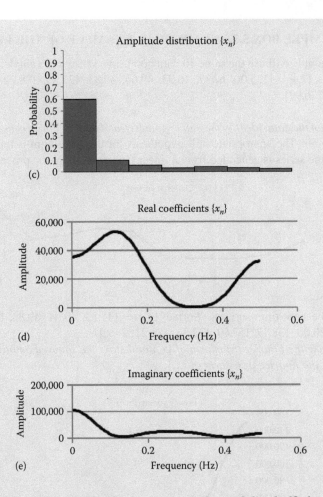

(c) Amplitude distribution $\{x_n\}$

(d) Real coefficients $\{x_n\}$

(e) Imaginary coefficients $\{x_n\}$

3. *Shuffle $\{x_n\}$ and take the Fourier transform of the shuffled series.*
   This series is called FTRandomized $\{x_n\}$. Shuffled $\{x_n\}$ = {49.64,
   276.97, 172.36, 188.22, 120.00, 46.33, 49.83, 157.40, 138.77, 67.37}.
   The FTRandomized $\{x_n\}$ results in the following real and imaginary
   coefficients:

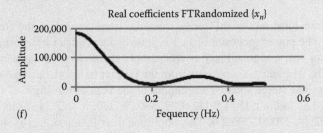

(f) Real coefficients FTRandomized $\{x_n\}$

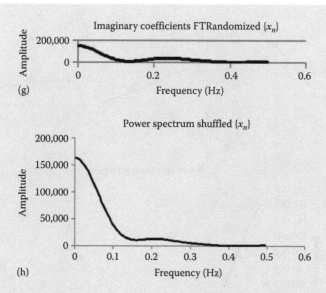

(g)

(h)

The power spectrum of Shuffled $\{x_n\}$ is different from the spectrum of $\{x_n\}$, so needs to be adjusted. However, the amplitude distribution Shuffled $\{x_n\}$ is similar with that of the $\{x_n\}$.

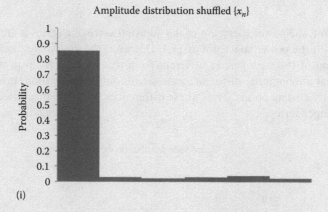

(i)

4. *The power spectrum is adjusted by replacing the squared amplitudes of FTRandomized* $\{x_n\}$ *with* $\{X_k^2\}$. This randomizes the series without changing the phases. Then, the series is transformed back by using the inverse Fourier transform. That results in a surrogate {102.19, 281.05, 185.90, 187.87, 139.30, 65.28, 13.55, 111.26, 107.20, 78.28}. This time series now looks like:

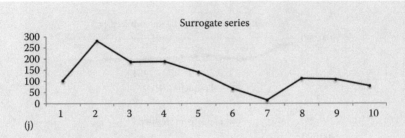

Surrogate series

(j)

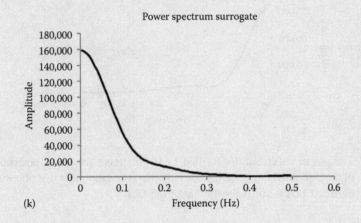

Power spectrum surrogate

(k)

Now, the power spectrum of the adjusted surrogate series is similar with the power spectrum as $\{x_n\}$. However, the amplitude distribution of the surrogate is different from that of $\{x_n\}$. Keep in mind that although the differences are small, our example time series is only 10 data points. Thus, these differences would be magnified for longer series.

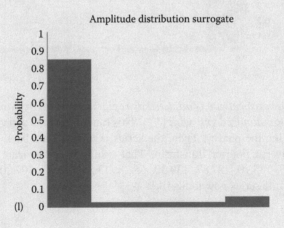

Amplitude distribution surrogate

(l)

5. *Adjust the amplitude distribution.* The procedure from Step 4 will change the amplitude distribution. The amplitudes are adjusted by ranking the values of the surrogate time series and replacing them by the values of Sorted_$\{x_n\}$. Rank order of the surrogate is {13.55, 65.28, 78.28, 102.19, 107.20, 111.26, 139.30, 185.90, 187.87, 281.05} which results in the Rank_surrogate = {7, 6, 10, 1, 9, 8, 5, 3, 4, 2}. Now, the rank is sorted and ranked according to its position. For example, you can see that rank number 1 of Rank_surrogate was in the 4th position, rank number 2 in the 10th position, etc., which results in Sorted_rank_surrogate = {4, 10, 8, 9, 7, 2, 1, 6, 5, 3}. The final part of this step is to replace them with the values of Sorted_$\{x_n\}$. From step 1, Sorted_$\{x_n\}$ = {46.33, 49.64, 49.83, 67.37, 120.00, 138.77, 157.40, 172.36, 188.22, 276.97}. When the Sorted_rank_surrogate is replaced with the values from Sorted_$\{x_n\}$, the 4th number from Sorted_$\{x_n\}$ is placed 1st in our new series, the 10th number from Sorted_$\{x_n\}$ 2nd, and so on, resulting in the Amplitude_adjusted_surrogate = {67.37, 276.97, 172.36, 188.22, 157.40, 49.64, 46.33, 138.77, 120.00, 49.83}.

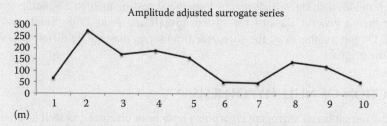

Amplitude adjusted surrogate series

(m)

6. *The procedure in step 5 may again alter the power spectrum. Thus, step 4 and step 5 are repeated until some convergence is achieved and both the power spectrum and the amplitude distribution are close to being preserved.* By examining the amplitude distribution shown in the following, it is clear that the amplitude distribution has changed and is (again) similar with $\{x_n\}$, but the power spectrum has changed (again). However, the differences between this power spectrum and $\{x_n\}$, are less than between the spectrum of Shuffled $\{x_n\}$ and $\{x_n\}$.

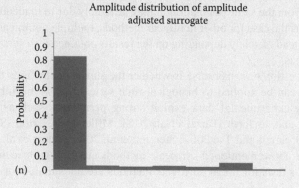

Amplitude distribution of amplitude adjusted surrogate

(n)

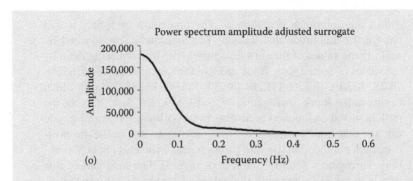

(o)

7. *Calculate the discriminant statistic.*
8. *Test for significance between discriminating statistic values of the original time series and the series of IAAFT surrogates.*

enough randomization, which makes hypothesis testing against a specific system rather than a general class of the system (Small and Judd 1998; Small and Tse 2002). Or, put another way, the surrogate time series may not be different enough from the original.

REJECTION OF NULL HYPOTHESIS

So far different linear surrogate algorithms have been discussed as well as how surrogate time series are generated by preserving some linear properties of an original time series while destroying other dynamics (Figures 5.11 and 5.12). The rejection of null hypothesis has also been discussed as being an indication of the presence of more complex dynamics than linear dynamics in the original time series. However, results of surrogate methods do not provide any definite answers regarding the exact nature of the underlying dynamics of the original data. The rejection of the null hypothesis only indicates that the underlying dynamics of the original time series are not consistent with the null hypothesis. In addition, even if there is no significant difference between the original and the surrogate time series, it cannot be concluded that they are from the same population. It may be simply due to inadequate statistics. Therefore, as is the case for other nonlinear methods, multiple nonlinear tools should be applied instead of solely depending on the results obtained by a surrogate method for data analysis.

Another question one may raise is whether the surrogate methods that were discussed so far can be applied to biological time series that exhibit inherent trends. In fact, many experimental data exhibit strong periodicity such as gait, human speech, ECG and so forth (Buzzi et al. 2003; Miller et al. 2006; Schreiber and Schmitz 2000; Small and Tse 2002; Stergiou et al. 2004; Zhang et al. 2007). What happens if the above mentioned surrogate methods are used with such time series? The hypothesis tests for linear surrogate methods are not suitable for a time series

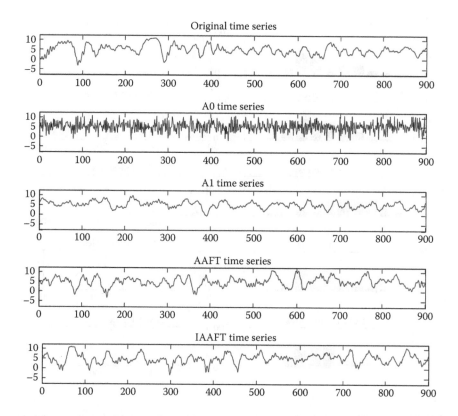

FIGURE 5.11   Original time series of center of pressure (COP) data from standing posture in the anterior–posterior (AP) direction and surrogate time series generated by different algorithms.

with periodicity: such time series are inconsistent with the null hypothesis of a linearly filtered noise. As a result, surrogate time series generated from a time series with periodicity by using linear surrogate methods have geometric structures different from that of the original time series (Figure 5.13). This would lead to a higher rejection rate of the null hypothesis than what should actually occur simply because the structure of the time series in the surrogate is changed (Algorithm 0 and 1) or because the surrogate has changed geometric structure (AAFT and IAAFT). Therefore, we need another testing hypothesis and surrogate algorithm for a time series with regular persistent fluctuations or underlying periodicity.

PSEUDOPERIODIC SURROGATE METHOD

Small et al. (2001) introduced a method called the pseudoperiodic surrogate (PPS) algorithm (Small et al. 2001). Pseudoperiodic time series are defined as time series that have a noisy periodic orbit perturbed by either dynamical noise or observational noise or have an oscillatory chaotic flow. The power spectrum of these time

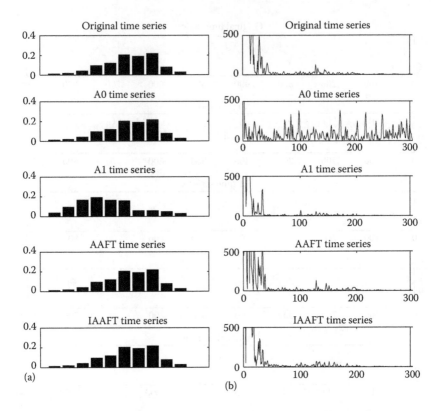

FIGURE 5.12 The probability distribution (a) and power spectra (b) of the original time series and all surrogate time series generated by the different algorithms from Figure 5.11.

series display clear spikes (Small 2005) (Figure 5.14) due to the dominant inherent frequencies. Since such a time series already exhibits a deterministic behavior, what is actually sought in this case is if there is any type of nonlinear structure on the fluctuations that are on top of these inherent dominant frequencies. A human electrocardiogram is an example of a signal with periodic orbits that result from successive heartbeats. However, there may be additional order within the dynamics of the sinus rhythm, or it could be consistent with uncorrelated noise (Small et al. 2001). Therefore, the null hypothesis of the PPS states that a time series is consistent with a periodic orbit perturbed by uncorrelated noise. To test this null hypothesis, the PPS generates a surrogate time series that keeps the large-scale behavior of the original time series but does not preserve any additional small-scale dynamics that can be regarded as chaotic, linear, or nonlinear deterministic structure. Therefore, intracycle dynamics, which are dynamic patterns within one period of a cyclic pattern, are preserved, while intercycle dynamics, which are dynamic patterns between different periods across a cyclic pattern of the time series, are altered. Two alternative hypotheses are suggested: (1) deterministic nonperiodic intercycle dynamics

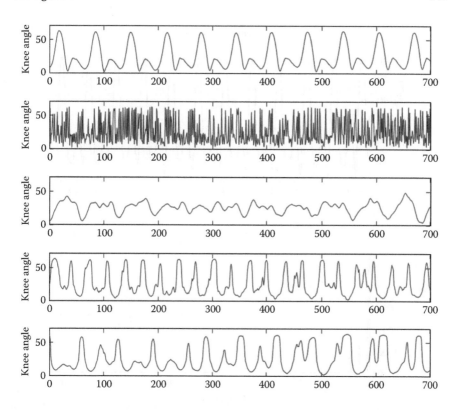

FIGURE 5.13 Applying linear surrogate methods is not suitable for time series with inherent periodicity. Knee flexion and extension angle data from human gait produces cycles that correspond to steps. Using Algorithms, A0 and A1 would result in false rejection of the null hypothesis because these methods change the structure of the time series. Similarly, AAFT and IAAFT algorithms change the geometric structure of the time series and would also lead to false rejection of the null.

and (2) a periodic orbit with correlated noise. In the case of the electrocardiogram, the application of the PPS algorithm showed that the sinus rhythm has deterministic nonperiodic intercycle dynamics (Small et al. 2001).

The first step of generating a surrogate time series by the PPS algorithm involves the reconstruction of the state space. Therefore, the embedding dimension (m) and the time lag (τ) need to be defined. The embedding parameters to compute discriminating statistics, which require the reconstruction of the state space, are usually set to be the same for the entire data sets. However, for generating a surrogate time series, the embedding parameters should be specific to each data set (Small and Tse 2002). The other parameter the PPS requires is the noise radius (ρ), which defines the amount of noise in a surrogate (Small et al. 2001). If noise radii are too large, then the surrogate time series will be too distinct from the original while if noise radii are too small, the original and surrogate time series will be too similar, which may result in a false positive result for the hypothesis testing (Figure 5.15). Noise radii should be

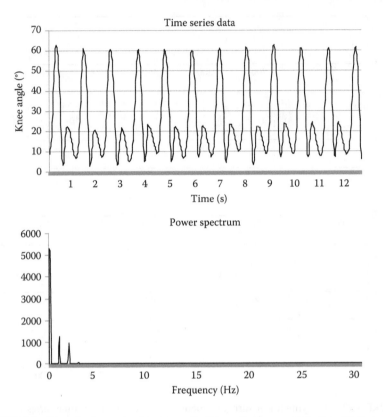

FIGURE 5.14   Knee flexion and extension angle time series have a periodic orbit that cycles with every step. The power spectrum displays a clear spike, which demonstrates the frequency of the dynamics in the time series. Such time series already exhibit deterministic behavior, so a different algorithm, the pseudoperiodic surrogate method, is required to identify whether additional determinism exists in the system.

chosen such that the fine intercycle dynamics are removed, but the intracycle dynamics are preserved. Small et al. (2001) suggested selecting a ρ that maximizes the number of short segments (length ≥2) that are the same for the original time series and the surrogate. These segments represent the amount of correlation between the surrogate and the original data sets (Small et al. 2001). If ρ is too large, surrogate time series will be too different from the original time series because the dynamics were poorly approximated. If ρ is too small, surrogate time series will be too similar to the original time series.

Let us look at the procedure of generating a surrogate time series with the PPS:

1. Select the embedding dimension (m) and time lag (τ) for time delay embedding reconstruction.
2. Randomly select an embedded point as an initial condition (Figure 5.16a). This embedded point is a delay vector that has m elements, and we call it v_1.

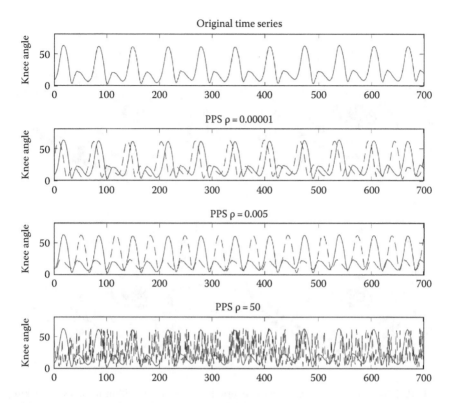

FIGURE 5.15 The noise radius is an important parameter for implementing the pseudoperiodic surrogate algorithm. If the noise radius is too small, the original and surrogate time series will be too similar. If the noise radius is too large, the surrogate time series will be too distinct from the original. Noise radii should be chosen such that the fine intercycle dynamics are removed, but the intracycle dynamics are preserved.

3. Randomly select a neighboring vector to v_1 and call it v_2 (Figure 5.16b). The neighbors are chosen with a certain probability equation.
4. Randomly select a neighboring vector to v_2 and call it v_3 (Figure 5.16c).
5. Repeat this procedure until the number of vectors that we select reaches the length of the original time series (Figure 5.16d).
6. A surrogate time series is generated by taking the first element of the selected delay vectors.

The surrogate time series generated by the PPS can be considered as a random walk on the attractor; therefore, it follows the same vector field as the original time series but is contaminated with dynamic noise (Figures 5.17 and 5.18). This addition of dynamic noise destroys subtle deterministic intercycle dynamics, including periodic dynamics with correlated noise, pseudoperiodic chaos or any deterministic nonperiodic intercycle dynamic behavior (Small and Tse 2002; Zhao et al. 2008). The PPS algorithm has been applied to gait kinematics data (Miller et al. 2006).

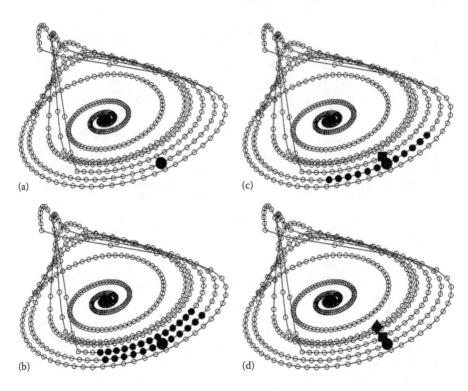

FIGURE 5.16 The process of the pseudoperiodic surrogate algorithm includes (a) picking an embedded point on the attractor as an initial condition, (b) identifying the neighbors within a certain probability equations, (c) randomly picking one neighboring vector and identifying its neighbors, and (d) randomly picking one neighbor's neighboring vector. This process is repeated until the number of vectors selected equals the length of the original time series. In (a), the initial condition is shown as a circle and its neighbors are diamonds in (b). The neighbors of a randomly selected neighboring vector are shown in (c) and one neighbor's neighboring vector is shown as a circle in (d).

Specifically, knee angle kinematic time series from healthy subjects were evaluated using the PPS algorithm, and Theiler et al. algorithm 0. The average time lag for the series was 9.833 and the average embedding dimension was 6.333. The noise radii that maximized the number of short segments that are the same for the original time series and the surrogate was 3.351. The paper demonstrated that Theiler et al. algorithm 0 destroyed the intracycle dynamics of the gait time series by changing the overall shape, which resulted in a false rejection of the null hypothesis. The PPS algorithm did not alter the intracycle dynamics of the original time series, which made it more appropriate to explore the presence of underlying processes within these dynamics. Example Box 5.1 shows the general surrogation procedure using the PPS algorithm. The data for a knee flexion and extension angle, along with one surrogate generated using the PPS algorithm are included in Appendix 5.A. The SampEn values of the original and surrogate series, along with the parameters used are included in Example Box 5.1.

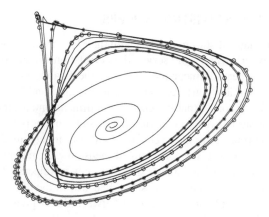

FIGURE 5.17 The phase portrait of the original Rossler attractor is plotted as a solid black line. The trajectories of the original attractor are indicated with open circles, while the trajectories of the pseudoperiodic surrogate attractor are indicated with asterisks. Clearly, the surrogate attractor follows the same vector field as the original, but since it has been contaminated with dynamic noise, the trajectory is not identical to that of the original attractor.

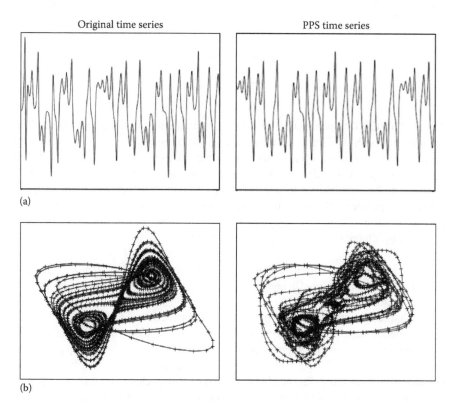

FIGURE 5.18 The plot of the original and pseudoperiodic surrogate time series (a) and two dimensional vector phase portraits (b) from the Lorenz attractor. The surrogate is a random walk in the same vector field as the original time series but is contaminated with dynamic noise.

DISCRIMINATING STATISTICS FOR PPS

As for discriminating statistics to be used with the PPS, it was reported that for both theoretical and experimental time series, the correlation dimension performed the best compared to other nonlinear tools such as the Shannon's entropy, prediction error, mutual information, kurtosis and skewness (Small and Tse 2002). However, Zhang et al. (2007) reported that the correlation dimension and the PPS algorithm failed to differentiate between a chaotic system and a noisy periodic orbit. In this study, a theoretical time series of the chaotic Rossler system (Equation 5.4) was used as the original time series. If the correlation dimension was an appropriate discriminating statistic, then the null hypothesis should have been rejected. However, the correlation dimension of the original time series lied within the dimension distribution of the surrogates and could not differentiate between the original and the surrogate time series. This is due to the fact that the correlation dimension characterizes the distribution of the points in the state space; however for the PPS algorithm, the distribution of the original and surrogate time series should follow the same pattern. Thus, an alternative discriminating statistic must be used when implementing PPS surrogation:

$$\dot{x} = -(y + z)$$

$$\dot{y} = x + ay \qquad\qquad (5.4)$$

$$\dot{z} = 2 + z(x - 4)$$

Zhang et al. (2007) introduced alternative new methods to be used as discriminating statistics with the PPS. Those methods do not require the reconstruction of the state space but take the cycle in the time series as the basic processing unit. The discriminating statistics depend on the correlation coefficient between cycles and are supposed to be more robust to nonstationarity in data and different kinds of noise. There are separate methods for detecting the temporal, or time index, correlation and the spatial, or configuration of cycles, correlation. The basic ideas of the methods proposed by Zhang et al. (2007) are the following:

1. Divide a pseudoperiodic time series into consecutive cycles C_i ($i = 1, 2,\ldots, m$).
2. Find correlation coefficients (ρ) between cycles as a measure of their distance in phase space.
3. Characterize the similarity of wave form between a pair of cycles. A large ρ means there is a higher level of similarity. Two cycles will also be close in the phase space with a higher ρ.

For chaotic systems, the distance between two nearby cycles will increase exponentially over time due to sensitivity to initial conditions, whereas the correlation will drop exponentially. More specifically, Zhang et al. presents two specific alternative surrogate methods. The first is average cycle divergence rate, which detects a correlation between the temporal cycles. For chaotic systems, the distance between two nearby cycles will increase exponentially over time, due to the sensitive dependence on initial conditions. The correlation between two cycles is expected to drop exponentially as the number of cycles increase. The second alternative method investigates the fluctuation of the degree of distribution of cycles in the phase space and is quantified through the variance of the normalized derivative. In this method, the degree distribution curve and the variance of the normalized derivative distribution are calculated. The degree distribution curve provides the distribution of cycles in the phase space. A chaotic system will show multiple distribution peaks, whereas a noisy periodic system will show a Poisson distribution of peaks. The peaks or smoothness of the distribution are quantified by the variance of the normalized derivative. A chaotic system will have a high value, and a noisy periodic system, which has more homogeneous smoothness, will have a low value.

A more recent surrogate method called the small shuffle surrogate was introduced by Nakamura and Small (2005) to investigate whether there are dynamics in irregular fluctuations (short term variability), even if the fluctuations are modulated by trends or periodicities. This algorithm generates surrogates that preserve long-term behaviors but destroys local structures. The null hypothesis is that irregular fluctuations are independently distributed (temporally uncorrelated) random variables. This algorithm changes the flow of information in the data and can be used to detect whether dynamics are present or not, regardless of whether the time series are linear or nonlinear. The authors propose that autocorrelation or average mutual information are appropriate to use as the discriminating techniques. The autocorrelation function and average mutual information answer the question regarding how much future data points are determined by past data points. To test the hypothesis, 39 surrogate time series are developed (two-sided test) and discriminating statistics calculated for the original and surrogate time series. If the values of the discriminating statistics of the original fall within the distribution of the surrogates, the null is not rejected. Time series with no dynamics (random process) have autocorrelation function, and average mutual information values fall within the distribution of the small surrogate shuffle distribution. Time series that contain dynamics will result in autocorrelation function and average mutual information values that are separate from the surrogate distribution. This method was robust in systems that contain long-term trends and those contaminated by stochastic noise.

One limitation of the small shuffle surrogate method is that it cannot distinguish between linear or nonlinear phenomena, as both types of systems exhibit some type of dynamics, which would lead to rejecting the null hypothesis. Nakamura et al. (2006) proposed a modification to the small shuffle surrogate that would test for the presence of nonlinearity in time series containing long-term trends and short-term fluctuations called truncated Fourier transform surrogate. This method assumes that the frequencies of irregular fluctuations are higher than the long-term trends and that when the data are linear, all phases can be treated as linear data when the power spectrum is preserved. The null hypothesis for this algorithm is that irregular fluctuations are generated by a stationary linear system. The algorithm destroys nonlinearity in the irregular fluctuations and preserves the trends or periodicities. This is done by randomizing those phases from the power spectrum in the higher-frequency domains while maintaining the low-frequency phases. Thus, the major difference from the previous small shuffle surrogate is that not all phases are randomized, but only those in the higher-frequency domain. This algorithm requires the selection of a parameter to determine which frequencies will be randomized. This limitation of the truncated Fourier transform surrogate led Rios et al. (2015) to develop two new methods using decomposition to improve the surrogation techniques. The new techniques are the empirical mode decomposition–Fourier transform and empirical mode decomposition–amplitude-adjusted Fourier transform. These techniques rely on decomposing the data into a set of monocomponents plus residuals, with the residuals demonstrating the time series trend. Next, traditional surrogate methods are applied on each monocomponent, which results in a set of monocomponent surrogates. Finally, the set of surrogates is combined and retrended by adding the residuals back into the time series from the first step. This algorithm allows testing for the presence of linear and nonlinear behaviors in both stationary and nonstationary time series.

SUMMARY

In this chapter, we have discussed surrogate methods, which take the form of hypothesis testing. We examined several different surrogate algorithms, four linear surrogate methods, the pseudoperiodic surrogate method, and the small shuffle surrogate. The linear surrogate methods are designed to be applied to a stationary irregular time series without any long-term trend or periodicity, while the pseudoperiodic is applied to time series with periodicity. The small shuffle surrogate provides information regarding dynamics in irregular fluctuations, even if the fluctuations are modulated by trends or periodicities. Each algorithm generates a surrogate time series, which is consistent with a specific null hypothesis. Surrogate methods are used as an indirect approach to identify the nature of a time series. They try to narrow down the possibility of what a time series is by eliminating the possibilities of what a time series is not. Surrogate methods can identify whether a "hidden" structure exists within the data, but not necessarily tell if chaos exists. A surrogate method alone cannot decide what the time series is but is an extremely helpful tool when used with other nonlinear tools.

EXERCISES

1. State the general procedure of conducting a surrogate test.
2. State the null hypothesis of Algorithm 0.
3. State the null hypothesis of Algorithm 1.
4. State the null hypothesis of Algorithm 2.
5. What is the difference between Algorithm 2 and IAAFT?
6. Can we use linear surrogate methods when a time series exhibits strong periodicity? Why or why not?

7. State the null hypothesis of the PPS algorithm.
8. What three parameters are necessary for the PPS algorithm?
9. Can you determine what a time series is by using surrogate methods?
10. Explain two kinds of discriminating criteria.

APPENDIX 5.A: KNEE JOINT FLEXION/EXTENSION ANGLE (DEGREES)

ORIGINAL SERIES

8.9612	12.578	25.092
9.7076	14.736	30.052
10.999	17.075	34.983
12.622	19.491	40.42
14.419	21.488	45.34
17.115	22.29	50.399
20.207	22.265	54.797
24.619	22.061	57.619
29.044	21.629	59.679
34.142	21.241	60.858
39.573	20.817	61.133
44.759	21.04	60.848
49.739	20.637	59.408
54.843	19.316	57.758
58.542	18.678	55.071
60.774	17.495	51.788
62.389	16.124	48.584
62.196	14.93	43.881
62.171	13.69	39.086
61.575	12.439	33.177
59.821	11.267	26.737
57.643	10.207	20.074
54.715	9.302	13.561
51.169	8.5962	8.1246
47.151	7.7525	4.782
42.075	7.2274	2.8538
35.762	6.8028	2.8926
29.722	6.6854	4.4985
23.035	7.0044	7.0089
16.215	7.5202	9.2506
11.144	8.3092	10.876
6.6787	9.5507	12.778
4.3748	10.634	15.692
3.4397	12.254	18.496
4.6151	14.471	20.266
7.3564	17.542	20.526
10.249	21.09	20.45

20.485	34.294	18.385
20.501	28.575	22.163
20.069	22.217	26.077
19.438	15.664	30.343
19.219	10.865	34.79
18.51	6.7063	39.653
17.474	4.36	44.762
16.718	3.2073	49.475
15.219	3.9469	54.155
14.25	6.542	56.516
13.251	8.452	58.711
12.093	11.194	59.818
11.015	13.136	60.459
9.7966	14.735	60.116
8.6375	16.063	58.864
8.0029	18.232	56.819
7.4718	19.856	54.73
7.0539	20.942	51.357
7.0923	21.685	47.767
7.624	21.156	43.319
7.991	20.515	38.25
8.9692	20.305	31.784
10.382	19.543	25.41
12.074	18.632	18.241
14.513	17.751	12.775
17.673	17.33	8.3107
21.398	15.568	5.7746
25.6	14.439	4.7991
30.065	12.788	5.4521
34.683	11.664	7.252
39.781	10.341	10.041
45.339	8.8039	12.566
49.923	7.7423	14.798
54.053	6.3726	17.933
57.503	5.5298	20.797
59.414	4.9179	23.074
60.413	4.9681	23.312
60.424	4.9942	22.75
60.287	5.4474	21.821
59.089	5.7399	21.809
56.91	6.7546	21.635
54.625	7.8583	21.346
51.825	9.234	20.976
47.954	11.085	20.004
44.343	13.089	18.694
39.828	15.602	17.514

16.833	6.172	59.904
15.748	8.7978	60.064
14.811	11.818	59.735
13.767	14.175	59.006
13.046	16.626	57.236
12.233	19.409	55.149
11.395	21.455	51.881
11.043	22.41	48.264
10.098	21.86	45.083
9.3043	21.326	40.315
8.6863	21.17	34.958
8.6412	20.953	29.086
8.9573	20.711	23.003
9.8134	19.943	17.55
11.062	19.012	12.304
13.032	17.888	8.9619
15.424	16.889	7.1428
18.64	15.826	6.5955
22.644	14.575	7.6152
26.84	13.611	9.3094
31.358	12.269	11.563
36.497	11.255	13.711
41.339	9.9009	15.32
46.514	9.164	18.008
51.32	7.9652	20.571
55.239	7.6236	22.131
58.468	6.8844	22.771
59.867	6.7978	22.457
60.618	6.8674	22.075
60.685	7.3732	21.818
59.528	8.0175	21.668
58.682	9.0707	21.053
56.665	10.739	20.497
54.062	12.226	20.088
51.362	14.413	19.105
47.681	17.15	17.911
43.842	20.42	16.509
38.084	24.323	15.515
32.691	28.578	14.619
26.653	33.036	14.001
20.583	37.901	12.752
14.562	43.144	11.41
10.1	47.896	10.876
6.719	52.56	9.6281
4.9821	55.894	8.833
4.8589	58.446	8.2302

7.1681	23.498	47.993
7.5316	23.151	42.995
7.6462	23.046	37.955
8.155	22.685	32.211
9.0405	22.416	25.922
10.48	22.112	19.329
12.019	21.613	13.066
14.143	20.718	8.1002
16.536	19.749	4.9102
19.937	18.704	3.4886
23.942	17.439	3.7459
28.48	16.742	5.4572
33.381	15.858	7.9289
38.509	15.029	10.387
43.778	13.786	12.289
48.795	13.241	14.95
53.255	12.462	18.168
57.514	11.624	20.786
59.803	11.14	22.191
60.379	10.688	22.535
60.745	10.094	22.263
61.129	10.217	22.175
59.998	10.508	21.973
58.18	11.127	21.959
56.05	12.127	21.603
52.888	13.695	21.213
49.539	15.538	20.607
45.418	17.848	19.525
40.387	20.735	18.82
35.095	24.59	17.654
28.6	28.798	16.639
22.251	33.379	15.502
15.247	38.638	14.507
10.352	43.54	13.862
6.2817	48.942	12.873
4.618	53.522	12.018
4.2304	57.697	10.793
5.4652	59.845	10.054
8.1121	61.454	9.0675
10.589	61.933	8.6673
12.855	61.578	8.6682
14.994	61.012	8.7991
17.341	59.332	9.3349
19.835	57.317	10.757
21.98	54.946	12.119
23.398	51.479	14.471

16.985	20.085	10.92
20.392	19.294	8.6063
24.368	17.772	7.0982
28.529	16.352	6.5939
33.403	15.246	8.1424
38.097	14.534	10.584
43.153	13.217	13.743
48.927	12.099	16.208
53.825	11.107	18.112
57.878	10.065	19.88
60.481	9.5547	22.265
61.898	9.081	23.548
62.526	8.6737	24.356
62.566	8.5694	23.884
61.809	8.8998	23.039
60.491	9.3981	22.423
58.281	10.395	21.961
55.879	11.618	21.158
52.87	13.484	20.332
49.361	15.74	19.148
45.07	18.586	17.707
40.907	21.849	16.558
35.457	25.907	15.607
29.854	30.262	14.216
23.848	34.676	13.369
17.678	39.309	12.272
13.003	44.134	11.467
9.3651	49.565	10.7
7.3227	53.917	9.7143
6.8289	57.409	8.8553
7.6683	59.772	8.6787
9.6401	60.752	7.9992
12.135	61.196	7.6539
14.628	61.22	7.8662
16.402	60.719	7.9757
18.799	59.112	8.4738
20.716	56.994	9.4577
22.589	54.797	10.94
23.685	51.513	12.879
23.955	47.928	15.348
23.613	43.74	18.331
23.391	38.666	21.913
22.926	33.049	26.323
22.43	27.394	30.906
21.814	21.394	35.439
21.437	15.337	40.819

46.206	24.454	16.796
50.497	23.568	19.678
54.896	23.362	23.314
58.094	22.61	27.119
59.928	22.823	32.058
60.787	21.783	37.112
61.003	20.661	42.176
60.438	19.748	47.556
59.521	18.595	52.439
57.651	17.153	56.779
55.088	16.45	59.074
51.606	14.902	60.953
48.204	13.894	61.25
44.285	13.174	61.654
39.07	12.133	60.786
33.371	10.818	59.582
27.034	10.144	57.577
20.331	9.6492	54.643
14.671	9.1698	51.619
10.459	8.8224	47.6
8.0987	8.5052	43.06
7.4885	8.4115	37.446
8.1968	8.2302	31.552
10.589	8.8595	24.704
13.886	8.9071	18.513
16.381	9.8471	12.488
18.542	10.919	8.4084
20.648	12.492	6.2972
23.207	14.368	

PPS Surrogate Series

16.558	6.6854	45.34
17.772	7.0044	49.475
16.352	7.5202	54.155
15.246	8.3092	56.516
12.269	9.5507	58.711
11.255	10.634	59.818
10.341	12.254	60.459
8.8039	14.471	60.116
7.7423	17.542	58.864
9.302	21.09	56.819
8.5962	25.092	54.73
7.7525	30.052	51.788
7.2274	34.983	48.584
6.8028	40.42	43.881

39.086	13.089	16.833
33.177	15.602	15.748
28.6	18.385	14.811
23.003	25.092	13.767
17.55	26.077	12.133
12.775	34.983	10.818
8.3107	40.42	10.144
4.782	45.34	9.6492
4.7991	50.399	9.1698
5.4521	54.797	8.8224
7.252	57.619	9.3043
10.041	59.679	8.6863
12.566	61.933	8.6412
14.798	61.578	8.9573
17.933	59.408	9.8134
20.797	57.758	8.9071
23.074	55.071	9.8471
23.312	51.788	10.48
22.75	48.584	12.879
21.821	43.881	18.64
21.809	39.086	22.644
21.635	33.177	26.84
21.346	26.737	31.358
20.976	20.331	36.497
20.004	14.562	41.339
19.105	10.1	46.514
17.911	6.2972	51.32
16.509	7.4885	55.239
15.515	8.1968	58.468
15.515	10.589	59.867
14.619	13.886	59.928
14.001	16.381	61.25
11.015	18.542	61.654
8.8039	20.648	59.089
7.7423	20.571	56.91
6.3726	22.131	54.625
5.5298	22.771	51.881
4.9179	22.457	48.264
4.9681	22.075	45.083
4.9942	21.818	40.315
5.4474	21.668	34.958
5.7399	21.053	28.6
6.7546	20.976	22.251
7.8583	20.004	15.247
9.234	18.694	10.459
11.085	17.514	8.0987

7.4885	57.409	8.2302
8.1968	59.772	8.2302
5.4572	60.752	7.3732
7.9289	61.196	8.0175
13.743	59.528	9.3349
16.208	60.719	10.395
18.112	59.582	11.618
19.88	57.577	13.484
22.265	55.071	15.74
22.589	51.788	12.254
23.685	48.584	14.471
23.955	40.315	17.542
23.039	34.958	21.09
22.423	27.034	25.092
21.961	20.331	30.052
21.158	13.561	34.983
20.332	10.865	40.42
19.148	6.7063	45.34
17.707	4.36	50.399
16.558	3.2073	54.797
15.607	3.9469	57.619
14.216	6.542	59.679
13.369	9.2506	60.858
12.272	10.876	60.459
11.467	12.778	60.116
10.876	14.735	59.582
9.6281	16.063	57.577
8.833	18.232	54.643
8.2302	23.398	48.584
7.1681	23.498	43.881
8.6673	23.151	39.086
8.6682	23.046	31.784
5.7399	21.959	25.41
9.4577	21.603	18.241
10.94	21.213	12.775
12.879	20.607	8.3107
15.348	19.525	5.7746
18.331	18.704	4.7991
21.913	17.439	5.4521
26.323	16.742	7.252
30.906	15.858	10.041
34.676	15.029	12.566
38.509	13.786	14.798
43.778	13.241	17.933
48.795	9.302	14.735
53.255	8.5962	16.063

18.232	54.73	18.64
19.856	51.357	22.644
20.45	47.767	26.84
20.45	43.319	31.358
20.485	40.315	36.497
20.501	34.958	41.339
20.515	29.086	46.514
20.305	23.003	51.32
19.543	17.55	55.239
18.632	12.304	58.468
17.751	8.9619	59.867
17.33	7.1428	60.618
15.219	6.5955	60.685
14.25	10.589	61.22
13.251	13.886	59.521
12.093	16.381	57.577
11.015	18.542	54.643
9.7966	20.648	51.513
7.7423	23.207	45.418
9.6281	24.454	40.387
8.833	23.568	37.955
8.2302	23.362	32.211
7.1681	22.61	25.922
7.5316	22.823	20.583
7.6462	21.783	14.671
8.155	20.661	10.459
9.0405	19.748	8.0987
10.48	18.595	7.3227
12.019	17.153	6.8289
14.143	16.45	7.6683
16.536	15.826	10.584
20.392	16.124	12.135
24.59	15.246	14.628
28.798	14.534	16.402
33.379	13.217	18.799
38.638	12.099	20.716
43.54	11.107	23.362
48.942	10.065	24.356
53.917	9.5547	23.884
57.409	9.081	23.039
59.772	7.6539	22.423
60.413	7.8662	21.961
60.424	7.0044	21.158
60.116	11.062	21.814
58.864	13.032	21.437
56.819	15.424	20.085

19.294	16.208	60.848
17.772	18.112	59.408
14.216	19.88	56.819
12.272	22.265	54.73
11.467	23.548	51.357
10.207	23.685	47.767
9.302	22.263	43.319
8.5962	22.175	38.25
9.0675	21.973	31.784
8.6673	21.959	25.41
8.6682	21.603	18.241
7.0044	21.213	12.775
6.7546	20.607	8.1246
12.226	16.889	6.2817
18.64	15.826	4.618
22.644	14.575	3.2073
26.84	13.611	6.172
31.358	13.767	8.7978
36.497	13.046	9.2506
41.339	12.233	10.876
46.514	11.395	14.994
51.32	11.043	18.008
55.239	10.098	20.571
58.468	9.3043	22.131
59.867	8.6863	22.771
60.752	8.6412	22.457
61.196	8.9573	22.075
59.528	9.8134	21.818
58.682	11.127	21.668
59.332	10.48	21.053
57.317	14.368	20.497
54.946	12.254	18.632
51.479	14.471	19.105
47.993	17.542	16.889
42.995	21.09	15.826
37.955	25.092	13.894
33.049	30.052	13.174
27.394	34.983	12.269
21.394	40.42	13.046
13.066	45.34	11.467
9.3651	50.399	10.7
7.3227	54.797	9.7143
6.8289	57.619	8.8553
7.6683	59.679	9.3043
10.584	60.858	8.6863
13.743	61.133	8.6412

7.5316	21.158	8.9619
8.8998	20.332	4.618
11.062	19.148	4.2304
13.032	19.525	5.4652
15.424	18.82	6.542
15.538	17.654	8.452
17.848	16.639	11.194
20.735	13.369	13.136
24.368	12.233	14.735
28.529	11.395	16.063
36.497	11.043	18.232
41.339	7.6236	19.856
46.514	8.2302	22.457
51.32	7.1681	21.821
55.239	8.6412	21.809
58.468	8.9573	21.635
59.867	9.8134	21.346
60.618	8.4738	20.976
59.528	9.4577	20.004
58.281	10.94	18.694
55.879	12.019	17.514
52.87	14.143	16.833
49.361	16.536	15.748
45.07	19.937	14.811
40.907	23.942	13.767
35.457	28.48	12.752
29.854	33.381	13.786
23.848	38.509	13.241
17.678	44.134	12.462
13.003	49.565	11.624
9.3651	53.522	11.14
7.3227	57.697	10.688
6.8289	59.845	10.094
7.6683	61.454	10.217
7.9289	61.933	11.127
10.387	61.578	12.127
12.289	61.012	13.695
14.95	58.281	15.538
18.168	52.888	17.848
20.786	49.539	20.735
22.191	45.418	24.368
23.498	40.387	28.529
23.884	35.095	33.403
23.039	28.6	38.097
22.423	23.003	43.153
21.961	14.562	48.927

53.825	58.682	38.084
57.878	56.665	32.691
60.481	54.062	26.653
61.898	51.825	20.583
61.196	47.954	14.562
61.22	43.842	

REFERENCES

Acharya, U. R., O. Faust, N. Kannathal, T. Chua, and S. Laxminarayan. (2005). Non-linear analysis of EEG signals at various sleep stages. *Computer Methods and Programs in Biomedicine* 80 (1): 37–45.

Amato, I. (June 26, 1992). Chaos breaks out at NIH, but order may come of it. *Science* 256 (5065): 1763–1764.

Barahona, M. and C. Poon. (May 16, 1996). Detection of nonlinear dynamics in short, noisy time series. *Nature* 381: 215–217.

Breakspear, M. and J. R. Terry. (2002). Nonlinear interdependence in neural systems: Motivation, theory, and relevance. *The International Journal of Neuroscience* 112 (10): 1263–1284.

Buchman, T. G., J. P. Cobb, A. S. Lapedes, and T. B. Kepler. (2001). Complex systems analysis: A tool for shock research. *Shock* 16 (4): 248–251.

Buzzi, U. H., N. Stergiou, M. J. Kurz, P. A. Hageman, and J. Heidel. (2003). Nonlinear dynamics indicates aging affects variability during gait. *Clinical Biomechanics* 18 (5): 435–443.

Cavanaugh, J. T., N. Kochi, and N. Stergiou. (2010). Nonlinear analysis of ambulatory activity patterns in community-dwelling older adults. *The Journals of Gerontology. Series A, Biological Sciences and Medical Sciences* 65 (2): 197–203.

Chang, T., S. J. Schiff, T. Sauer, J. P. Gossard, and R. E. Burke. (1994). Stochastic versus deterministic variability in simple neuronal circuits: I. monosynaptic spinal cord reflexes. *Biophysical Journal* 67 (2): 671–683.

Cignetti, F., F. Schena, and A. Rouard. (2009). Effects of fatigue on inter-cycle variability in cross-country skiing. *Journal of Biomechanics* 42 (10): 1452–1459.

Collins, J. J. and C. J. De Luca. (1995). The effects of visual input on open-loop and closed-loop postural control mechanisms. *Experimental Brain Research* 103 (1): 151–163.

Costa, M. D., T. Henriques, M. N. Munshi, A. R. Segal, and A. L. Goldberger. (2014). Dynamical glucometry: Use of multiscale entropy analysis in diabetes. *Chaos* 24 (3): 033139.

Diks, C. (1996). Estimating invariants of noisy attractors. *Physical Review E, Statistical Physics, Plasmas, Fluids, and Related Interdisciplinary Topics* 53 (5): R4263–R4266.

Dingwell, J. B. and J. P. Cusumano. (2000). Nonlinear time series analysis of normal and pathological human walking. *Chaos* 10 (4): 848–863.

Ehlers, C. L., J. Havstad, D. Prichard, and J. Theiler. (1998). Low doses of ethanol reduce evidence for nonlinear structure in brain activity. *The Journal of Neuroscience* 18 (18): 7474–7486.

Garfinkel, A., M. L. Spano, W. L. Ditto, and J. N. Weiss. (Aug 28, 1992). Controlling cardiac chaos. *Science* 257 (5074): 1230–1235.

Georgoulis, A. D., C. Moraiti, S. Ristanis, and N. Stergiou. (2006). A novel approach to measure variability in the anterior cruciate ligament deficient knee during walking: The use of the approximate entropy in orthopaedics. *Journal of Clinical Monitoring and Computing* 20 (1): 11–18.

Goldstein, B., D. Toweill, S. Lai, K. Sonnenthal, and B. Kimberly. (1998). Uncoupling of the autonomic and cardiovascular systems in acute brain injury. *The American Journal of Physiology* 275 (4 Pt 2): R1287–R1292.

Govindan, R. B., K. Narayanan, and M. S. Gopinathan. (1998). On the evidence of deterministic chaos in ECG: Surrogate and predictability analysis. *Chaos* 8 (2): 495–502.

Grassberger, P. and I. Procaccia. (1983). Measuring the strangeness of strange attractors. *Physica D* 9: 189–208.

Hausdorff, J. M., C. K. Peng, Z. Ladin, J. Y. Wei, and A. L. Goldberger. (1995). Is walking a random walk? Evidence for long-range correlations in stride interval of human gait. *Journal of Applied Physiology* 78 (1): 349–358.

Ivanov, D. K., H. A. Posch, and C. Stumpf. (1996). Statistical measures derived from the correlation integrals of physiological time series. *Chaos* 6 (2): 243–253.

Janjarasjitt, S., M. S. Scher, and K. A. Loparo. (2008). Nonlinear dynamical analysis of the neonatal EEG time series: The relationship between sleep state and complexity. *Clinical Neurophysiology* 119 (8): 1812–1823.

Kantz, H. and T. Schreiber. (1997). *Nonlinear Time-Series Analysis.* Cambridge, U.K.: Cambridge University Press.

Kaplan, D. and L. Glass. (1995). *Understanding Nonlinear Dynamics.* New York: Springer-Verlag.

Keenan, D. (1985). A Tukey non-additivity type test of time series nonlinearity. *Biometrika* 72 (1): 39–44.

Kugiumtzis, D. (1999). Test your surrogate data before you test for nonlinearity. *Physical Review E, Statistical Physics, Plasmas, Fluids, and Related Interdisciplinary Topics* 60 (3): 2808–2816.

Kugiumtzis, D. (2001). On the reliability of the surrogate data test for nonlinearity in the analysis of noisy time series. *International Journal of Bifurcation and Chaos* 11 (7): 1881–1896.

Kunhimangalam, R., P. K. Joseph, and O. K. Sujith. (2008). Nonlinear analysis of EEG signals: Surrogate data analysis. *IRBM* 29 (4): 239–244.

Kurz, M. J., T. N. Judkins, C. Arellano, and M. Scott-Pandorf. (2008). A passive dynamic walking robot that has a deterministic nonlinear gait. *Journal of Biomechanics* 41 (6): 1310–1316.

Ladislao, L. and S. Fioretti. (2007). Nonlinear analysis of posturographic data. *Medical & Biological Engineering & Computing* 45 (7): 679–688.

Lamoth, C. J., E. Ainsworth, W. Polomski, and H. Houdijk. (2010). Variability and stability analysis of walking of transfemoral amputees. *Medical Engineering & Physics* 32 (9): 1009–1014.

Lamoth, C. J., F. J. van Deudekom, J. P. van Campen, B. A. Appels, O. J. de Vries, and M. Pijnappels. (2011). Gait stability and variability measures show effects of impaired cognition and dual tasking in frail people. *Journal of Neuroengineering and Rehabilitation* 17 (8): 2.

Lehnertz, K., R. G. Andrzejak, J. Arnhold, T. Kreuz, F. Mormann, C. Rieke, G. Widman, and C. E. Elger. (2001). Nonlinear EEG analysis in epilepsy: Its possible use for interictal focus localization, seizure anticipation, and prevention. *Journal of Clinical Neurophysiology* 18 (3): 209–222.

Little, M. A., P. E. McSharry, I. M. Moroz, and S. J. Roberts (2006). Testing the assumptions of linear prediction analysis in normal vowels. *The Journal of the Acoustical Society of America* 119 (1): 549–558.

Martinerie, J., C. Adam, M. Le Van Quyen, M. Baulac, S. Clemenceau, B. Renault, and F. J. Varela. (1998). Epileptic seizures can be anticipated by non-linear analysis. *Nature Medicine* 4 (10): 1173–1176.

Miller, D. J., N. Stergiou, and M. J. Kurz. (2006). An improved surrogate method for detecting the presence of chaos in gait. *Journal of Biomechanics* 39 (15): 2873–2876.

Mitra, S., M. A. Riley, and M. T. Turvey. (1997). Chaos in human rhythmic movement. *Journal of Motor Behavior* 29 (3): 195–198.

Myers, S. A., J. M. Johanning, I. I. Pipinos, K. K. Schmid, and N. Stergiou. (2012). Vascular occlusion affects gait variability patterns of healthy younger and older individuals. *Annals of Biomedical Engineering.*

Myers, S. A., J. M. Johanning, I. I. Pipinos, K. K. Schmid, and N. Stergiou. (Aug, 2013). Vascular occlusion affects gait variability patterns of healthy younger and older individuals. *Annals of Biomedical Engineering* 41 (8): 1692–1702.

Nakamura, T. and M. Small. (2005). Small-shuffle surrogate data: Testing for dynamics in fluctuating data with trends. *Physical Review E, Statistical, Nonlinear, and Soft Matter Physics* 72 (5 Pt 2): 056216.

Nakamura, T., M. Small, and Y. Hirata. (2006). Testing for nonlinearity in irregular fluctuations with long-term trends. *Physical Review E* 74: 026205.

Nurujjaman, M. D., R. Narayanan, and A. N. S. Iyengar. (2009). Comparative study of nonlinear properties of EEG signals of normal persons and epileptic patients. *Nonlinear Biomedical Physics* 3: 6.

Orsucci, F. F. (2006). The paradigm of complexity in clinical neurocognitive science. *The Neuroscientist* 12 (5): 390–397.

Osborne, A. and A. Provencale. (1989). Finite correlation dimension for stochastic systems with power-law spectra. *Physica D* 35: 357–381.

Palus, M. (1995). Testing for nonlinearity using redundancies: Quantitative and qualitative aspects. *Physica D* 80: 186–205.

Palus, M. (1996). Nonlinearity in normal human EEG: Cycles, temporal asymmetry, nonstationarity and randomness, not chaos. *Biological Cybernetics* 75 (5): 389–396.

Peng, C. K., S. Havlin, H. E. Stanley, and A. L. Goldberger. (1995). Quantification of scaling exponents and crossover phenomena in nonstationary heartbeat time series. *Chaos* 5 (1): 82–87.

Pincus, S. M. (1991). Approximate entropy as a measure of system complexity. *Proceedings of the National Academy of Sciences of the United States of America* 88 (6): 2297–2301.

Pincus, S. M., I. M. Gladstone, and R. A. Ehrenkranz (1991). A regularity statistic for medical data analysis. *Journal of Clinical Monitoring* 7 (4): 335–345.

Poggi, D., A. Porporato, L. Ridolfi, J. Albertson, and G. Katul. (2004). Interaction between large and small scales in the canopy sublayer. *Geophysical Research Letters* 31 (5): L05102.

Pompe, B. (1993). Measuring statistical dependences in a time series. *Journal of Statistical Physics* 73 (3/4): 587–610.

Porta, A., S. Guzzetti, R. Furlan, T. Gnecchi-Ruscone, N. Montano, and A. Malliani. (2007). Complexity and nonlinearity in short-term heart period variability: Comparison of methods based on local nonlinear prediction. *IEEE Transactions on Bio-Medical Engineering* 54 (1): 94–106.

Preatoni, E., M. Ferrario, G. Donà, J. Hamill, and R. Rodano. (2010). Motor variability in sports: A non-linear analysis of race walking. *Journal of Sports Sciences* 28 (12): 1327–1336.

Prichard, D. and J. Theiler. (1995). Generalized redundancies for time series analysis. *Physica D* 84 (476): 493.

Rapp, P. E., A. M. Albano, T. I. Schmah, and L. A. Farwell. (1993). Filtered noise can mimic low-dimensional chaotic attractors. *Physical Review E, Statistical Physics, Plasmas, Fluids, and Related Interdisciplinary Topics* 47 (4): 2289–2297.

Rathleff, M. S., A. Samani, C. G. Olesen, U. G. Kersting, and P. Madeleine. (2011). Inverse relationship between the complexity of midfoot kinematics and muscle activation in patients with medial tibial stress syndrome. *Journal of Electromyography and Kinesiology* 21 (4): 638–644.

Rieke, C., F. Mormann, R. G. Andrzejak, T. Kreuz, P. David, C. E. Elger, and K. Lehnertz. (2003). Discerning nonstationarity from nonlinearity in seizure-free and pre-seizure EEG recordings from epilepsy patients. *IEEE Transactions on Bio-Medical Engineering* 50 (5): 634–639.

Rios, R., M. Small, and R. de Mello. (2015). Testing for linear and nonlinear Gaussian processes in nonstationary time series. *International Journal of Bifurcation and Chaos* 25 (1): 155013.

Rombouts, S., R. Keunen, and C. Stam. (1995). Investigation of nonlinear structure in multichannel EEG. *Physics Letters A* 202: 352–358.

Schreiber, T. and A. Schmitz. (1997). Classification of time series data with nonlinear similarity measures. *Physical Review Letters* 79: 1475.

Schreiber, T. and A. Schmitz. (2000). Surrogate time series. *Physica D* 142: 346–382.

Slutzky, M. W., P. Cvitanovic, and D. J. Mogul. (2001). Deterministic chaos and noise in three in vitro hippocampal models of epilepsy. *Annals of Biomedical Engineering* 29 (7): 607–618.

Small, M. (2005). *Applied Nonlinear Time Series Analysis: Application in Physics, Physiology and Finance*. Singapore: World Scientific Publishing.

Small, M. and K. Judd. (1998). Comparison of new nonlinear modelling techniques with applications to infant respiration. *Physica D* 117: 283–298.

Small, M. and C. K. Tse. (2002). Minimum description length neural networks for time series prediction. *Physical Review E, Statistical, Nonlinear, and Soft Matter Physics* 66 (6 Pt 2): 066701.

Small, M., D. Yu, and R. G. Harrison. (2001). Surrogate test for pseudoperiodic time series data. *Physical Review Letters* 87 (18): 188101.

Stam, C. J., T. C. van Woerkom, and R. W. Keunen. (1997). Non-linear analysis of the electroencephalogram in Creutzfeldt-Jakob disease. *Biological Cybernetics* 77 (4): 247–256.

Stergiou, N., U. H. Buzzi, M. J. Kurz, and J. Heidel. (2004). Nonlinear tools in human movement. In *Innovative Analyses of Human Movement*, ed. N. Stergiou, pp. 63–90. Champaign, IL: Human Kinetics Publ.

Theiler, J., S. Eubank, A. Longtin, B. Galdrikian, and J. D. Farmer. (1992). Testing for nonlinearity in time series: The method of surrogate data. *Physica D* 58: 77–94.

Theiler, J. and P. E. Rapp. (1996). Re-examination of the evidence for low-dimensional, nonlinear structure in the human electroencephalogram. *Electroencephalography and Clinical Neurophysiology* 98 (3): 213–222.

Toweill, D. L. and B. Goldstein. (1998). Linear and nonlinear dynamics and the pathophysiology of shock. *New Horizons* 6 (2): 155–168.

Tsay, R. (1986). Nonlinearity tests for time series. *Biometrika* 73: 461–466.

Wagner, C. D., B. Nafz, and P. B. Persson. (1996). Chaos in blood pressure control. *Cardiovascular Research* 31 (3): 380–387.

Wolf, A., J. B. Swift, H. L. Swinney, and J. A. Vastano. (1985). Determining Lyapunov exponents from a time series. *Physica* 16D: 285–317.

Wurdeman, S. R., S. A. Myers, and N. Stergiou. (2014). Amputation effects on the underlying complexity within transtibial amputee ankle motion. *Chaos* 24 (1): 013140.

Yentes, J. M., N. Hunt, K. K. Schmid, J. P. Kaipust, D. McGrath, and N. Stergiou. (Feb, 2013). The appropriate use of approximate entropy and sample entropy with short data sets. *Annals of Biomedical Engineering* 41 (2): 349–365.

Yu, D., M. Small, R. G. Harrison, and C. Diks. (2000). Efficient implementation of the Gaussian kernel algorithm in estimating invariants and noise level from noisy time series data. *Physical Review E, Statistical Physics, Plasmas, Fluids, and Related Interdisciplinary Topics* 61 (4 Pt A): 3750–3756.

Zhang, J., X. Luo, T. Nakamura, J. Sun, and M. Small. (2007). Detecting temporal and spatial correlations in pseudoperiodic time series. *Physical Review E, Statistical, Nonlinear, and Soft Matter Physics* 75 (1 Pt 2): 016218.

Zhao, Y., J. Sun, and M. Small. (2008). Evidence consistent with deterministic chaos in human cardiac data: Surrogate and nonlinear dynamical modeling. *International Journal of Bifurcation and Chaos* 18 (1): 141.

6 Entropy

Jennifer M. Yentes

CONTENTS

What is Entropy?... 174
Entropy Measures for Time Series Data 178
  Approximate Entropy.. 178
    Calculation of Approximate Entropy 179
    Parameter Selection.. 185
    Approximate Entropy Normalization... 186
    Uses of Approximate Entropy 187
  Sample Entropy 190
    Calculation of Sample Entropy 191
    Parameter Selection.. 195
    Uses of Sample Entropy 196
    Comparison to Approximate Entropy... 197
  Multiscale Entropy 198
    Calculation of Multiscale Entropy 198
    Uses of Multiscale Entropy 204
  Symbolic Entropy...205
    Calculation of Symbolic Entropy 205
    Uses of Symbolic Entropy..208
  Other Entropy Measures 208
  Cross Entropy Algorithms...212
  Considerations for All Algorithms 212
Exercises 213
  Data Set 213
References..219
Reading List: Cardiology...229
Reading List: Respiration 238
Reading List: Endocrinology 239
Reading List: Psychology/Neuroscience 252
Reading List: Biomechanics/Gait/Posture 257
Reading List: Other Topics 259

For most of my life, one of the persons most baffled by my own work was myself.

Benoit Mandelbrot (1924–2010)

WHAT IS ENTROPY?

Before discussing the application of entropy concepts to biological time series, a historical perspective on entropy is presented to develop an understanding of what it is intended to measure. The concept of entropy was first developed in classical thermodynamics, where it grew out of the work by Carnot (1824) on steam engines, to develop an understanding of the limits of mechanical work that could be produced by such engines. The term "entropy" was introduced to the vocabulary of classical thermodynamics by Clausius (1867). In classical thermodynamics, entropy is a state function that quantifies the energy in a system that cannot be used to perform work. The study of statistical thermodynamics, first published by Boltzmann (1896), gave further insight into the concept of entropy, by using probability concepts to describe entropy on a molecular scale. Thermal energy is associated with the movement of atoms and molecules, which results in an increased variability in position and velocity of those atoms and molecules. Statistical thermodynamics views entropy as the amount of microscopic variability that a system has for a given macroscopically observable state and is based on the distribution of microscopic configurations that can give rise to the macroscopic state. Boltzmann quantified the concept of entropy as follows:

$$S = -k \sum_i p_i \log p_i \qquad (6.1)$$

where
   S is the entropy
   p_i is the probability of the system being in microscopic configuration i
   k is the Boltzmann constant, 1.38065×10^{-23} J K^{-1}

The Boltzmann entropy can be conceptualized as a measure of the randomness of the system, where "randomness" refers to a lack of correlation between the different configurations and does not imply a lack of determinism.

Entropy considerations are fundamental to our understanding of emergent properties in complex systems. The equations of classical mechanics, quantum mechanics, and relativity are time invariant, meaning that time could run forward or backward with no apparent consequences. For example, one could watch a video of a ball accelerating as it rolls down a hill, losing potential energy and gaining kinetic energy. If the video was played in reverse, the ball would have an initial high velocity and low potential energy, the ball would appear to slow down as it rolled up the hill, with the expected trade-off between kinetic and potential energy. Both the forward movie and the backward movie would make sense based on the laws of classical mechanics. However, processes that involve significant changes in entropy do not have this time-invariant quality. Mixing is an example of a process that increases the entropy of the system. Watch a video of milk mixing into a cup of coffee and then play the video in reverse. The reverse video does not make sense, because the milk would appear to separate out from the coffee. The second law of thermodynamics says that in an isolated system, the only allowable changes are ones that involve an increase in entropy. The separation of the milk back out of the coffee would involve a decrease in entropy and therefore would not make sense to someone watching the reversed video. Thus, it is entropy that determines the so-called "arrow of time" in physical systems (Kondepudi and Prigogine 1998).

The "arrow of time" is important in emergent behavior in complex systems, because self-organization occurs in one time direction and not in the reverse. For example, if one were to watch a time-lapsed video of the development of an infant as it grows and matures and then play the video in reverse, it would not make sense. Just as the milk-mixing video would not make sense in reverse. Of course, the infant is not an isolated system by any means, so one should not assume that the entropy of the infant increases. It is the entropy of the infant plus environment that must increase according to the second law of thermodynamics, so it is the increasing entropy of the infant plus environment that defines the arrow of time. While entropy is an interesting concept in emergent behavior of complex systems, specific predictions about entropy for complex, open systems are nontrivial. An open system, such as a biological organism, exchanges matter and energy with its environment, allowing for the possibility that entropy may decrease as self-organizing processes occur.

The concept of entropy has also been widely used in the field of information theory. *Entropy* is defined as the loss of information in a time series or signal. In other words, it is based on what you know about the current state of a time series or signal, how well can you predict the next state of the system? If a system has very low entropy, the next state of the system is very predictable. However, high entropy would indicate a higher level of uncertainty in what the next state will be. Determining the information content of a signal, and therefore how much it could be compressed, is important in communication technology. Shannon (1948a,b), working at Bell Laboratories, previously known as Bell Telephone Laboratories, Inc., applied the concept of entropy to information theory. The Shannon Entropy, H_S, is calculated as follows:

$$H_S = -\sum_i p_i \log p_i \qquad (6.2)$$

where p_i is the probability of the symbol i being present in the string. Note the similarity to Equation 6.1, but no Boltzmann constant is necessary to convert the units as in Equation 6.1. Instead the units are bits of information. Shannon entropy is a specific value of H_R, the more general Rényi entropy (Rényi 1961):

$$H_\alpha = \frac{1}{1-\alpha} \log \sum_i p_i^\alpha \qquad (6.3)$$

The Shannon entropy is the limit of the Rényi entropy as the general continuous parameter α approaches the value of 1. Other typically used α values are 0 and 2, where H_2 is the extension entropy, and H_0 is a count of the nonzero probabilities in the probability vector p (Zyczkowski, 2003).

The highest entropy values are for a uniform probability distribution. If all the states are visited with equal probability, then the entropy is high. However, if most of the time the system is in a few favored states, then the entropy is low. One can envision this on the atomic level, with entropy as a measure of the randomness in position and velocity of molecules being characterized. Alternatively, one can apply the concept to time series data, in order to investigate the randomness in the dynamics of whatever signal is being evaluated.

The use of the word "randomness" may be problematic for some readers because they may have been taught that something is either random or not, with no shades of gray allowed. Randomness implies a lack of predictability. Either one can or cannot predict an event, again with no shades of gray allowed. But let us examine this notion a bit more carefully. If randomness implies a lack of predictability, should the converse hold true, that is, does a lack of predictability imply randomness? An event can be predictable to a "smart" observer (e.g., one who understands the mechanism generating the result) and at the same time be unpredictable to a second "ignorant" observer. In this scenario, is the event random? Although people may not agree on this definition, the tendency is to say that if the event is predictable by anyone, then it is not random. An observer's ignorance does not make an event random, even though it may make it unpredictable by that particular observer. However, this leads to a bit of a dilemma in trying to figure out if a given event is predictable by anyone, or will ever be predictable by anyone. Philosophically, if one believes in a deterministic world, nothing is random, and in fact, it is difficult, if not impossible, to find an example of a natural process that is random (Stewart 2002). In many cases, modeling a process as random can be useful, but the fact that a random model is convenient is in no way a proof that the underlying process is actually random.

In examining a series of numbers, if one finds a repeating pattern such that one can correctly predict additional numbers in the series, then the series is not random. But not finding a pattern may mean that the observer was just not smart enough to figure out the pattern. Mathematically proving that a series of numbers is random is not thought to be possible (Chaitin 1975). This concept of random variable is useful as a model, but this theoretical ideal may not represent reality. There is no such thing as a time series that can be proven to be random. Thus, we should not get confused in interpretation of the results of any measure of entropy. Entropy of a time series is a measure of how difficult it is to compress the time series by finding repeating patterns in it, and we will use the word "randomness" to denote that the particular algorithm we are using is not finding many repeated patterns in the data. Finding a high entropy value for a time series should not be interpreted as a lack of determinism in the physical process that was measured to generate the time series. Entropy can be interpreted in various ways depending on the context in which it is used. For the purposes of discussion on biological time series, entropy provides us with the probability that similar patterns of behavior will not be followed by additional similar patterns. Therefore, it provides us with a measure of unpredictability or irregularity of the time series.

Furthermore, one should not confuse entropy with complexity, either. This will be discussed at length later in the chapter but should be noted here as well. Very periodic states (e.g., easily predicted) and highly random states (e.g., difficult to predict) are both very low in complexity (Costa et al. 2002; Stergiou et al. 2006). The majority of entropy algorithms provide insight into the predictability on only one time scale. A proper investigation into the complexity of a time series includes analysis over multiple time scales.

In summary, patterns in data may be predictable or not based on the observer's knowledge of the system dynamics, but regardless of how well the system can be predicted, it is possible to examine the structure of the data for patterns. Figure 6.1 demonstrates the concept of randomness versus highly ordered structure visually. Figure 6.1a has spots that do not have a discernable pattern, and they have been generated randomly. Figure 6.1b shows some order to the spots, but unless you happen to be familiar with the Henon map and know the starting points exactly, you couldn't predict where additional spots will be located. Figure 6.1c shows spots in a highly ordered pattern, a pattern that could easily be continued because it is so predictable.

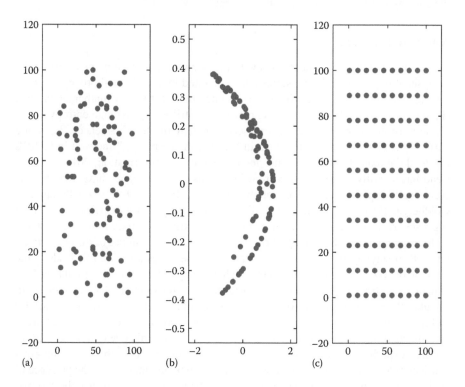

FIGURE 6.1 Visual representation of system organization: (a) dots spaced randomly (high entropy), (b) dots loosely ordered (medium entropy), and (c) dots rigidly ordered (low entropy).

ENTROPY MEASURES FOR TIME SERIES DATA

There are a number of different algorithms that have been used to estimate entropy of a time series. Historically, the most popular was approximate entropy, so it will be discussed in some detail. In addition to being popular, other techniques such as sample entropy and multiscale entropy are built upon the approximate entropy algorithm, so understanding approximate entropy in some detail is worthwhile. This does not mean that approximate entropy is the "best" entropy measure to be applied to all data. There are several items that must be carefully considered before choosing the correct entropy measure to answer a research question.

Symbolic entropy is the basis for another class of techniques that involve coding the time series data as symbols, and then performing analysis on those symbols. Thus, it can be tailored to many different data types by altering the process used to generate the symbols, so it is also worth understanding in some detail. Other entropy measures will be highlighted as well. One measure that will not be included is the entropy measure from recurrence quantification analysis. This measure is the Shannon entropy of the segment line lengths in a recurrence plot (Riley et al. 1999) and is only applicable to a recurrence plot. In this case, entropy measures the probability that a line length on a recurrence plot will occur again on the same recurrence plot. It is based upon the distribution of line lengths within the recurrence plot, not the entropy of the time series as we have previously described.

APPROXIMATE ENTROPY

Approximate entropy was developed with the intention that it might be useful in the analysis of experimental time series data generated by a biological process, in contrast to some other measures that were designed more for purely mathematical data (Pincus et al. 1991). Because of its experimental utility, approximate entropy is one of the most popular measures of time series entropy in the life sciences. There are currently over 890 papers, that contain "approximate entropy," indexed in NCBI's PubMed database (National Center for Biotechnology Information, 2015), and the trend has steadily increased (Figure 6.2). Pincus and colleagues have written several excellent papers on the use of this measure (Pincus 1991, 1998; Pincus and Goldberger 1994), and the following discussion is based on these articles, which are suggested reading for anyone wishing to use approximate entropy in their own work.

Entropy quantifies the tendency of the system to visit a number of different states, rather than staying in a few preferred states. In time series analysis, this leads to the question of how long you have to wait to see how many states it will occupy, that is, how long does the time series need to be to determine the distribution of states visited? To calculate the true entropy of a system exactly, one would need an infinite time series. By calling this measure "approximate" entropy, Pincus is emphasizing that the measure is an estimate of the actual entropy based on a time series of limited length (Pincus 1991). Because experimental time series are necessarily of finite length, this is an important consideration. Another important consideration in experimental data is the presence of "noise," contamination of the signal of interest with measurement error, and the approximate entropy algorithm can deal with this explicitly, as described in detail later (i.e., lag).

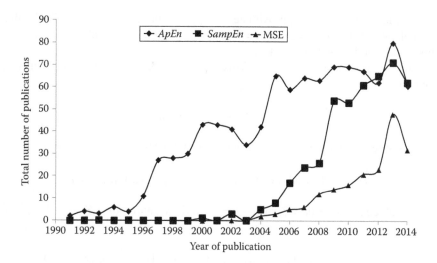

FIGURE 6.2 Number of publications indexed in PubMed that contain "approximate entropy" (*ApEn*), "sample entropy" (*SampEn*), or "multiscale entropy" (MSE) for each year since 1991, the year approximate entropy was introduced (Pincus et al. 1991).

Calculation of Approximate Entropy

The approximate entropy algorithm takes as input the time series data of length N, a tolerance radius r, a vector length m (sometimes called pattern length, segment length, or pattern window), and, if needed, a lag. The time series of length N is divided into short vectors of length m. Then, for each of these vectors, one counts how many of the other vectors are similar to each other. To determine whether two vectors are similar, one compares each element in the vector with the corresponding element in the second vector. The two are considered to be similar if the differences are below the radius r of the entire time series. The process is repeated, but now the vectors are one longer, that is, length of $m + 1$. The similar vectors of length m are counted and the log average found, and then similar vectors of length $m + 1$ are counted and log average found. If the time series jumps around randomly, then there will be a lot fewer similar vectors of length $m + 1$ than there are of length m. If the time series has a repeating pattern to it, then there will be just as many similar vectors of length $m + 1$ as there are of length m, that is, the length of the vector is not so important if the time series repeats exactly. For the analysis of a time series with unknown structure, the idea is to compare the number of similar vectors of length m with the number of similar vectors of length $m + 1$ and use the result as a measure of the randomness of the time series.

Let us start with a time series of length N, $\{x_1, x_2, x_3, \ldots, x_N\}$ and an m of 2. The lag parameter is the distance skipped when creating the vectors. For example, a lag of 1 would result in $\{x_1, x_2\}$, $\{x_2, x_3\}$, etc., whereas a lag of 2 would result in $\{x_1, x_3\}$, $\{x_2, x_4\}$, etc. A lag of 1 is most often used, but there are instances where different lag values can be useful. For example, a data set acquired at 240 Hz was contaminated with 60 Hz noise. By using a lag of 4, each vector created had data points taken at the same point in the 60 Hz noise cycle.

Now, let us look at the approximate entropy calculation in more detail. For this example, we will choose lag = 1, $N = 8$ and $m = 2$. For a numerical example of how this works, see Example Box 6.1.

Time series of length N ($N = 8$). This is a time-ordered list of numbers; that is, your data:

$$\{x_1, x_2, x_3, x_4, x_5, x_6, x_7, x_8\}$$

Vectors of length m ($m = 2$). Note we get $N - m + 1 = 8 - 2 + 1 = 7$ vectors:

$$\{x_1, x_2\}, \{x_2, x_3\}, \{x_3, x_4\}, \{x_4, x_5\}, \{x_5, x_6\}, \{x_6, x_7\}, \{x_7, x_8\}$$

Vectors of length $m + 1$ ($m = 2$, so $m + 1 = 3$). Note we get $N - (m + 1) + 1 = N - m = 6$ vectors:

$$\{x_1, x_2, x_3\}, \{x_2, x_3, x_4\}, \{x_3, x_4, x_5\}, \{x_4, x_5, x_6\}, \{x_5, x_6, x_7\}, \{x_6, x_7, x_8\}$$

Therefore, now that we have our vectors, we are ready to count how many are similar. For the vectors of length 2, we look at the vector #1, $\{x_1, x_2\}$, and see how many of the length 2 vectors, $\{x_a, x_b\}$, are similar. We judge similarity by seeing if x_a is within distance r of x_1, and if x_b is within distance r of x_2. If both values are similar (within radius r), then we add one to our count and make the next comparison. The count of similar vectors is divided by the number of vectors with which the comparisons were made to get the conditional probabilities denoted C_i^m. For example, C_i^2 denotes the probability of finding vectors similar to the first vector ($i = 1$) among the vectors of length m, that is, number of vectors similar to the first one divided by the total number of vectors compared. Note the m value is not an exponential power to which C is to be raised, that is, C_i^2 is not squared, the 2 just means $m = 2$.

We continue counting for all combinations of vectors of length m. Then, we repeat the entire process for our vectors of length $m + 1$. For the case of the $m + 1$ vectors, we have one less vector with which to compare, but we now have three numbers to compare for each vector, and all three need to be within radius r to be counted as being similar. The vector being used as the comparison vector, corresponding to the index i, is always found as being similar to itself in the counting process, so the lowest values for any of the counts will be 1, not 0. This may seem a bit odd at first—why bother counting that a vector is the same as itself? This is done because later in the calculation we will be taking the logarithm, and this self-counting means we never have to be concerned with taking the logarithm of zero, which is not defined.

One thing to consider in making the comparison of C_i^m and C_i^{m+1} is that one can make more of the shorter vectors than of the longer $m + 1$ vectors. In our example, there were 7 of the vectors of length 2, but only 6 of the vectors of length 3. In a random time series, just because there are more shorter ones with which to compare, by chance there will likely be more similar short ones, that is, if you have 6 other vectors with which to compare, you have a better chance of finding a match than if there are only five other vectors with which to compare. But since you know how many vectors you have for each length ($N - m + 1$ for length m vectors, and $N - m$

EXAMPLE BOX 6.1   APPROXIMATE ENTROPY

Using the RANDBETWEEN function in Excel, the following time series was generated for data points between 0 and 10. Twenty-six data points were generated.

Time series: {9 4 8 1 2 4 5 8 7 7 0 2 1 5 9 8 8 0 1 0 4 2 10 0 0 1}

1. *Plot the data*: This is a critical, yet frequently overlooked, step to all time series analysis. Plotting the data will allow you to visualize how periodic or random the data look. Typically, we cannot tell what entropy value it will have, but it will give us an indication of repeating patterns, outliers, and/or other data treatment issues.

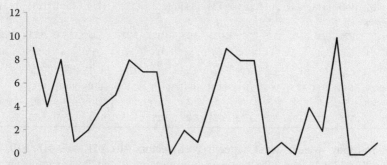

2. *Choose your parameters*: In our case, $N = 26$. However, if you have many different trials and each one is of different length, you must cut them all to be the same length. Approximate entropy is very sensitive to data length so having different length time series will affect the results. Based on typically chosen values, we will set the parameters to be $m = 2$. Choosing r can be difficult in this case; because the example is all integer numbers, we will arbitrarily set $r = 1$. This will make the math in the example easier and should not be a reason for a parameter choice when analyzing biological data. (*Note*: this is not 1*the standard deviation, just the number 1.)

3. *Divide our time series into "vector lengths" of 2 points ($m = 2$)*: We get 25 vectors of length 2:

   {9 4} {4 8} {8 1} {1 2} {2 4} {4 5} {5 8} {8 7} {7 7} {7 0} {0 2} {2 1} {1 5}
   {5 9} {9 8} {8 8} {8 0} {0 1} {1 0} {0 4} {4 2} {2 10} {10 0} {0 0} {0 1}

4. *Count the number of similar vector lengths ($m = 2$) that fall within a tolerance of ± 1 (r) and the conditional probability (C_i^m)*: Taking the very first vector, {9 4}, we will look for any other vectors that fall within {9 ± 1, 4 ± 1}, or simply, that the first number has to be between 8–10 and second number is between 3–5. There are no such matches, but we still count a self-match. So for the first vector, we count one match. To calculate its conditional probability, we place the number of matches over the number of total comparisons made, or 1/25.

Let us look at the second vector, {4 8}. We need to look for vectors that have a first number between 3–5 and second number between 7–9. We find vector #7, {5 8}, and #14, {5 9}. This means that for the second vector, we have three matches (self-match plus two). To calculate the conditional probability, we place the number of matches, 3, over the total number of comparisons, 25. If you continue comparing all of the vectors, you get the following number of matches:

#	1	2	3	4	5	6	7	8	9	10	11	12	13
C_i^m #	C_1^2	C_2^2	C_3^2	C_4^2	C_5^2	C_6^2	C_7^2	C_8^2	C_9^2	C_{10}^2	C_{11}^2	C_{12}^2	C_{13}^2
Vector	{9 4}	{4 8}	{8 1}	{1 2}	{2 4}	{4 5}	{5 8}	{8 7}	{7 7}	{7 0}	{0 2}	{2 1}	{1 5}
Matches	1	3	3	5	2	1	3	4	3	3	4	3	3
C_i^m	1/25	3/25	3/25	5/25	2/25	1/25	3/25	4/25	3/25	3/25	4/25	3/25	3/25

#	14	15	16	17	18	19	20	21	22	23	24	25
C_i^m #	C_{14}^2	C_{15}^2	C_{16}^2	C_{17}^2	C_{18}^2	C_{19}^2	C_{20}^2	C_{21}^2	C_{22}^2	C_{23}^2	C_{24}^2	C_{25}^2
Vector	{5 9}	{9 8}	{8 8}	{8 0}	{0 1}	{1 0}	{0 4}	{4 2}	{2 10}	{10 0}	{0 0}	{0 1}
Matches	3	3	4	3	6	5	2	1	1	1	4	6
C_i^m	3/25	3/25	4/25	3/25	6/25	5/25	2/25	1/25	1/25	1/25	4/25	6/25

You may wonder, what happens with vectors #10, #11, #17, #18, #19, #20, #23, #24, and #25? These vectors contain a 0, and if we examine an r of 1 that would give us a range of −1 to 1. However, since our example does not contain negative numbers, we will consider something to be a like vector if it has a range from 0 to 1.

Note: Remember that when you are applying this algorithm to your data, r is usually 0.10–0.25* the standard deviation of the entire data set. The number of significant digits, or precision of your data, may also have an effect on your results.

5. *Count the number of similar vector lengths (m + 1 = 3) that fall within a tolerance of ± 1 (r) and the conditional probability (C_i^{m+1})*: Taking the very first vector, {9 4 8}, we will look for any vectors that fall within {9 ± 1, 4 ± 1, 8 ± 1}, or simply, that the first number has to be between 8–10 and second number is between 3–5 and the third number between 7–9. There are no such matches, but we still count a self-match. So for the first vector, we count one match. Thus, the conditional probability is 1/24. Only one match was found for 24 comparisons.

Look at a vector that does have more than its own self-match, #3, {8 1 2}. You will find that vector #10 and vector #17 are matches. The first number falls between 7–9, second number between 0–2 and the third between 1–3. This means that for the third vector, we have three matches (self-match plus two). This makes the conditional probability 3/24 (3 matches over 24 comparisons). If you continue comparing all of the vectors, you get the following number of matches:

#	1	2	3	4	5	6	7	8	9	10	11	12	13
C_i^{m+1} #	C_1^3	C_2^3	C_3^3	C_4^3	C_5^3	C_6^3	C_7^3	C_8^3	C_9^3	C_{10}^3	C_{11}^3	C_{12}^3	C_{13}^3
Vector	{9 4 8}	{4 8 1}	{8 1 2}	{1 2 4}	{2 4 5}	{4 5 8}	{5 8 7}	{8 7 7}	{7 7 0}	{7 0 2}	{0 2 1}	{2 1 5}	{1 5 9}
Matches	1	1	3	2	1	1	2	2	2	3	2	3	1
C_i^{m+1}	1/24	1/24	3/24	2/24	1/24	1/24	2/24	2/24	2/24	3/24	2/24	3/24	1/24

#	14	15	16	17	18	19	20	21	22	23	24
C_i^{m+1} #	C_{14}^3	C_{15}^3	C_{16}^3	C_{17}^3	C_{18}^3	C_{19}^3	C_{20}^3	C_{21}^3	C_{22}^3	C_{23}^3	C_{24}^3
Vector	{5 9 8}	{9 8 8}	{8 8 0}	{8 0 1}	{0 1 0}	{1 0 4}	{0 4 2}	{4 2 10}	{2 10 0}	{10 0 0}	{0 0 1}
Matches	2	2	2	3	3	2	1	1	1	1	2
C_i^{m+1}	2/24	2/24	2/24	3/24	3/24	2/24	1/24	1/24	1/24	1/24	2/24

6. *Calculate the natural log for each conditional probability for both*
   m and m + 1
   $$m = 2$$

C_i^2 #	C_1^2	C_2^2	C_3^2	C_4^2	C_5^2	C_6^2	C_7^2	C_8^2	C_9^2	C_{10}^2	C_{11}^2	C_{12}^2	C_{13}^2
C_i^m	1/25	3/25	3/25	5/25	2/25	1/25	3/25	4/25	3/25	3/25	4/25	3/25	3/25
$\ln C_i^m$	−3.219	−2.120	−2.120	−1.609	−2.526	−3.219	−2.120	−1.833	−2.120	−2.120	−1.833	−2.120	−2.120
C_i^2 #	C_{14}^2	C_{15}^2	C_{16}^2	C_{17}^2	C_{18}^2	C_{19}^2	C_{20}^2	C_{21}^2	C_{22}^2	C_{23}^2	C_{24}^2	C_{25}^2	
C_i^m	3/25	3/25	4/25	3/25	6/25	5/25	2/25	1/25	1/25	1/25	4/25	6/25	
$\ln C_i^m$	−2.120	−2.120	−1.833	−2.120	−1.427	−1.609	−2.526	−3.219	−3.219	−3.219	−1.833	−1.427	

   $$m + 1 = 3$$

C_i^{m+1} #	C_1^3	C_2^3	C_3^3	C_4^3	C_5^3	C_6^3	C_7^3	C_8^3	C_9^3	C_{10}^3	C_{11}^3	C_{12}^3	C_{13}^3
C_i^{m+1}	1/24	1/24	3/24	2/24	1/24	1/24	2/24	2/24	2/24	3/24	2/24	3/24	1/24
$\ln C_i^{m+1}$	−3.178	−3.178	−2.079	−2.485	−3.178	−3.178	−2.485	−2.485	−2.485	−2.079	−2.485	−2.079	−3.178
C_i^{m+1} #	C_{14}^3	C_{15}^3	C_{16}^3	C_{17}^3	C_{18}^3	C_{19}^3	C_{20}^3	C_{21}^3	C_{22}^3	C_{23}^3	C_{24}^3		
C_i^{m+1}	2/24	2/24	2/24	3/24	3/24	2/24	1/24	1/24	1/24	1/24	2/24		
$\ln C_i^{m+1}$	−2.485	−2.485	−2.485	−2.079	−2.079	−2.485	−3.178	−3.178	−3.178	−3.178	−2.485		

7. *Sum up all the natural logs of conditional probabilities for m and*
   m + 1: For *m*, the sum is −55.751 and for *m* + 1, −63.847.

8. *Calculate* Φ^m *and* Φ^{m+1}: To calculate Φ^m, divide the sum found in
   Step 7 by $N - m + 1$. If you recall, in this example, N is 26 and m is 2.
   So we would divide as follows:

$$\frac{-55.751}{(26-2+1)} \rightarrow \frac{-55.751}{25} \rightarrow -2.23004$$

To calculate Φ^{m+1}, divide the sum found in Step 7 by $N - m$.

$$\frac{-63.847}{(26-2)} \rightarrow \frac{-63.847}{24} \rightarrow -2.66029$$

9. *Calculate approximate entropy*: To calculate approximate entropy, subtract Φ^m and Φ^{m+1}.

$$-2.23004 - (-2.66029) = 0.43025$$

You may ask, why the algorithm returned a value close to zero when we know that the numbers were randomly generated?
Should not this value be closer to 2? Technically, yes. However, there are several limitations to approximate entropy that are discussed in the chapter. One is time series length. We know that the 26 data points are not nearly enough to give a clear picture of the dynamics of the system. In addition, we do not know if the choice of a different m, r, or lag would have given us a different value. As an additional exercise, you should take the time to recalculate the approximate entropy of this example using a (1) m of 3, (2) r of 2 or (3) lag of 2. You will find that the resulting value differs depending on your choice of parameters. Extreme caution must be used if employing approximate entropy with biological data. Care must be given to correctly choose your parameters. Relative consistency, as discussed in the chapter, is of utmost importance. This will provide the evidence that your findings are true and not an artifact of parameter choice.

for length $m + 1$ vectors), one can correct for this statistically in the approximate entropy calculation.

Now, we are ready to calculate the approximate entropy. The method used by Pincus in the approximate entropy calculation to compare the counts for the different vector lengths is to calculate the function Φ, one for vectors of length m (Φ^m) (Equation 6.4) and the other for vectors of length $m + 1$ (Φ^{m+1}) (Equation 6.5), then subtract them to find the approximate entropy. Again, the m or $m + 1$ just denotes the vector length used in calculating the Φ, and is not to be taken as indicating an exponent. Note that just as the C's depend on the filtering radius r that was used, the Φ's will also depend on the r value used (see the section "Parameter Selection").

Calculation of the Φ values involves logarithm summation of all the C's for that particular vector length and then division by the number of vectors that can be formed from that vector length. This is expressed mathematically as follows:

$$\Phi^m = \frac{1}{N-m+1} \sum_{i=1}^{N-m+1} \ln C_i^m \tag{6.4}$$

$$\Phi^{m+1} = \frac{1}{N-m} \sum_{i=1}^{N-m} \ln C_i^{m+1} \tag{6.5}$$

The calculation of the approximate entropy is then given by the difference:

$$ApEn = \Phi^m - \Phi^{m+1} \tag{6.6}$$

As discussed earlier, if the count of similar vectors is the same for both m length vectors and for $m + 1$ length vectors, as might happen in the time series formed by perfectly repeated patterns, then Φ^m and Φ^{m+1} will be very similar, and the entropy value will be very close to zero. If, however, the time series is quite random, then while some of the shorter vectors will be similar just by chance, by comparison considerably fewer of the longer vectors will be similar by chance, resulting in a positive value for $\Phi^m - \Phi^{m+1}$. Thus, approximate entropy cannot be negative—this would mean that there are more similar vectors of the longer length than there are similar vectors of the shorter length, which is not possible.

Values of approximate entropy will range from 0 to 2. Zero represents no entropy or a perfectly repeatable time series, that is, sine wave. Two represents a perfectly random time series, that is, white noise. After calculating the approximate entropy, one must interpret the results. Typically, the measure is applied to data sets from two or more conditions, or populations, or some other type of comparison is being made. One can say that the condition or population with the lower approximate entropy has more regularity in its dynamics. Some authors have attempted to interpret the results as indicating deterministic chaos, and Pincus and Goldberger (1994) explicitly warn against this interpretation because different stochastic mathematical models can be seen to differ in approximate entropy values just as deterministic ones do.

Parameter Selection

A key consideration in the application of the approximate entropy algorithm to experimental time series data is the selection of appropriate parameters for your data set. These include the r and m values and, determining how long the time series needs to be, what N value is needed. Many papers have been written on this topic and a full consideration of parameter choice should be made before applying this tool to data. Typically, m is set to a value of 2 or 3. Consideration should be given to what exactly the parameter m represents when choosing the correct value for the research question being asked. For instance, if the data set was a series of spatial gait variables, such as step length, then an m of 2 would represent two consecutive step lengths. Therefore, thoughtful consideration is required when choosing the m parameter value, bearing in mind what the choice of m represents in biological terms with respect to individual data sets (Yentes et al. 2013).

Recall that r is the allowable difference when determining similarity between elements in the vectors. If the r value is too small, then the counts are thrown off because similar data points are not seen as similar. If r is too large, then details of the system dynamics are lost. If one knows the experimental error, it might be appropriate to set the r value at three times larger than the noise amplitude (Pincus and Goldberger 1994). That way, two measured values of x_i will be certain to be counted as similar if they are within the experimental error in the measurement. However, often the noise component of the measurement is not well characterized. Thus, a more common method for selecting the r value is to base it on the standard deviation of the time series data, and Pincus and Goldberger have suggested that a value of about 0.10–0.25 times the standard deviation in the data. Finally, there are some situations where one is using the

approximate entropy as descriptive statistic to separate two (or more) populations, for example, a pathologic population from a healthy population, or performance of devices near failure from unused devices. One might have some
training data and that training data are to be used to develop a statistic that can
be applied for classification of individuals into one or the other of the two groups.
In this case, one might simply choose to maximize the difference in the results
from the two populations by adjusting the values of r. Other suggestions for the
selection of r include a value that either minimizes or maximizes the entropy
error and conditional probability (Lake et al. 2002) to provide a maximum value
of entropy (Lu et al. 2008; Chon et al. 2009) or using a fixed tolerance value that
does not depend on the standard deviation of each vector during comparison
(Sarlabous et al. 2010). Choosing the value of r is quite debatable, and thought
and consideration should be given before choosing a value.

The value selected for m depends on the length of the data series (N), where
the N needs to be "at least 10^m, and ideally 30^m" (Pincus and Goldberger 1994,
p. H1647). For example, for $m = 2$, 30^2 implies 900 or more data points are ideal.
Early suggestions were that N should be set at 1000 (Pincus and Huang 1992)
and could be as short as 75 data points (Pincus and Huang 1992; Pincus 1995).
Yet, this has been found to be too short for the use of approximate entropy (Chen
et al. 2005; Yentes et al. 2013). It is essential that the reader understands that the
length of the time series has an enormous effect on the calculation of approximate entropy. Further, nonstationarity or drift in the data is typically present and
drift will increase as N is increased, thus affecting approximate entropy calculations (Costa et al. 2005). The reader may want to review Chapter 2 for a discussion on sampling rate and time series length, before deciding on an experimental
protocol to acquire the time series data for approximate entropy calculations, if
sampling rate is an adjustable parameter in the protocol. For example, sampling
at 10,000 Hz for a fraction of a second when the system dynamics has time
constants on the order of seconds is not going to provide sufficient information
for the dynamics to be well characterized by approximate entropy, or any other
method.

Approximate Entropy Normalization
There have been varying methods proposed to normalize approximate entropy
to allow for comparison across different time series lengths or across studies.
Approximate entropy could be normalized to different time lengths by the following
method:

$$\frac{(\Phi^m - \Phi^{m+1})}{N} \tag{6.7}$$

where N is the data length for that particular time series. This will allow one to make
comparisons of different entropy values for different length data sets; however, this
has not been formally tested. Further, doing normalization like this should be done
with extreme caution. As stated earlier, approximate entropy is very sensitive to data

length and normalization such as this may not be correct for the inherent issues of having varying data lengths.

Another form of normalization that has been suggested is that of "ratio" approximate entropy (Fonseca et al. 2012). Essentially, this is the ratio of the approximate entropy from the original data divided by the approximate entropy of a random (or shuffled) data set of the same N as the original data set. This is done by generating a random data set that is the same length as the experimental (original) data set. Then, the approximate entropy of the random data set is calculated:

$$\frac{ApEn_{original}}{ApEn_{random}} \tag{6.8}$$

Again, this normalization method has not been fully tested, therefore caution should be used when applying this type of normalization to biological data. Further, one must consider why they would need to complete normalization. For instance, is normalization needed for the research question you are asking?

Uses of Approximate Entropy

Now, we have developed an understanding of approximate entropy, and let us examine some examples from the literature. Likely, there are other papers with approximate entropy from nonmedical/biological disciplines that are not included in this discussion. One of the first papers (Pincus 1991) published on approximate entropy was titled "Approximate entropy as a measure of system complexity." However, the use of the word "complexity" in the literature needs to be addressed. A completely rigid structure in a system would result in low entropy, whereas randomness or a complete lack of control would result in high entropy. Often in physical systems, and especially in physiological systems, the desired level of structure is somewhere in between these extremes. A physiological control system needs a certain level of structure in order to pursue a desired goal state, but a too rigid structure can be costly to maintain and may reduce adaptability to unexpected events in the environment. In cases where the control structure has become nonoptimal, such as in pathology or aging, the change in entropy measures may be an increase if the system control has become more random than optimal, or it may be a decrease if the system control has become too rigid. Historically, examples of pathology associated with decreases in entropy were found first, resulting in what was called a "loss of complexity" description of pathology, where "complexity" was used synonymously with approximate entropy (Goldberger et al. 2002). It is now recognized that pathology can exist at both the ends of the control spectrum, with pathologic control being either too structured or not structured enough (Stergiou et al. 2006; Stergiou and Decker 2011). Some authors have now adopted a second meaning for the word "complexity" to mean the optimal level of entropy for a given system. With this new definition, entropy is no longer a measure of complexity for these authors because maximal complexity occurs at intermediate values of entropy. However, there is no *a priori* reason to believe that the optimal amount of entropy for heart rate is same as the optimal amount of entropy for postural control or that either of these is the optimal amount of entropy for growth hormone secretion. Thus, finding a general measure for this second type of complexity, optimal entropy, is difficult. Even further, some authors now define complexity as richness in data across multiple time scales. Using this definition, most entropy algorithms would not be applicable but rather fractal type algorithms would provide quantification of complexity. We have avoided using the word "complexity" because of these conflicting definitions (Goldberger et al. 2002; Vaillancourt and Newell 2002a,b). In reading the literature, the reader should be very careful to check what a given author means by the word "complexity" especially if it is used in the context of a discussion of entropy.

Here, six categories will be discussed: (1) cardiology, (2) respiration, (3) endocrinology, (4) psychology/neuroscience, (5) biomechanics/gait/posture, and (6) other topics. A few papers from each are discussed in the text to give the reader a sample of the work in that category, and then, in order to demonstrate the wide variety of different uses for approximate entropy in each category, the reader is referred to the six reading lists at the end of the chapter.

Cardiology

The use of nonlinear analysis, and approximate entropy in particular, is common in the analysis of heart rate variability. Control of heart rate is a complex interaction of several control mechanisms, including both sympathetic and parasympathetic neural control, as well as cardiac rhythm generated within the heart itself. The variability in inter-heartbeat interval, or time between heartbeats, has been shown to give clues to the health of the heart as the interplay between these various autonomic control mechanisms changes with pathology. Many authors have found that an increase in the regularity of heart rate, as indicated by a decrease in the approximate entropy, is associated with poor health over a wide age range of different pathologies. Decrease in approximate entropy is an indicator of atrial fibrillation (Shin et al. 2006). Patients in a persistent vegetative state were found to have lower approximate entropy of heart rate than controls (Sara et al. 2008). Approximate entropy is lower in fetuses that are small for their age as compared to typical (Hoh et al. 2007).

Respiration

Like heart rate variability, respiration is another pseudoperiodic activity with interesting variability patterns, and regularity has been characterized using approximate entropy. Approximate entropy of respiration interval has been shown to be changed during sleep and depends on the stage of sleep (Burioka et al. 2002, 2003; Dragomir et al. 2008). Approximate entropy of breath times may be a useful predictor of breathing difficulties after surgery, with lower values of approximate entropy associated with higher incidence of respiratory apnea (Sleigh 1999). Patients with asthma also show lower approximate entropy in airflow patterns as compared to healthy controls demonstrating a reduction in the adaptability of the respiratory system (Veiga et al. 2011).

Endocrinology

Approximate entropy in endocrinology is widely used as it is in cardiology. The regularity of hormone secretion can be altered in pathological conditions, and the regularity of secretion of a number of different hormones has been characterized by approximate entropy, and growth hormone has been particularly well studied. Women are found to have a much more irregular secretion of growth hormone than do men, and tumors of hormone-producing tissue are often associated with decreased regularity of secretion (Veldhuis and Pincus 1998). Those with growth hormone deficiency and treated with growth hormone as adolescents were also found to have decreased regularity of blood levels of growth hormone as adults, as compared to controls (Svensson et al. 2006). A decrease in the regularity of growth hormone secretion (Misra et al. 2003), but not cortisol secretion (Misra et al. 2004) was found in adolescent girls with anorexia nervosa, as compared to controls. The secretion of growth hormone and prolactin is found to be more irregular in patients with Cushing's disease (Veldman et al. 2000). The entropy of growth hormone, cortisol, and leptin secretion also demonstrates different profiles in elderly patients with different body composition phenotypes (Waters et al. 2008).

Psychology/Neuroscience

Approximate entropy has been applied to electroencephalograph (EEG) data, and may be useful in predicting epileptic seizures (Abasolo et al. 2007), and has been shown to drop during a seizure (Bhattacharya 2000; Burioka et al. 2005). Approximate entropy of EEG data may be useful in characterizing states of consciousness, such as sleep or awake (Acharya et al. 2005), or response to anesthesia (Schneider et al. 2005; Esmaeili et al. 2007). Approximate entropy also decreases during memory retrieval (Talebi et al. 2012). Approximate entropy can also be applied to more traditional psychological research by using subject response time series, such as mood in bipolar disorder, where regularity of mood decreases prior to onset of a manic or depressive episode, especially for a manic episode (Glenn et al. 2006), and regularity of mood ratings were significantly higher for pemoline treatment as compared to both fluoxetine and placebo (Yeragani et al. 2003). Recently, approximate entropy has been used to differentiate between normal and alcoholic EEG signals (Acharya et al. 2012).

Biomechanics of Gait and Posture

Approximate entropy has been used to study variability in gait parameters during walking. For example, approximate entropy of minimum foot clearance in treadmill walking in elderly may be useful in predicting potential for falling, which is important because falling is a major cause of injury in the elderly (Karmakar et al. 2007; Khandoker et al. 2008). Subjects who have had injury to their anterior cruciate ligament have been shown to have lower approximate entropy than controls (Georgoulis et al. 2006). The same approximate entropy profile has been observed in patients with multiple sclerosis as compared to healthy controls (Kaipust et al. 2012). High-heeled walking leads to a greater approximate entropy, or a less predictable pattern, in the ankle joint as compared to barefoot walking (Alkjær et al. 2012). Further, approximate entropy has been applied to virtual reality, Parkinson's disease, and vascular occlusion (Katsavelis et al. 2010; Kurz and Hou 2010; Myers et al. 2010).

Approximate entropy has also been used in studying postural control. Postural sway, the subtle movements that the body makes in maintaining upright posture, can give insight into the functioning of the neuromuscular system. Several authors have used approximate entropy from postural sway measurements to characterize the randomness in postural control. Approximate entropy has been shown to decrease in postural sway of athletes after mild traumatic brain injury (Cavanaugh et al. 2005; Sosnoff et al. 2011). The measure is so sensitive that posture can be seen to be more random depending on whether the subject is preoccupied with a cognitive task or not (Cavanaugh et al. 2007). Approximate entropy has been found to either increase or decrease when subjects have eyes closed, depending on whether they are standing with one foot in front of the other (approximate entropy increased with eyes closed) or standing normally with feet side-by-side (approximate entropy decreased) (Hong et al. 2007). The measure has also been applied to infant sitting posture to find changes in postural control with development in infants born premature and in children with developmental delays (Harbourne and Stergiou 2003; Deffeyes et al. 2009; Dusing et al. 2009). It has been applied to postural control in pathology such as multiple sclerosis (Huisinga et al. 2012).

Other Topics

There are a number of other interesting uses of approximate entropy. For example, body temperature is often used to say whether a patient has a fever or not, but a time series of body temperature can give insight into the health of the control system. Nonsurviving patients with multiple organ failure have lower approximate entropy of body temperature than do survivors (Varela et al. 2005, 2006; Cuesta et al. 2007). Approximate entropy of body temperature time series decreases with age (Varela et al. 2003). A decrease in approximate entropy of menstrual cycles is an indicator of approaching menopause (Weinstein et al. 2003).

In nonphysiological time series analysis, approximate entropy has been used to investigate whether the digits of square root of three are less random than the digits of pi (Pincus and Kalman 1997; Rukhin 2000). It has also been applied to seismic data with the hopes of better earthquake prediction (Karamanos et al. 2006).

SAMPLE ENTROPY

Sample entropy is very similar to approximate entropy and attempts to rectify some of the shortcomings of the approximate entropy algorithm. As discussed earlier, in calculating approximate entropy, each vector m is counted as being similar to itself in order to avoid the issue of having to take the log of 0, which is undefined. However, as discussed by Richman and Moorman (2000), this leads to entropy values that are biased toward regularity. This is especially an issue in short data sets. To look at an extreme example, if we have a short time series with five vectors of length m, then 1/5 will be counted as similar, that is, 20%, due to counting of the vector as similar to itself, even if there is no repetition of any pattern at all. In a long time series with 1000 vectors, only 1/1000 are counted as similar, that is, 0.1%, even if there is no repetition of any pattern at all. Thus, the bias is more significant when the count of similar vectors is low, as would occur in time series with low similarity and/or shorter time series. While in many applications, this bias in the final numerical result for the approximate entropy is small and may lead to inconsistency in the results (Pincus 1995; Richman and Moorman 2000).

Further, approximate entropy lacks relative consistency or simply, the stability of the measure (Pincus 1995). This means that as the input parameters m, r, and N are changed, the results may "flip." An example that has been shown over and over is between white noise and a sine wave. It is known that the sine wave should have a lower approximate entropy value than white noise; however, if one of the input parameters is set at a small value, white noise has a smaller approximate entropy value than the sine wave. As the input parameters are altered, this will lead to a "flip" and the approximate entropy value in the white noise will become greater than the sine wave. This is a very important problem to consider when examining biological data. If parameter choices are made incorrectly, results that are reported regarding an experiment could in fact be the result of parameter choice artifact and not truly a difference in conditions or between groups. Therefore, authors are encouraged to report entropy values using neighboring parameter values in their supplementary data. This will increase the transparency of parameter choice and ensure that reported results are not the artifact of parameter choice (Yentes et al. 2013).

The third issue with approximate entropy is that the m, r, and N parameters should be the same when fixed. When comparing data, this can only be done when the input parameters are the same (Pincus 1995). This is because the approximate entropy algorithm is extremely sensitive to the choice of input parameters and data length (Richman and Moorman 2000; Lake et al. 2002). Sample entropy was developed to overcome these problems.

Sample entropy is very similar to approximate entropy in the approach, yet it does not count self-matches, thus eliminating the regularity bias that is present in approximate entropy. It is still a probability measure and is defined as the "negative natural logarithm of the conditional probabilities that two sequences similar for m points remain similar at the next point" (Richman and Moorman 2000, p. H2039). Sample entropy differs from approximate entropy in that sample entropy: (1) eliminates the counting of self-matches and (2) takes the logarithm of the sum of conditional probabilities rather than the logarithm of each individual conditional property as approximate entropy does. On the other hand, it has been suggested that sample entropy is highly dependent on the relationship between sampling frequency and Nyquist rate as well as the signal-to-noise ratio (Costa et al. 2005; Aboy et al. 2007). Similar to approximate entropy, a time series with similar distances between data points would result in a lower sample entropy value and large differences would result in greater sample entropy values with no upper limit. Thus, a perfectly repeatable time series elicited a sample entropy value ~0 and a perfectly random time series elicited a sample entropy value converging toward infinity.

Calculation of Sample Entropy

Data treatment for sample entropy is very similar to that of approximate entropy. The number of similar vectors is counted for length m and their conditional probabilities are summed and divided by $N - m$. This represents the value A_i. This step is then repeated for vector length of $m + 1$ and represents the value B_i. Sample entropy is truly defined as follows:

$$\lim_{N \to \infty} - \ln \frac{A_i}{B_i} \tag{6.9}$$

However, to resolve the limit, sample entropy is truly calculated as follows:

$$- \ln \frac{A}{B} \tag{6.10}$$

where

$$A = \frac{(N - m - 1)(N - m)}{2} A_i \tag{6.11}$$

and

$$B = \frac{(N - m - 1)(N - m)}{2} B_i \tag{6.12}$$

For a full example of how to calculate sample entropy, please see Example Box 6.2. The sample entropy is not defined for $A = 0$ (log of zero is undefined), and for $B = 0$ (division by zero is undefined). Thus, the bias that was introduced into the approximate entropy algorithm by self-counting is not present in sample entropy, but those cases where there are no matches other than self-matches are now undefined.

EXAMPLE BOX 6.2   SAMPLE ENTROPY

Using the same data from Example Box 6.1, the following sample entropy calculation can be done. The first three steps are the same as well:

1. *Plot the data.*
2. *Choose your parameters.*
3. *Divide our time series into "vector lengths" of 2 points ($m = 2$).*
4. *Count the number of similar vector lengths ($m = 2$) that fall within a tolerance of ± 1 (r). Calculate the conditional probability (C_i^m). The sum of C_i^m divided by $N - m$ will be defined as B_i: Taking the very first vector, {9 4}, we will look for any other vectors that fall within {9 $\pm$ 1, 4 $\pm$ 1}, or simply, that the first number has to be between 8–10 and second number is between 3–5. There are no such matches, so we count this as a 0. Remember there are no self-matches in sample entropy.*

Let us look at the second vector, {4 8}. We need to look for vectors that have a first number between 3–5 and second number between 7–9. We find vector #7, {5 8}, and #14, {5 9}. This means that for the second vector, we have two matches.

Notice that as compared to approximate entropy in Example Box 6.1, you have one less comparison, so your conditional probability is out of 24 comparisons not 25. This is because you do not perform a self-match. If you continue comparing all of the vectors, you get the following number of matches:

#	1	2	3	4	5	6	7	8	9	10	11	12	13
C_i^m #	C_1^2	C_2^2	C_3^2	C_4^2	C_5^2	C_6^2	C_7^2	C_8^2	C_9^2	C_{10}^2	C_{11}^2	C_{12}^2	C_{13}^2
Vector	{9 4}	{4 8}	{8 1}	{1 2}	{2 4}	{4 5}	{5 8}	{8 7}	{7 7}	{7 0}	{0 2}	{2 1}	{1 5}
Matches	0	2	2	4	1	0	2	3	2	2	3	2	2
C_i^m	0/24	2/24	2/24	4/24	1/24	0/24	2/24	3/24	2/24	2/24	3/24	2/24	2/24

#	14	15	16	17	18	19	20	21	22	23	24	25
C_i^m #	C_{14}^2	C_{15}^2	C_{16}^2	C_{17}^2	C_{18}^2	C_{19}^2	C_{20}^2	C_{21}^2	C_{22}^2	C_{23}^2	C_{24}^2	C_{25}^2
Vector	{5 9}	{9 8}	{8 8}	{8 0}	{0 1}	{1 0}	{0 4}	{4 2}	{2 10}	{10 0}	{0 0}	{0 1}
Matches	2	2	3	2	5	4	1	0	0	0	3	5
C_i^m	2/24	2/24	3/24	2/24	5/24	4/24	1/24	0/24	0/24	0/24	3/24	5/24

We now take the sum of all of the conditional probabilities and divide by $N - m$ to get B_i:

$$B_i = \frac{\left[\begin{array}{c} 0/24 + 2/24 + 2/24 + 4/24 + 1/24 + 0/24 + 2/24 + 3/24 + 2/24 + 2/24 + 3/24 + 2/24 + 2/24 \\ + 2/24 + 2/24 + 3/24 + 2/24 + 5/24 + 4/24 + 1/24 + 0/24 + 0/24 + 0/24 + 3/24 + 5/24 \end{array}\right]}{(26 - 2)}$$

$$B_i = \frac{(52/24)}{(24)} = 0.0903$$

5. *Count the number of similar vector lengths ($m + 1 = 3$) that fall within a tolerance of ± 1 (r). Calculate the conditional probability (C_i^{m+1}). The sum of C_i^{m+1} divided by $N - m$ will be defined as A_i:*
Taking the very first vector, {9 4 8}, we will look for any vectors that fall within {9 ± 1, 4 ± 1, 8 ± 1}, or simply, that the first number has to be between 8–10 and second number is between 3–5 and the third number between 7–9. There are no such matches. Thus, the conditional probability is 0/23.

Look at a vector that does have more than its own self-match, #3, {8 1 2}. You will find that vector #10 and vector #17 are matches. The first number falls between 7–9, second number between 0–2 and the third between 1–3. This means that for the third vector, we have two matches. This makes the conditional probability 2/23 (two matches over 23 comparisons). If you continue comparing all of the vectors, you get the following number of matches:

#	1	2	3	4	5	6	7	8	9	10	11	12
C_i^{m+1} #	C_1^3	C_2^3	C_3^3	C_4^3	C_5^3	C_6^3	C_7^3	C_8^3	C_9^3	C_{10}^3	C_{11}^3	C_{12}^3
Vector	{9 4 8}	{4 8 1}	{8 1 2}	{1 2 4}	{2 4 5}	{4 5 8}	{5 8 7}	{8 7 7}	{7 7 0}	{7 0 2}	{0 2 1}	{2 1 5}
Matches	0	0	2	1	0	0	1	1	1	2	1	2
C_i^{m+1}	0/23	0/23	2/23	1/23	0/23	0/23	1/23	1/23	1/23	2/23	1/23	2/23
#	13	14	15	16	17	18	19	20	21	22	23	24
C_i^{m+1} #	C_{13}^3	C_{14}^3	C_{15}^3	C_{16}^3	C_{17}^3	C_{18}^3	C_{19}^3	C_{20}^3	C_{21}^3	C_{22}^3	C_{23}^3	C_{24}^3
Vector	{1 5 9}	{5 9 8}	{9 8 8}	{8 8 0}	{8 0 1}	{0 1 0}	{1 0 4}	{0 4 2}	{4 2 10}	{2 10 0}	{10 0 0}	{0 0 1}
Matches	0	1	1	1	2	2	1	0	0	0	0	1
C_i^{m+1}	0/23	1/23	1/23	1/23	2/23	2/23	1/23	0/23	0/23	0/23	0/23	1/23

We now take the sum of all of the conditional probabilities and divide by $N - m$ to get A_i.

$$A_i = \frac{\left[\begin{array}{c} 0/23 + 0/23 + 2/23 + 1/23 + 0/23 + 0/23 + 1/23 + 1/23 + 1/23 + 2/23 + 1/23 + 2/23 \\ + 0/23 + 1/23 + 1/23 + 1/23 + 2/23 + 2/23 + 1/23 + 0/23 + 0/23 + 0/23 + 0/23 + 1/23 \end{array}\right]}{(26 - 2)}$$

$$A_i = \frac{(20/23)}{(24)} = 0.0362$$

6. *Calculate sample entropy*: Sample entropy is defined as $\lim_{N \to \infty} \{-\ln(A_i/B_i)\}$. However, in order to resolve the limit, you calculate sample entropy as:

$$A = \frac{(N - m - 1)(N - m)}{2} A_i$$

$$\text{so } A = \frac{(26 - 2 - 1)(26 - 2)}{2} 0.0362 = 276 \times 0.0362 = 9.9912$$

$$B = \frac{(N - m - 1)(N - m)}{2} B_i$$

$$\text{so } B = \frac{(26 - 2 - 1)(26 - 2)}{2} 0.0903 = 276 \times 0.0903 = 24.9228$$

$$\text{Sample entropy} = -\ln\left(\frac{A}{B}\right) = -\ln\left(\frac{9.9912}{24.9228}\right) = -\ln(0.40089) = 0.9141$$

Parameter Selection

The selection of data length or N for sample entropy is a clear advantage of sample entropy over approximate entropy. Sample entropy has been suggested to be independent of data length and demonstrates relative consistency (Richman and Moorman 2000). However, Richman and Moorman (2000) did state that when using data sets of less than 100, sample entropy diverged from their predictions. A recent study examining different parameter choices using sample entropy did in fact find that sample entropy was independent of data length, even for shorter data sets (Yentes et al. 2013). Yet, the authors suggest using as long of a data set as possible because relative consistency may still be an issue at very small r values.

In the case of approximate entropy, the numerical result depends on the length of the time series, leading to the problem that is difficult to compare results from different experimental protocols. For example, Research Lab A studies the entropy of knee flexion angle during walking in patients with Parkinson's disease. Research Lab B studies the entropy of knee flexion angle during walking in patients with peripheral arterial disease. It would be nice to be able to compare the entropy results between these two populations. Sample entropy may be a better choice for this reason, since it does not have the dependence on length of the time series, as does the approximate entropy.

The methodology for selecting the m and r parameters in the sample entropy are more clearly defined than with approximate entropy (Lake et al. 2002); nevertheless, there is still much debate on correct parameter selection with sample entropy. According to Lake et al. (2002), the m parameter is set by looking at an autoregressive model of the data and finding how many time steps get included in the optimal model, that is, the order of the model. An m of 2 has also been utilized in even the earliest papers reporting SampEn (Richman and Moorman 2000). Yet, an m of 3 has been found to be acceptable for analysis using SampEn (Lake et al. 2002). Consideration with the vector length, m, should not go without consideration of the r value. Sample entropy does not have an upper limit and if the m is too large and r is small, the entropy value may converge toward infinity.

The r parameter is chosen by finding a value that minimizes the relative error of sample entropy and the relative error of conditional probability (Lake et al. 2002). The logic is that too small of an r will result in no matches being found, while too large of an r will result in too many matches being found and thus not be sensitive to differences between time series. Recall that r is a parameter that defines how closely the points in two vectors have to be in order to be counted as similar. With sample entropy for time series that are random or nearly so, the selection of the r value is driven by the requirement that one needs to find similar vectors to avoid the log(0) problem. In a time series that really is not characterized by repeating patterns, the sample entropy procedure forces the r value to be large enough that some of the patterns are characterized as being similar. In other words, for time series with no repeating patterns, both sample entropy and approximate entropy have to create some type of similarity by either self counting or increasing the r value to force matches to be made. Thus, each method has its weaknesses, especially with data sets that are random or nearly random.

How exactly should one go about choosing parameter values? Based on the current discussion, as well as past studies, it appears that there is no set combination of parameters that will work every time. Time and care will have to be devoted to parameter choice when piloting a project, and it is suggested that a range of parameter combinations be examined before data collection. For a full review of how parameter choices affect both approximate and sample entropy calculations, please see Yentes et al. (2013). The results of this study demonstrate that both *ApEn* and *SampEn* are extremely sensitive to parameter choices, especially for very short data sets ($N \leq 200$; Yentes et al. 2013). It was suggested to use an N larger than 200, an m of 2 and examine several r values before selecting your parameters. It appeared that *SampEn* was less sensitive to changes in data length and demonstrated fewer problems with relative consistency.

Uses of Sample Entropy

Cardiology

Heart rate dynamics are particularly popular for sample entropy analysis. Over 100 studies have been conducted looking at heart rate dynamics or other cardiology topics and sample entropy. Most notable are the earliest studies using sample entropy by Richman and Moorman (2000) and Lake et al. (2002). Sample entropy has been used extensively with heart rate and exercise topics (Heffernan et al. 2007; Platisa et al. 2008; Millar et al. 2009). Post-exercise cardiac deceleration is related to post-exercise recovery heart rate sample entropy yet is independent of sample entropy during the rest period (Javorka et al. 2002). Vuksanović and Gal (2005) have demonstrated that posture has an effect on heart rate variability using sample entropy. Posture influences heart rate variability more so than the effect of aging from adolescence to adulthood. Sample entropy of heart rate has also been utilized with different pathologies such as anorexia nervosa (Platisa et al. 2006) and schizophrenia (Chang et al. 2009). Bornas et al. (2006b) have found sample entropy of short ECG recordings to be useful in distinguishing between fearful and nonfearful flyers. Sample entropy has further been used to investigate the effect of treatment therapy for flight phobia (Bornas et al. 2012).

Respiration

Few studies have used sample entropy to analyze respiratory time series. Sample entropy has been used to explore respiratory maturation in premature neonates (Engoren et al. 2009). For intubated patients, a more irregular (higher sample entropy) interbreath interval was observed in patients who successfully separated from mechanical ventilation as compared to those who did not (White et al. 2010). Sample entropy has also been used to determine respiratory pattern complexity during surgery to assist in outcome prognosis (Papaioannou et al. 2011) and the effect of different anesthesia on respiratory pattern complexity (Chung et al. 2013). Sample entropy has been utilized in studying sleep apnea (Yamauchi et al. 2011). Jin et al. (2008) proposed an automatic wheeze detection method from respiratory sound signals that uses sample entropy.

Psychology/Neuroscience

Sample entropy has been used to detect sleepiness in EEG of automobile drivers (Chouvarda et al. 2007; Tran et al. 2008). Sample entropy holds promise for monitoring the depth of anesthesia utilizing EEG in a rapid and more accurate manner (Shalbaf et al. 2013). Song et al. (2012) have proposed automatic seizure detection in epilepsy using EEG signals and sample entropy. Using EEG and MEG sample entropy may prove to be helpful in diagnosing Alzheimer's disease (Hornero et al. 2009). Brain activity has also been explored using sample entropy in attention deficit hyperactivity disorder (Sokunbi et al. 2013).

Biomechanics of Gait and Posture

Within the past 10 years or so, sample entropy has been used extensively with gait and postural control data. With respect to gait, sample entropy has been found to discriminate foot types for proper footwear selection (Mei et al. 2013), can be sensitive to changes in conditions during walking (Lamoth et al. 2010; Decker et al. 2012), or during dual task conditions (Lamoth et al. 2011). Sample entropy has also been used to determine that children with cerebral palsy have a more regular postural sway than typical children (Donker et al. 2008). Lamoth et al. (2009) have demonstrated that sample entropy is useful in discriminating levels of athletic skill in postural sway time series. Similarly, sample entropy of postural sway is useful in determining different pathologies from controls (Perlmutter et al. 2010; Lamoth and van Heuvelen 2012; Schniepp et al. 2013). Sample entropy is also sensitive to the amount of attention given to postural control as well (Donker et al. 2007; Stins et al. 2009; Kuczyński et al. 2011).

Other Topics

Sample entropy has been shown to be potentially useful in predicting sepsis in neonates (Cao et al. 2004) and to characterize climate temperature dynamics (Li et al. 2006). Sample entropy of the spatial layout of cancer cells versus normal cells has been investigated (Pham and Ichikawa 2013). Sample entropy may also be a useful tool in determining team synchronization during soccer gameplay (Duarte et al. 2013). Interestingly enough, sample entropy has been indicated as a useful triage tool after a blast injury based upon the Boston Marathon bombing in 2013 (Peev et al. 2013).

Comparison to Approximate Entropy

How does sample entropy compare to approximate entropy? Several studies have used both approximate entropy and sample entropy on the same data sets, which allow us to compare the two methods. Both approximate entropy and sample entropy are sensitive to spikes in the data and amount of variance such as nonstationarity (Molina-Picó et al. 2011). A study investigating body temperature in patients with multiple organ failure concluded that approximate entropy provided better discrimination between two groups as compared to sample entropy (Cuesta-Frau et al. 2009). Chua et al. (2008) find approximate entropy to be a better measure of cardiac pathology than sample entropy. Conversely, Chen et al. (2005) demonstrate that sample entropy yields more consistent results than approximate entropy for respiratory signals. Signorini et al. (2006) find sample entropy and approximate entropy perform similarly for comparing control subjects with subjects who have congestive heart failure, especially for longer 60 min time series, but that approximate entropy had a slightly lower p value for comparing shorter 15 min time series, although it was not reported as to whether the difference was significant. Batchinsky et al. (2007) found a high correlation ($r = 0.99$) between the sample entropy and approximate entropy in heart rate interval analysis of trauma patients. However, sample entropy has been shown to work better on random, computer-generated data and to be less sensitive to the length of the time series (Richman and Moorman 2000). A recent investigation examining both walking data sets and theoretical data sets concluded sample entropy was less sensitive to changes in data length, demonstrated fewer problems with relative consistency and did not contain the inherent bias associated with the approximate entropy algorithm (Yentes et al. 2013).

Multiscale Entropy

Multiscale entropy is an extension of the sample entropy concept, but here the entropy of the system is considered on multiple time scales rather than on a single time scale (Costa et al. 2002). Costa et al. (2005) state that complexity is coupled with structural richness across multiple time scales and that this richness is meaningful. Entropy measures that have been presented thus far only quantify one time scale and increase linearly in entropy as randomness increases, leading to maximum values reflective of white noise or uncorrelated signals. White noise is an unpredictable state and conversely, very low in complexity because it lacks meaningful richness. The same is true for the opposite instance, sine wave, in which something is perfectly repeatable and is low in complexity. Hence, multiscale entropy is designed to investigate entropy across multiple scales.

Calculation of Multiscale Entropy

For multiscale entropy, windows of various sizes are created (see Example Box 6.3), and data are averaged within these windows to create multiple new time series, a process called "coarse graining." Once the coarse graining has been performed on the original time series data to create a new time series, an entropy measure, such as approximate entropy or sample entropy, is used to assess the entropy of the course-grained data. More often than not, it is sample entropy that is utilized as the entropy measure. The bias of approximate entropy towards smaller values for shorter time series makes sample entropy more widely used for multiscale entropy calculations than approximate entropy. As an example of sample entropy analysis (Figure 6.3), the dynamics of white noise appear different than dynamics of brown noise as a function of changing window size. Note that the time scaling behavior of the system dynamics can also be addressed by fractal measures, such as the Hurst exponent or detrended fluctuation analysis. Finally, entropy is plotted as a function of the scale factor used to coarse grain the original time series and analysis of the multiscale entropy curve profiles is

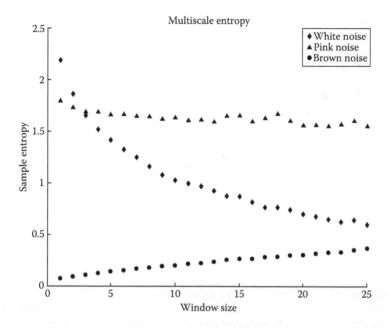

FIGURE 6.3 Multiscale entropy analysis of white noise, pink noise, and brown noise using sample entropy. Note the change in entropy, as a function of window size used in the coarse-graining for white noise is different than that for brown noise. Brown noise increases in entropy as the window sizes increase, whereas white noise decreases. Pink noise is consistent no matter the window size. $N = 5000$, $m = 2$, $r = 0.2 \times$ std.

then completed. It should be noted, that if comparison is to be done between two different time series, normalization of the time series should be completed before coarse-graining occurs.

The following guidelines have been established to compare complexity, as defined by Costa et al. (2005) between time series: (1) if one signal demonstrates a higher entropy for the majority of the time scales as compared to the other signal, the signal with higher entropy is considered more complex and (2) if a signal demonstrates a linear decrease in entropy with each increase in time scale, the signal is considered to contain information only on the smallest scale(s) (Costa et al. 2005, p. 5). Analysis of the curves themselves is what the developers of this tool encourage (Costa et al. 2005), rather than looking for one particular entropy value. However, the use of the "complexity index" has been identified, which is the area under the curve (Kang et al. 2009) and thus has been used as one value to represent the multiscale entropy. However, using the complexity index can be problematic as the area under the curve can be equivalent for two different types of signals (Figure 6.4), thus losing the ability to differentiate between deterministic and nondeterministic signals.

A potential problem in calculating multiscale entropy is using a constant m and r for the calculation of entropy for each course-grained time series. However, the selection of m and r is influenced by data length and standard deviation of time series.

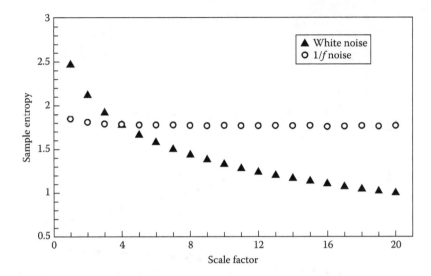

FIGURE 6.4 Multiscale entropy of white noise and pink noise (1/f noise) using sample entropy for scales from 1 to 20. As can be seen in the figure, the complexity index or area under the curve will be nearly equivalent for both white noise and 1/f noise, thus demonstrating no difference between the two signals.

Given that the data length and standard deviation vary with levels of scale factor, specific m and r for each coarse-grained time series could possibly be applied based on the data length and standard deviation. Another potential problem with multiscale entropy is that averaging the data to create the course-grained time series may destroy the temporal structure of the data. A potential alternative is to simply downsample the data to different scales to generate the coarse-grained data sets. Any data treatment outside of the specified algorithmic instructions should be tested and justified.

EXAMPLE BOX 6.3   MULTISCALE ENTROPY

Multiscale entropy is essentially the same as sample entropy but done over different time scales. Just like approximate and sample entropy, multiscale entropy also relies on the parameter choice of N, m and r. Specifically, one will perform the sample entropy of a time scale of 1 or simply, the original time series. Then one will perform sample entropy of a time scale of 2 and so forth. The time scale factors range from 1 to N/τ. In this case, tau, τ, represents non-overlapping window lengths. The data within each of these window lengths are averaged to generate a new time series. Each of these time series are referred to as coarse-grained time series. The sample entropy from each coarse-grained time series is plotted as a function of scale factor. Then one can analyze the multiscale entropy curve.

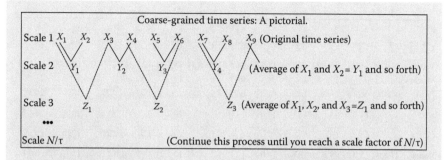

Coarse-grained time series: A pictorial.

Scale 1 X_1 X_2 X_3 X_4 X_5 X_6 X_7 X_8 X_9 (Original time series)

Scale 2 Y_1 Y_2 Y_3 Y_4 (Average of X_1 and $X_2 = Y_1$ and so forth)

Scale 3 Z_1 Z_2 Z_3 (Average of X_1, X_2, and $X_3 = Z_1$ and so forth)

•••

Scale N/τ (Continue this process until you reach a scale factor of N/τ)

To calculate the sample entropy of scale factor 1, the procedure is the same as it was in Example Box 6.2.

Time series: {9 4 8 1 2 4 5 8 7 7 0 2 1 5 9 8 8 0 1 0 4 2 10 0 0 1}

1. *Plot the data*: See Example Box 6.1.
2. *Choose your parameters*: See Example Box 6.1.
3. *Divide our time series into "vector lengths" of 2 points (m = 2)*:
   We get 25 vectors of length 2: {9 4} {4 8} {8 1} {1 2} {2 4} {4 5} {5 8}
   {8 7} {7 7} {7 0} {0 2} {2 1} {1 5} {5 9} {9 8} {8 8} {8 0} {0 1} {1 0}
   {0 4} {4 2} {2 10} {10 0} {0 0} {0 1}
4. *Count the number of similar vector lengths (m = 2) that fall within a tolerance of ± 1 (r). Calculate the conditional probability (C_i^m). The sum of C_i^m divided by N − m will be defined as B_i.*

#	1	2	3	4	5	6	7	8	9	10	11	12	13
C_i^m #	C_1^2	C_2^2	C_3^2	C_4^2	C_5^2	C_6^2	C_7^2	C_8^2	C_9^2	C_{10}^2	C_{11}^2	C_{12}^2	C_{13}^2
Vector	{9 4}	{4 8}	{8 1}	{1 2}	{2 4}	{4 5}	{5 8}	{8 7}	{7 7}	{7 0}	{0 2}	{2 1}	{1 5}
Matches	0	2	2	4	1	0	2	3	2	2	3	2	2
C_i^m	0/24	2/24	2/24	4/24	1/24	0/24	2/24	3/24	2/24	2/24	3/24	2/24	2/24
#	14	15	16	17	18	19	20	21	22	23	24	25	
C_i^m #	C_{14}^2	C_{15}^2	C_{16}^2	C_{17}^2	C_{18}^2	C_{19}^2	C_{20}^2	C_{21}^2	C_{22}^2	C_{23}^2	C_{24}^2	C_{25}^2	
Vector	{5 9}	{9 8}	{8 8}	{8 0}	{0 1}	{1 0}	{0 4}	{4 2}	{2 10}	{10 0}	{0 0}	{0 1}	
Matches	2	2	3	2	5	4	1	0	0	0	3	5	
C_i^m	2/24	2/24	3/24	2/24	5/24	4/24	1/24	0/24	0/24	0/24	3/24	5/24	

$$B_i = \frac{\left[\begin{array}{l} 0/24 + 2/24 + 2/24 + 4/24 + 1/24 + 0/24 + 2/24 + 3/24 + 2/24 + 2/24 + 3/24 + 2/24 + 2/24 \\ + 2/24 + 2/24 + 3/24 + 2/24 + 5/24 + 4/24 + 1/24 + 0/24 + 0/24 + 0/24 + 3/24 + 5/24 \end{array}\right]}{(26-2)}$$

$$B_i = \frac{(52/24)}{(24)} = 0.0903$$

5. *Count the number of similar vector lengths (m + 1 = 3) that fall within a tolerance of ± 1 (r). Calculate the conditional probability (C_i^{m+1}). The sum of C_i^{m+1} divided by N − m will be defined as A_i.*

#	1	2	3	4	5	6	7	8	9	10	11	12
C_i^{m+1}	C_1^3	C_2^3	C_3^3	C_4^3	C_5^3	C_6^3	C_7^3	C_8^3	C_9^3	C_{10}^3	C_{11}^3	C_{12}^3
Vector	{9 4 8}	{4 8 1}	{8 1 2}	{1 2 4}	{2 4 5}	{4 5 8}	{5 8 7}	{8 7 7}	{7 7 0}	{7 0 2}	{0 2 1}	{2 1 5}
Matches	0	0	2	1	0	0	1	1	1	2	1	2
C_i^{m+1}	0/23	0/23	2/23	1/23	0/23	0/23	1/23	1/23	1/23	2/23	1/23	2/23
#	13	14	15	16	17	18	19	20	21	22	23	24
C_i^{m+1}	C_{13}^3	C_{14}^3	C_{15}^3	C_{16}^3	C_{17}^3	C_{18}^3	C_{19}^3	C_{20}^3	C_{21}^3	C_{22}^3	C_{23}^3	C_{24}^3
Vector	{1 5 9}	{5 9 8}	{9 8 8}	{8 8 0}	{8 0 1}	{0 1 0}	{1 0 4}	{0 4 2}	{4 2 10}	{2 10 0}	{10 0 0}	{0 0 1}
Matches	0	1	1	1	2	2	1	0	0	0	0	1
C_i^{m+1}	0/23	1/23	1/23	1/23	2/23	2/23	1/23	0/23	0/23	0/23	0/23	1/23

$$A_i = \frac{\left[\begin{array}{c} 0/23+0/23+2/23+1/23+0/23+0/23+1/23+1/23+1/23+2/23+1/23+2/23 \\ +0/23+1/23+1/23+1/23+2/23+2/23+1/23+0/23+0/23+0/23+0/23+1/23 \end{array}\right]}{(26-2)}$$

$$A_i = \frac{(20/23)}{(24)} = 0.0362$$

6. *Calculate sample entropy*

$$A = \frac{(N-m-1)(N-m)}{2} A_i \quad \text{so } A = \frac{(26-2-1)(26-2)}{2} \; 0.0362 = 276 \times 0.0362 = 9.9912$$

$$B = \frac{(N-m-1)(N-m)}{2} B_i \quad \text{so } B = \frac{(26-2-1)(26-2)}{2} \; 0.0903 = 276 \times 0.0903 = 24.9228$$

$$\text{Sample entropy} = -\ln\left(\frac{A}{B}\right) = -\ln\left(\frac{9.9912}{24.9228}\right) = -\ln(0.40089) = 0.9141$$

7. *Plot the value of sample entropy for scale factor 1*: See plot at the end of the example box.
8. *Coarse-grain the time series to the new scale factor*:
   Original time series: {9 4 8 1 2 4 5 8 7 7 0 2 1 5 9 8 8 0 1 0 4 2 10 0 0 1}
   Scale factor 2 time series: {6.5 4.5 3 6.5 7 1 3 8.5 4.5 3 5.5}
9. *Repeat the steps 4–7 above for the new scale factor*: {6.5 4.5} {4.5 3} {3 6.5} {6.5 7} {7 1} {1 3} {3 8.5} {8.5 4} {4.5} {.5 3} {3 5} {5.5}

#	1	2	3	4	5	6	7	8	9	10	11	12
C_i^m #	C_1^2	C_2^2	C_3^2	C_4^2	C_5^2	C_6^2	C_7^2	C_8^2	C_9^2	C_{10}^2	C_{11}^2	C_{12}^2
Vector	{6.5 4.5}	{4.5 3}	{3 6.5}	{6.5 7}	{7 1}	{1 3}	{3 8.5}	{8.5 4}	{4.5}	{.5 3}	{3 5}	{5.5}
Matches	0	0	0	0	0	1	0	0	1	1	0	1
C_i^m	0/11	0/11	0/11	0/11	0/11	1/11	0/11	0/11	1/11	1/11	0/11	1/11

$$B_i = \frac{\left[0/11+0/11+0/11+0/11+0/11+1/11+0/11+0/11+1/11+1/11+0/11+1/11\right]}{(13-2)}$$

$$B_i = \frac{(4/11)}{(11)} = 0.0331$$

#	1	2	3	4	5	6	7	8	9	10	11
C_i^{m+1} #	C_1^3	C_2^3	C_3^3	C_4^3	C_5^3	C_6^3	C_7^3	C_8^3	C_9^3	C_{10}^3	C_{11}^3
Vector	{6.5 4.5 3}	{4.5 3 6.5}	{3 6.5 7}	{6.5 7 1}	{7 1 3}	{1 3 8.5}	{3 8.5 4}	{8.5 4.5}	{4.5 3}	{.5 3 5}	{3 5.5}
Matches	0	0	0	0	0	0	0	0	0	0	0
C_i^{m+1}	0/10	0/10	0/10	0/10	0/10	0/10	0/10	0/10	0/10	0/10	0/10

$$A_i = \frac{\left[0/10+0/10+0/10+0/10+0/10+0/10+0/10+0/10+0/10+0/10+0/10\right]}{(13-2)}$$

$$A_i = \frac{(0/10)}{(11)} = 0.000$$

$$A = \frac{(N-m-1)(N-m)}{2}A_i \quad \text{so } A = \frac{(13-2-1)(13-2)}{2} \quad 0.000 = 55 \times 0.000 = 0.000$$

$$B = \frac{(N-m-1)(N-m)}{2}B_i \quad \text{so } B = \frac{(13-2-1)(13-2)}{2} \quad 0.0331 = 55 \times 0.0331 = 1.821$$

$$\text{Sample entropy} = -\ln\left(\frac{A}{B}\right) = -\ln\left(\frac{0.000}{1.821}\right) = -\ln(0) = 0 \text{ (undefined)}$$

In this case, since our time series was too short from the outset, we were unable to find a match when $m + 1 = 3$.
10. *Repeat steps 8 and 9 for each scale factor up to N/τ.*
11. *Analyze the curve profiles from the plots.*

Note: In the graph below, only the data point for scale factor 1 is an actual data point from the example box.

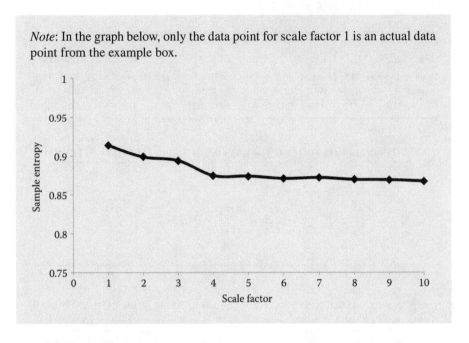

Uses of Multiscale Entropy

Multiscale entropy analysis on heart rate interval data has been reported by several authors. The concept was originally developed for use with heart rate data (Costa et al. 2002) and has been suggested to be useful in a number of different cardiopathologies (Costa et al. 2006). Multiscale entropy has been used to show that patients with diabetes mellitus type I have lower randomness in heart rate and blood pressure than controls (Javorka et al. 2008; Trunkvalterova et al. 2008). Patients with chronic heart failure have been found to have lower entropy than controls (Angelini et al. 2007) and multiscale entropy has been used in patients with congestive heart failure (Signorini et al. 2006). Multiscale entropy may also be used for monitoring the heart of a fetus (Ferrario et al. 2006a, 2009). Multiscale entropy has shown a reduction in the entropy of heart rate data in those with fear of flying when confronted with flight-related stimuli (Bornas et al. 2006a). Multiscale entropy of heart rate data has been shown to predict death in critically ill patients (Norris et al. 2008).

Multiscale entropy has also been used in other fields of medicine and physiology. Randomness of DNA sequences has been characterized using multiscale entropy (Costa et al. 2005). Multiscale entropy has been used with laser Doppler flowmetry signals and may be a useful signature of these signals (Humeau et al. 2010). Renal sympathetic nerve activity has been shown to have different entropy-scaling behavior in rats using multiscale entropy depending on whether the rats were anesthetized or conscious (Li et al. 2008a,b). Multiscale entropy has been used to study magneto-encephalogram data in patients with Alzheimer's disease, finding that lower entropy values are correlated with Alzheimer's pathology (Escudero et al. 2006; Gomez et al. 2007). Multiscale entropy has been used to study gait data (Costa et al. 2003), in postural sway of elderly (Costa et al. 2007; Manor et al. 2010), and during dual-task situations (Kang et al. 2009). Multiscale entropy revealed an altered postural control strategy in overweight children carrying a backpack leading to reduced balance (Pau et al. 2012). Endogenous spiking activity of neurons was shown to have long-range correlations using multiscale entropy, along with detrended fluctuation analysis (Bhattacharya et al. 2005).

SYMBOLIC ENTROPY

The overall, big picture of the symbolic entropy method is that the time series is first converted to a series of a relatively small number of symbols, and then, some type of entropy analysis is performed on the symbols. Thus, one needs a set of rules for mapping the time series data into the symbols and an entropy analysis technique to use on the symbols. The symbolic entropy discussed in detail here is that of Aziz and Arif (2006), which is a threshold-dependent symbolic entropy. One desirable aspect of this approach is that the result does not depend on the length of the time series, that is, the entropy remains within a well-defined range, regardless of the length of the time series. This could facilitate comparisons between different populations with data acquired in different laboratories.

Calculation of Symbolic Entropy

Calculation of symbolic entropy is described in Example Box 6.4 using the methodology presented by Aziz and Arif (2006). Some relevant points should be noted. First is that the threshold value is a key aspect of the process, as points in the time series are either above or below the threshold value. The selection of too low of a threshold produces more ones than zeros, with a correspondingly high number of words with mostly ones. Conversely, selecting too high a threshold value results in more zeros in the symbol series with a correspondingly high number of words with mostly zeros. If the symbol series is mostly ones (or mostly zeros), the corresponding entropy will be low, and the predictability of the time series will not be appropriately captured in the result. Thus, the selection of a threshold value must be done carefully. One choice might be to select the median value for the time series, thereby ensuring that half of the symbols will be zeros and half of them will be ones (Figure 6.5). The entropy value calculated with this approach will then be a reflection of the time series data crossing back and forth past this mean value. The important question is whether this reflects a meaningful measure or not.

It is this process of conversion to symbols that is critical to finding relevant patterns in the time series. Control of the system near the average value may not be the most sensitive measure of function in a control system. It may be that control toward the extreme values, that is, extreme high values and extreme low values, where there is a greater likelihood of adverse consequences, would be more important measure. With just a single threshold value in the symbolic entropy, this cannot really be explored fully. Extending the technique of Aziz and Arif (2006), a method of calculating the symbolic entropy, can be devised with two threshold values using three symbols to indicate the three different regions (Figure 6.6).

EXAMPLE BOX 6.4   SYMBOLIC ENTROPY

Example time series: {0.6773 0.8768 0.0129 0.3104 0.7791 0.3073 0.9267 0.6787 0.5163 0.4582}

1. *Plot the data.*
2. *Convert the time series into a binary symbol series based on a threshold value. Time series data points below the threshold are replaced by 0 and those above the threshold value are replaced by 1:* With a threshold of 0.5 is converted to the following symbol series:
   Symbol series: {1 1 0 0 1 0 1 1 1 0}
3. *Words are formed from the symbols, each with a word length, L (Figure 6.4, bottom). For our example, using a word length of three:* which is then be represented as a word series:
   Word series: {(110) (100) (001) (010) (101) (011) (111) (110)}
4. *The word series can be transformed by conversion of the binary into decimal: (110 = 6, 100 = 4, etc.) into a word symbol series:* {6 4 1 2 5 3 7 6}
5. *Shannon's entropy can be calculated from this word symbol series, where the index i runs from 0 to 7, since there are 8 possible states, and p is the probability of each state:* In the word series above, notice that the number six occurs twice, that is, 2/8, and all of the other six numbers occur only once in the data set, that is, 1/8. Therefore, we calculate the Shannon's entropy based on these occurrences:

$$H_S = -\sum p_i \log_2 p_i = -\left(6 * \frac{1}{8} * \log_2\left(\frac{1}{8}\right) + 1 * \frac{2}{8} * \log_2\left(\frac{2}{8}\right)\right) = 2.75$$

   Note that the $\log_2$ means a base 2 log, and that 6 states ($i = 1, 2, 3, 4, 5, 7$) have $p_i = 1/8$, and that one state has $p_i = 2/8$ ($i = 6$). The state $i = 0$ has zero probability (meaning 0 does not occur in the series). The log(0) is not defined, so states with zero probability are not counted.
6. *Note that the Shannon entropy values will depend on the length of the time series, so the result is then corrected and normalized as described by Aziz and Arif (2006):* The corrected Shannon entropy ($H_{S,corrected}$) is calculated as follows:

$$H_{S,corrected} = H_S + \frac{N_{words,actual} - 1}{2 \times N_{words,possible}} \frac{1}{\ln 2} = 2.75 + 0.54 = 3.29$$

   where
   $N_{words,actual}$ is the number of words actually present in the time series (7 in our example)
   $N_{words,possible}$ is the possible number of possible states or words that could occur (8 in our example)

Next the corrected Shannon entropy is divided by the maximum entropy of the time series to normalize it, where the maximum entropy is achieved if all states have an equal probability.

$$H_{max,corrected} = -\log_2\left(\frac{1}{N_{words,possible}}\right) + \left(\frac{N_{words,possible} - 1}{2 \times N_{words,possible} \ln 2}\right) = 3 + 0.54 = 3.54$$

$$SymbolicEntropy = \frac{H_{S,corrected}}{H_{max,corrected}} = \frac{3.29}{3.54} = 0.929$$

What if we use two threshold values?
Using the previous example time series, and choosing values of 0.2 and 0.8 for the threshold values, the time series
    {0.6773 0.8768 0.0129 0.3104 0.7791 0.3073 0.9267 0.6787 0.5163 0.4582}
is converted to the symbol series:
    {1 2 0 1 1 1 2 1 1 1}
where 0 indicates a data point below the lower threshold, 2 indicates a data point above the upper threshold, and 1 indicates a data point in between the thresholds. Again, using a word length of three, the following words are obtained:
    {(120), (201), (011), (111), (112), (121), (211), (111)}
With a word length of three and three symbols possible, there are $3^3 = 27$ possible words, coded from 0 to 26 as follows:

000 = 0	100 = 9	200 = 18
001 = 1	101 = 10	201 = 19
002 = 2	102 = 11	202 = 20
010 = 3	110 = 12	210 = 21
011 = 4	111 = 13	211 = 22
012 = 5	112 = 14	212 = 23
020 = 6	120 = 15	220 = 24
021 = 7	121 = 16	221 = 25
022 = 8	122 = 17	222 = 26

Therefore, the word series formed is:
    {15, 19, 4, 13, 14, 16, 22, 13}
As with the single threshold symbolic entropy, Shannon's entropy is calculated from the word series as before, but now the index i runs from 0 to 26:
    Probability = 0/27 for 0, 1, 2, 3, 5, 6, 7, 8, 9, 10, 11, 12, 17, 18, 20, 21, 23, 24, 25, 26
    Probability = 1/27 for 4, 14, 15, 16, 19, 22
    Probability = 2/27 for 13

$$H_S = -\sum p_i \log_2 p_i = -\left(6 * \frac{1}{27} * \log_2 \left(\frac{1}{27} \right) + 1 * \frac{2}{8} * \log_2 \left(\frac{2}{27} \right) \right) = 1.995$$

and then the normalized corrected Shannon's entropy is calculated. In this case now, the actual words arc 7 and the words possible are 27:

$$H_{S,corrected} = H_S + \frac{N_{words,actual} - 1}{2 \times N_{words,possible} \ln 2} = 1.995 + 0.160 = 2.155$$

$$H_{max,corrected} = -\log_2 \left(\frac{1}{N_{words,possible}} \right) + \left(\frac{N_{words,possible} - 1}{2 \times N_{words,possible} \ln 2} \right) = 4.755 + 0.160 = 4.915$$

$$SymbolicEntropy = \frac{H_{S,corrected}}{H_{max,corrected}} = \frac{2.155}{4.915} = 0.438$$

Uses of Symbolic Entropy

The use of symbolic entropy is not quite as popular as the other methods discussed earlier. Symbolic entropy has been successfully used to investigate infant sitting postural control (Deffeyes et al. 2009). Sitting postural sway of infants diagnosed with cerebral palsy or developmentally delayed and at risk for cerebral palsy was found to differ from sitting postural sway of infants with typical development. The symbolic entropy approach provided slightly better distinction between the two populations than did approximate entropy. Additionally, symbolic entropy has been used to investigate differences in gait between healthy individuals and individuals with neurodegenerative disease (Aziz and Arif 2006). Symbolic entropy analysis has also been applied to EEG signals (Liu et al. 2005). On the other hand, one can combine symbolic entropy and approximate entropy by translating the time series into symbols, and then calculating the approximate entropy on the resulting time series, to show that regularity of heart rate changes with fetal development (van Leeuwen et al. 2006, 2007).

OTHER ENTROPY MEASURES

Additionally, there are many other entropy algorithms that have been used, and some may offer an improvement over the more commonly used ones discussed earlier. There is no shortage of different entropy analysis methods, and new methods are still being developed as researchers try to characterize different aspects of regularity in time series data. There is even an entire journal devoted to studying entropy, *Entropy*.

Kolmogorov entropy is one of the first methods developed to calculate entropy and one of the first to be applied to biological data (Kolmogorov 1958). Historically,

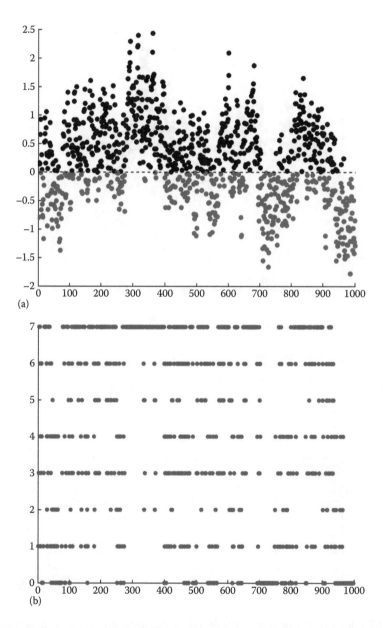

FIGURE 6.5 Use of a single threshold for calculating symbolic entropy. A pink noise time series (a) ($N = 1000$) above the threshold is assigned a value of 1 (black), whereas time series data points below the threshold are assigned a value of 0 (gray). Then using a word length of three in this example, values of 0–7 are assigned based on each word (b).

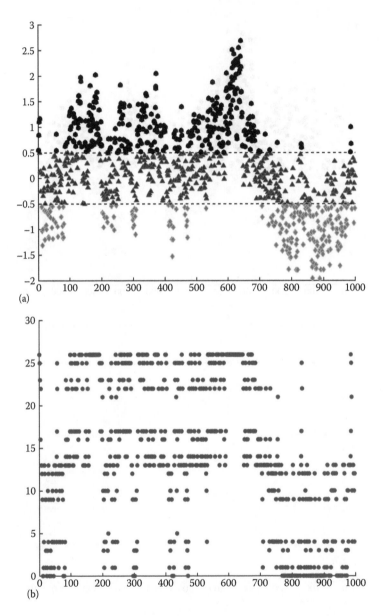

(a)

(b)

FIGURE 6.6 Use of a two thresholds for calculating symbolic entropy. A pink noise time series (a) ($N = 1000$) above the top threshold is assigned a value of 2 (black circle); time series between the two thresholds is assigned a value of 1 (gray triangle); time series data points below the lower threshold are assigned a value of 0 (light gray diamond). Then using a word length of three in this example, values of 0–26 are assigned based on each word (b).

it has been used along with the largest Lyapunov exponent to describe a deterministic, dynamical system. There are many variations of the Kolmogorov entropy algorithm, since it is designed for extremely long time series, most notably the Kolmogorov–Sinai entropy (K2 entropy). For a full review of the Komogorov–Sinai entropy see Costa, et al. (2005). Babloyantz and Destexhe (1988) determined that the normal heart rate in a healthy human is not a perfect oscillator using Kolmogorov entropy. Kolmogorov entropy has been used on EEG data (Dünki 1991) and furthermore, for epileptic seizure prediction (van Drongelen et al. 2003), dementia and Parkinson's disease (Stam et al. 1995), under emotional conditions (Aftanas et al. 1997), during imagined movement (Popivanov et al. 2001), and during voluntary movement (Dushanova 2001). Moreover, in EEG during motor imagery tasks, it has been found that Kolmogorov entropy accurately identifies event-related desynchronization and synchronization and effectively quantifies these dynamic processes (Gao et al. 2013).

Lempel and Ziv (1976) also developed an algorithm to calculate entropy in finite-sized time series to provide an entropy rate estimate. Originally developed as an algorithm for data compression (e.g., zip files), this algorithm relies on counting patterns and their rate of occurrence within a data sequence. It must be noted though that the use of Lempel–Ziv's algorithm alone cannot be interpreted as complexity from a deterministic component. Surrogate analysis must be used along with the Lempel–Ziv entropy (Nagarajan 2002). Lempel–Ziv entropy (also known as Lempel–Ziv complexity) has been shown to be sensitive to the health of a fetus (Ferrario et al. 2006b). Much like other entropy algorithms, Lempel–Ziv complexity has also been applied to heart rate dynamics (Heffernan et al. 2007), EEG recordings (Zhang and Roy 1999), as well as various other signals. Importantly, caution should be taken with application and interpretation of Lempel–Ziv complexity as has been suggested by several authors (Aboy et al. 2006; Hu et al. 2006).

Various other entropy algorithms include the following: (a) The corrected conditional entropy (Porta et al. 1998), which is a correction to the bias of regularity in the conditional entropy algorithm that is based upon the Shannon entropy. This algorithm has not been used quite as often as some of the others but has proven to be useful in the analysis of heart rate variability (Guzzetti et al. 2000; Tobaldini et al. 2008; Faes et al. 2013). (b) The von Neumann entropy (von Neumann 1996), originally derived for quantum mechanics applications, has been applied to EEG data (Kamousi et al. 2007). (c) Spectral entropy or the entropy of power spectra from a time series has been used extensively in neuroscience. (d) Fuzzy entropy, introduced by De Luca and Termini (1972), is a measure of the "quantity of information which is not necessarily related to random experiences" (p. 301) and is typically utilized for feature selection or image thresholding. Fuzzy entropy has been applied to EMG signals (Chen et al. 2007), radiographic images (Mir 2007), and heart rate variability (Liu et al. 2013). (e) Pemutation entropy (Bandt and Pompe 2002) has also been recently developed and utilized. Permutation entropy measures information within a time series based on a comparison to neighboring values and looking for patterns of increasing or decreasing values or simply, the temporal order for comparing similar or dissimilar vectors (Riedl et al. 2013). Given that similarity between elements in vectors is estimated by combination of sequence order, the permutation entropy does not consider how the elements in vector are different or equal to other elements in vector. For example, permutation entropy would consider vectors {1 7} similar to vector {102 1098} because both vectors demonstrate the same permutation, or increase in sequence. However, just looking at the two vectors, one would realize that the values of {1 7} are not similar to the values of {102 1098} and should not be considered similar. Moreover, if noise is included in the time series data and the data are very unstable, the permutation entropy may not detect these differences.

CROSS ENTROPY ALGORITHMS

Entropy can also be calculated between two separate time series. Cross-approximate entropy and cross-sample entropy have been developed to compare the asynchrony between the two time series (Pincus and Singer 1995; Pincus et al. 1996; Richman and Moorman 2000). Essentially, it is the same algorithm as presented previously except the "template" is chosen from one time series (template time series) and compared with the vectors or segment windows in the other time series (target time series). Cross-approximate entropy has an advantage over approximate entropy in which no self-matches are counted. Therefore, the inherent bias in approximate entropy is not observed in cross-approximate entropy. However, this introduces the issue of what happens when no like vectors are found, as there is an undefined conditional probability. Thus, cross-sample entropy has a clear advantage over cross-approximate entropy. Richman and Moorman (2000) have introduced two correction factors that may be used to negate this issue from cross-approximate entropy. One other consideration to cross-approximate entropy is that it is direction-dependent. This means that if you define the template time series as j and the target time series as k, cross-approximate entropy of j compared to k will be unequal to the cross-approximate entropy of k compared to j. This is not a consideration for cross-sample entropy (Richman and Moorman 2000).

CONSIDERATIONS FOR ALL ALGORITHMS

There are many things to consider before applying any entropy algorithm to your time series. First, it is the type of data that you have collected. All of the work that has been done thus far on entropy algorithms has been on non-phasic data. Whether or not it is appropriate to use entropy algorithms on phasic data (e.g., EMG data) has yet to be determined. Moreover, one should always plot his data before doing any data treatment. Spikes and outliers will have a very large effect on entropy calculation, as well as nonstationarity present in the time series.

In addition, you must consider the research question you are asking and whether or not entropy analysis, combined with the type of data that you have, will answer these questions. Entropy analysis provides information regarding regularity of movement. Pincus and Huang have warned that entropy analysis is not truly an algorithm to certify chaos but rather to distinguish between two systems (Pincus and Huang 1992). Thus, it is important to always have a 'reference' or control group in order to compare the entropy between the two groups.

Lastly, take into consideration matters such as equipment noise, sampling frequency, and filtering of data. The length of the time series is also of importance as well as the selection of other parameters. Review Chapter 2 in order to familiarize with these topics before collecting data and applying an entropy algorithm.

EXERCISES

Approximate Entropy

1. Given the time series {1, 2, 3, 4, 1, 2, 3, 4}, calculate the approximate entropy using $m = 2$, $r = 0.2$, and lag = 1. Examine the time series. Does there appear to be a repeating pattern? Does the result of your mathematical calculation of the approximate entropy agree with your observation?
2. Given the time series {1.05, 2.11, 2.95, 4.03, 0.93, 1.97, 3.04, 4.17}, calculate the approximate entropy using $m = 2$, $r = 0.2$, and lag = 1. Compare this time series with the time series from question 1. How do the results of your calculation of approximate entropy compare between the two time series? Explain this result. If r had been set at $r = 0.02$ instead of $r = 0.2$, would the results of your calculation of approximate entropy be different for the two time series? Why is r described as a filtering radius?

Sample Entropy and Multiscale Entropy

3. What is the feature of sample entropy over approximate entropy that makes it suited to use with multiscale entropy?
4. Calculate the sample entropy of the following time series {1 2 3 4 1 2 3 4} with $r = 0.1$ and $m = 2$. How does this compare with the approximate entropy result from problem 1?
5. For the time series {1 2 3 2 1 8 4 5 1 2 3 0}, calculate coarse-grained time series for window sizes 2, 3, and 4.

Symbolic Entropy

6. Convert each of the times series from questions 1 to 5 above to the symbols 0 and 1, based on a threshold of the mean value for the time series. Form words of length 2 calculate Shannon's entropy for the symbols.

DATA SET

Two time series are provided for your own calculation (Table 6.1). Software for both approximate entropy and sample entropy can be downloaded from http://www. physionet.org/. (However, we caution that you verify any codes downloaded before their use. For example, the approximate entropy code available on physionet [at the time of writing] contains a normalization and does not perform the last vector match in its calculation.) The approximate and sample entropies of the two time series are also provided for your reference.

These two time series, one from a healthy young adult (female; aged 26 years) and one from a healthy older adult (female; aged 70 years), are consecutive step widths (mm) while walking on a treadmill. The time series have been cut to match in length

TABLE 6.1
Sample Step Width (mm) Time Series, One from a Healthy Young Adult (Column 1) and One from a Healthy Older Adult (Column 2) while Walking on a Treadmill

Young	Older
78	86
79	94
75	88
73	89
74	90
76	92
73	91
76	87
75	90
75	92
74	90
75	92
75	93
77	91
75	94
74	89
76	90
74	91
78	90
77	97
76	94
74	95
78	89
77	88
77	90
75	89
73	93
74	95
76	95
74	93
75	94
76	94
73	90
77	87
75	93
72	94
73	93
76	89
76	92

(Continued)

TABLE 6.1 (*Continued*)
**Sample Step Width (mm) Time Series, One
from a Healthy Young Adult (Column 1)
and One from a Healthy Older Adult
(Column 2) while Walking on a Treadmill**

Young	Older
74	93
74	88
74	95
75	95
72	88
76	90
76	92
76	90
74	90
73	90
75	95
75	93
75	92
74	89
76	94
76	85
73	92
75	101
77	93
77	96
75	99
77	86
76	88
76	90
77	90
75	90
74	88
75	89
75	91
75	87
75	88
76	87
75	91
76	95
75	94
76	100
76	82
76	92
73	90

(*Continued*)

TABLE 6.1 (*Continued*)
Sample Step Width (mm) Time Series, One from a Healthy Young Adult (Column 1) and One from a Healthy Older Adult (Column 2) while Walking on a Treadmill

Young	Older
75	87
72	87
73	93
74	89
73	91
72	95
74	94
75	93
74	90
74	87
73	90
72	90
76	91
72	94
75	96
73	90
74	95
72	90
75	93
75	92
73	92
76	92
75	94
73	88
75	92
73	87
74	85
76	90
75	92
74	91
77	96
76	90
74	99
75	89
75	98
75	90
76	92
74	89
75	90

(*Continued*)

TABLE 6.1 *(Continued)*

Sample Step Width (mm) Time Series, One from a Healthy Young Adult (Column 1) and One from a Healthy Older Adult (Column 2) while Walking on a Treadmill

Young	Older
76	93
77	94
76	92
75	88
74	90
77	89
73	90
76	92
73	97
75	83
73	91
75	93
72	85
71	89
75	87
72	84
77	89
74	92
76	89
77	94
75	97
74	90
73	96
75	91
77	93
75	96
73	92
73	89
73	90
74	91
75	91
76	89
75	89
77	95
75	94
74	94
77	88
74	83
75	86

(Continued)

TABLE 6.1 (*Continued*)
Sample Step Width (mm) Time Series, One from a Healthy Young Adult (Column 1) and One from a Healthy Older Adult (Column 2) while Walking on a Treadmill

Young	Older
74	89
75	86
76	93
72	88
74	86
76	91
74	88
75	99
75	87
74	93
75	86
73	92
76	87
75	88
75	85
73	88
75	87
79	84
74	86
75	94
73	96
76	87
77	86
77	84
76	86
75	88
75	87
74	89
77	86
75	92
76	96
76	89
74	85
74	87
77	89
77	92
77	89
73	87
75	84

(*Continued*)

TABLE 6.1 (*Continued*)
Sample Step Width (mm) Time Series, One from a Healthy Young Adult (Column 1) and One from a Healthy Older Adult (Column 2) while Walking on a Treadmill

Young	Older
75	86
73	87
76	88
73	88
75	87

TABLE 6.2

Approximate Entropy and Sample Entropy Values for the Sample Time Series in Table 6.1

	Approximate Entropy		Sample Entropy	
	$r = 0.25$	$r = 0.30$	$r = 0.25$	$r = 0.30$
Young	1.217	1.217	1.701	1.701
Older	0.552	1.185	2.504	1.395

Parameters used were $N = 200$, $m = 2$, and $r = 0.25$ and 0.3 times the standard deviation of the entire time series.

(200 data points). The time series were run with an $m = 2$, $N = 200$, and two different r values. The two different r values used were 0.25 and 0.3 times the standard deviation of the entire time series. These two time series were chosen in particular, as the entropy of the two time series is significantly different from each other under one set of parameter choices. When the tolerance, or r, is changed just slightly, they are no longer significantly different from each other (Table 6.2). The healthy young adult's entropy does not vary much with the change in parameter choice, yet the healthy older adult's entropy changes drastically from $r = 0.25$ to $r = 0.3$. This example should emphasize the point that transparency is key in reporting entropy values. A range of values should be tested, and reported values should demonstrate an actual finding and not an arbitrary finding due to parameter choice.

REFERENCES

Abasolo, D., James, C.J., and Hornero, R. (2007). Non-linear analysis of intracranial electro-encephalogram recordings with approximate entropy and Lempel-Ziv complexity for epileptic seizure detection. *Conference Proceedings of IEEE Engineering in Medicine and Biology Society,* Lyon, *2007*, pp. 1953–1956.

Aboy, M., Cuesta-Frau, D., Austin, D., and Mico-Tormos, P. (2007). Characterization of sample entropy in the context of biomedical signal analysis. *Conference Proceedings of IEEE Engineering in Medicine and Biology Society,* Lyon, *2007*, pp. 5943–5946.

Aboy, M., Hornero, R., Abásolo, D., and Alvarez, D. (2006). Interpretation of the Lempel-Ziv complexity measure in the context of biomedical signal analysis. *IEEE Transactions in Biomedical Engineering, 53(11)*, 2282–2288.

Acharya, U.R., Faust, O., Kannathal, N., Chua, T., and Laxminarayan, S. (2005). Non-linear analysis of EEG signals at various sleep stages. *Computer Methods and Programs in Biomedicine, 80(1)*, 37–45.

Acharya, U.R., Sree, S.V., Chattopadhyay, S., and Suri, J.S. (2012). Automated diagnosis of normal and alcoholic EEG signals. *International Journal of Neural Systems, 22(3)*, 1250011.

Aftanas, L.I., Lotova, N.V., Koshkarov, V.I., Pokrovskaja, V.L., Popov, S.A., and Makhev, V.P. (1997). Non-linear analysis of emotion EEG: Calculation of Kolmogorov entropy and the principal Lyapunov exponent. *Neuroscience Letters, 226(1)*, 13–16.

Alkjær, T., Paffalt, P., Petersen, N.C., and Simonsen, E.B. (2012). Movement behavior of high-heeled walking: How does the nervous system control the ankle joint during an unstable walking condition? *PLoS One, 7(5)*, e37390.

Angelini, L., Maestri, R., Marinazzo, D., Nitti, L., Pellicoro, M., Pinna, G.D., Stramaglia, S., and Tupputi, S.A. (2007). Multiscale analysis of short term heart beat interval, arterial blood pressure, and instantaneous lung volume time series. *Artificial Intelligence in Medicine, 41(3)*, 237–250.

Aziz, W. and Arif, M. (2006). Complexity analysis of stride interval time series by threshold dependent symbolic entropy. *European Journal of Applied Physiology*, 98, 30–40.

Babloyzntz, A. and Destexhe, A. (1988). Is the normal heart rate a periodic oscillator? *Biological Cybernetics, 58(3)*, 203–211.

Bandt, C. and Pompe, B. (2002). Permutation entropy: A natural complexity measure for time series. *Physical Review Letters, 88(17)*, 174102.

Batchinsky, A.I., Cancio, L.C., Salinas, J., Kuusela, T., Cooke, W.H., Wang, J.J., Boehme, M., Convertino, V.A., and Holcomb, J.B. (2007). Prehospital loss of R-to-R interval complexity is associated with mortality in trauma patients. *Journal of Trauma, 63(3)*, 512–518.

Bhattacharya, J. (2000). Complexity analysis of spontaneous EEG. *Acta Neurobiologiae Experimentalis, 60(4)*, 495–501.

Bhattacharya, J., Edwards, J., Mamelak, A.N., and Schuman, E.M. (2005). Long-range temporal correlations in the spontaneous spiking of neurons in the hippocampal-amygdala complex of humans. *Neuroscience, 131(2)*, 547–555.

Boltzmann, L. (1896). As cited in Kondepudi and Prigogine (1998).

Bornas, X., Llabres, J., Noguera, M., Lopez, A.M., Gelabert, J.M., and Vila, I. (2006a). Fear induced complexity loss in the electrocardiogram of flight phobics: A multiscale entropy analysis. *Biological Psychology, 73(3)*, 272–279.

Bornas, X., Llabres, J., Noguera, M., and Pez, A. (2006b). Sample entropy of ECG time series of fearful flyers: Preliminary results. *Nonlinear Dynamics, Psychology, and Life Sciences, 10(3)*, 301–318.

Bornas, X., Riera del Amo, A., Tortella-Feliu, M., and Llabrés, J. (2012). Heart rate variability profiles and exposure therapy treatment outcome in flight phobia. *Applied Psychophysiology and Biofeedback, 37(1)*, 53–62.

Burioka, N., Cornélissen, G., Halberg, F., Kaplan, D.T., Suyama, H., Sako, T., and Shimizu, E. (2003). Approximate entropy of human respiratory movement during eye-closed waking and different sleep stages. *Chest, 123(1)*, 80–86.

Burioka, N., Cornélissen, G., Maegaki, Y., Halberg, F., Kaplan, D.T., Miyata, M., Fukuoka, Y., Endo, M., Suyama, H., Tomita, Y., and Shimizu, E. (2005). Approximate entropy of the electroencephalogram in healthy awake subjects and absence epilepsy patients. *Clinical EEG and Neuroscience, 36(3)*, 188–193.

Burioka, N., Suyama, H., Sako, T., Miyata, M., Takeshima, T., Endo, M., Kurai, J. et al. (2002). Non-linear dynamics applied to human respiratory movement during sleep. *Biomedicine & Pharmacotherapy, 56(Suppl 2)*, 370s–373s.

Cao, H., Lake, D.E., Griffin, M.P., and Moorman, J.R. (2004). Increased nonstationarity of neonatal heart rate before the clinical diagnosis of sepsis. *Annals of Biomedical Engineering, 32(2)*, 233–244.

Carnot, S. (1824). *Reflections on the Motive Force of Fire and on the Machines Fitted to Develop that Power.* As cited in Kondepudi and Prigogine (1998).

Cavanaugh, J.T., Guskiewicz, K.M., Giuliani, C., Marshall S., Mercer V.S., and Stergiou, N. (2006). Recovery of postural control after cerebral concussion: New insights using approximate entropy. *Journal of Athletic Training, 41(3)*, 305–313.

Chaitin, G.J. (1975). Randomness and mathematical proof. *Scientific American, 232(5)*, 47–52.

Chang, J.S., Yoo, C.S., Yi, S.H., Hong, K.H., Oh, H.S., Hwang, J.Y., Kim, S.G., Ahn, Y.M., and Kim, Y.S. (2009). Differential pattern of heart rate variability in patients with schizophrenia. *Progress in Neuro-Psychopharmacology & Biological Psychiatry, 33(6)*, 991–995.

Chen, W., Wang, Z., Xie, H., and Yu, W. (2007). Characterization of surface EMG signal based on fuzzy entropy. *IEEE Transactions on Neural Systems and Rehabilitation Engineering, 15(2)*, 266–272.

Chen, X., Solomon, I., and Chon, K. (2005). Comparison of the use of approximate entropy and sample entropy: Applications to neural respiratory signal. *Conference Proceedings of IEEE Engineering in Medicine and Biology Society*, Shanghai, Vol. 4, pp. 4212–4215.

Chon, K., Scully, C.G., and Lu, S. (2009). Approximate entropy for all signals. *IEEE Engineering in Medicine and Biology Magazine, 28*, 18–23.

Chouvarda, I., Papadelis, C., Kourtidou-Papadeli, C., Bamidis, P.D., Koufogiannis, D., Bekiaris, E., and Maglaveras, N. (2007). Non-linear analysis for the sleepy drivers problem. *Studies in Health Technology and Informatics, 129(Pt 2)*, 1294–1298.

Chua, K.C., Chandran, V., Acharya, U.R., and Lim, C.M. (2008). Computer-based analysis of cardiac state using entropies, recurrence plots and Poincare geometry. *Journal of Medical Engineering & Technology, 32(4)*, 263–272.

Chung, A., Fishman, M., Dasenbrook, E.C., Loparo, K.A., Dick, T.E., and Jacono, F.J. (2013). Isoflurane and ketamine anesthesia have different effects on ventilator pattern variability in rats. *Respiratory Physiology and Neurobiology, 185(3)*, 659–664.

Clausius, R. (1867). *Mechanical Theory of Heat.* As cited in Kondepudi and Prigogine (1998).

Costa, M., Cygankiewicz, I., Zareba, W., Bayes de Luna, A., Goldberger, A.L., and Lobodzinski, S. (2006). Multiscale complexity analysis of heart rate dynamics in heart failure: Preliminary findings from the MUSIC study. *Computers in Cardiology, 33*, 101–103.

Costa, M., Goldberger, A.L., and Peng, C.K. (2002). Multiscale entropy analysis of complex physiologic time series. *Physical Review Letters, 89(6)*, 068102-1–068102-4.

Costa, M., Goldberger, A.L., and Peng, C.K. (2005). Multiscale entropy analysis of biological signals. *Physical Review E, 71(2 Pt 1)*, 021906.

Costa, M., Peng, C.K., Goldberger, A.L., and Hausdorff, J.M. (2003). Multiscale entropy analysis of human gait dynamics. *Physica A, 330*, 53–60.

Costa, M., Priplata, A.A., Lipsitz, L.A., Wu, Z., Huang, N.E., Goldberger, A.L., and Peng, C.K. (2007). Noise and poise: Enhancement of postural complexity in the elderly with a stochastic-resonance-based therapy. *Europhysics Letters, 77*, 68008.

Cuesta, D., Varela, M., Miró, P., Galdós, P., Abásolo, D., Hornero, R., and Aboy, M. (2007). Predicting survival in critical patients by use of body temperature regularity measurement based on approximate entropy. *Medical and Biological Engineering and Computing, 45(7)*, 671–678.

Cuesta-Frau, D., Miró-Martínez, P., Oltra-Crespo, S., Varela-Entrecanales, M., Aboy, M., Novak, D., and Austin, D. (2009). Measuring body temperature time series regularity using approximate entropy and sample entropy. *Conference Proceedings of IEEE Engineering in Medicine and Biology Society*, Minneapolis, MN, *2009*, pp. 3461–3464.

De Luca, A. and Termini, S. (1972). A definition of nonprobabilistic entropy in the setting of fuzzy sets theory. *Information and Control, 20*, 301–312.

Decker, L.M., Cignetti, F., and Stergiou, N. (2012). Wearing a safety harness during treadmill walking influences lower extremity kinematics mainly through changes in ankle regularity and local stability. *Journal of Neuroengineering and Rehabilitation, 9*, 8.

Deffeyes, J.E., Harbourne, R.T., DeJong, S.L., Kyvelidou, A., Stuberg, W.A., and Stergiou, N. (2009). Use of information entropy measures of sitting postural sway to quantify developmental delay in infants. *Journal of Neuroengineering and Rehabilitation, 6*, 34.

Donker, S.F., Ledebt, A., Roerdink, M., Savelsbergh, G.J., and Beek, P.J. (2008). Children with cerebral palsy exhibit greater and more regular postural sway than typically developing children. *Experimental Brain Research, 184(3)*, 363–370.

Donker, S.F., Roerdink, M., Greven, A.J., and Beek, P.J. (2007). Regularity of center-of-pressure trajectories depends on the amount of attention invested in postural control. *Experimental Brain Research, 181(1)*, 1–11.

Dragomir, A., Akay, Y., Curran, A.K., and Akay, M. (2008). Complexity measures of the central respiratory networks during wakefulness and sleep. *Journal of Neural Engineering, 5(2)*, 254–261.

Duarte, R., Araújo, D., Correia, V., Davids, K., Marques, P., and Richardson, M.J. (2013). Competing together: Assessing the dynamics of team-team and player-team synchrony in professional association football. *Human Movement Science, 32(4)*, 555–566.

Dünki, R.M. (1991). The estimation of the Kolmogorov entropy from a time series and its limitations when performed on EEG. *Bulletin of Mathematical Biology, 53(5)*, 665–678.

Dushanova, J. (2001). Does the Kolmogorov entropy give more information about the organization of the voluntary movement? *Acta Physiologica et Pharmacologica Bulgarica, 26(1–2)*, 93–96.

Dusing, S.C., Kyvelidou, A., Mercer, V.S., and Stergiou, N. (2009). Infants born preterm exhibit different patterns of center-of-pressure movement than infants born at full term. *Physical Therapy, 89(12)*, 1354–1362.

Engoren, M., Courtney, S.E., and Habib, R.H. (2009). Effect of weight and age on respiratory complexity in premature neonates. *Journal of Applied Physiology, 106(3)*, 766–773.

Escudero, J., Abásolo, D., Hornero, R., Espino, P., and López, M. (2006). Analysis of electroencephalograms in Alzheimer's disease patients with multiscale entropy. *Physiological Measurement, 27(11)*, 1091–1106.

Esmaeili, V., Shamsollahi, M.B., Arefian, N.M., and Assareh, A. (2007). Classifying depth of anesthesia using EEG features, a comparison. *Conference Proceedings of IEEE Engineering in Medicine and Biology Society,* Lyon, *2007*, pp. 4106–4109.

Faes, L., Nollo, G., and Porta, A. (2013). Mechanisms of causal interaction between short-term RR interval and systolic arterial pressure oscillations during orthostatic challenge. *Journal of Applied Physiology, 114(12)*, 1657–1667.

Ferrario, M., Signorini, M.G., and Magenes, G. (2006a). New indexes from the fetal heart rate analysis for the identification of severe intrauterine growth restricted fetuses. *Conference Proceedings of IEEE Engineering in Medicine and Biology Society*, New York, NY, Vol. 1, pp. 1458–1461.

Ferrario, M., Signorini, M.G., Magenes, G., and Cerutti, S. (2006b). Comparison of entropy-based regularity estimators: Application to the fetal heart rate signal for the identification of fetal distress. *IEEE Transactions on Biomedical Engineering, 53(1)*, 119–125.

Ferrario, M., Signorini, M.G., and Magenes, G. (2009). Complexity analysis of the fetal heart rate variability: Early identification of severe intrauterine growth-restricted fetuses. *Medical & Biological Engineering & Computing, 47(9)*, 911–919.

Fonseca, S., Milho, J., Passos, P., Araújo, and D., Davids, K. (2012). Approximate entropy normalized measures for analyzing social neurobiological systems. *Journal of Motor Behavior, 44(3)*, 179–183.

Gao, L., Wang, J., and Chen, L. (2013). Event-related desynchronization and synchronization quantification in motor-related EEG by Kolmogorov entropy. *Journal of Neural Engineering, 10(3)*, 036023.

Georgoulis, A.D., Moraiti, C., Ristanis, S., and Stergiou, N. (2006). A novel approach to measure variability in the anterior cruciate ligament deficient knee during walking: The use of the approximate entropy in orthopaedics. *Journal of Clinical Monitoring and Computing, 20(1)*, 11–18.

Glenn, T., Whybrow, P.C., Rasgon, N., Grof, P., Alda, M., Baethge, C., and Bauer, M. (2006). Approximate entropy of self-reported mood prior to episodes in bipolar disorder. *Bipolar Disorders, 8(5 Pt 1)*, 424–429.

Goldberger, A.L., Peng, C.K., and Lipsitz, L.A. (2002). What is physiologic complexity and how does it change with aging and disease? *Neurobiology of Aging, 23(1)*, 23–26.

Gomez, C., Hornero, R., Abásolo, D., Fernández, A., and Escudero, J. (2007). Analysis of MEG recordings from Alzheimer's disease patients with sample and multiscale entropies. *Conference Proceedings of IEEE Engineering in Medicine and Biology Society*, Lyon, *2007*, pp. 6184–6187.

Guzzetti, S., Mezzetti, S., Magatelli, R., Porta, A., De Angelis, G., Rovelli, G., and Malliani, A. (2000). Linear and non-linear 24 h heart rate variability in chronic heart failure. *Autonomic Neuroscience, 86(1–2)*, 114–119.

Harbourne, R.T. and Stergiou, N. (2003). Nonlinear analysis of the development of sitting postural control. *Developmental Psychobiology, 42*, 368–377.

Heffernan, K.S., Fahs, C.A., Shinsako, K.K., Jae, S.Y., and Fernhall, B. (2007). Heart rate recovery and heart rate complexity following resistance exercise training and detraining in young men. *American Journal of Physiology: Heart and Circulatory Physiology, 293(5)*, H3180–H3186.

Hoh, J.K., Park, Y.S., Cha, K.J., Oh, J.E., Lee, H.J., Lee, G.T., and Park, M.I. (2007). Chaotic indices and canonical ensemble of heart rate patterns in small-for-gestational age fetuses. *Journal of Perinatal Medicine, 35(3)*, 210–216.

Hornero, R., Abásolo, D., Escudero, J., and Gómez, C. (2009). Nonlinear analysis of electro-encephalogram and magnetoencephalogram recordings in patients with Alzheimer's disease. *Philosophical Transactions, Series A: Mathematical, Physical, and Engineering Sciences, 367(1887)*, 317–336.

Hu, J., Gao, J., and Principe, J.C. (2006). Analysis of biomedical signals by the Lempel-Ziv complexity: The effect of finite data size. *IEEE Transactions in Biomedical Engineering, 53(12 Part 2)*, 2606–2609.

Huisinga, J.M., Yentes, J.M., Filipi, M.L., and Stergiou, N. (2012). Postural control strategy during standing is altered in patients with multiple sclerosis. *Neuroscience Letters, 524(2)*, 124–128.

Humeau, A., Buard, B., Mahé, G., Rousseau, D., Chapeau-Blondeau, F., and Abraham, P. (2010). Multiscale entropy of laser Doppler flowmetry signals in healthy human subjects. *Medical Physics, 37(12)*, 6142–6146.

Javorka, M., Trunkvalterova, Z., Tonhajzerova, I., Javorkova, J., Javorka, K., and Baumert, M. (2008). Short-term heart rate complexity is reduced in patients with type 1 diabetes mellitus. *Clinical Neurophysiology, 119(5)*, 1071–1081.

Javorka, M., Zila, I., Balhárek, T., and Javorka, K. (2002). Heart rate recovery after exercise: Relations to heart rate variability and complexity. *Brazilian Journal of Medical and Biological Research, 35(8)*, 991–1000.

Jin, F., Sattar, F., and Goh, D.Y. (2008). Automatic wheeze detection using histograms of sample entropy. *Conference Proceedings of IEEE Engineering in Medicine and Biology Society,* Vancouver, BC, *2008,* pp. 1890–1893.

Kaipust, J.P., Huisinga, J.M., Filipi, M., and Stergiou, N. (2012). Gait variability measures reveal differences between multiple sclerosis patients and healthy controls. *Motor Control, 16*(2), 229–244.

Kamousi, B., Amini, A.N., and He, B. (2007). Classification of motor imagery by means of cortical current density estimation and Von Neuman entropy. *Journal of Neural Engineering, 4,* 17–25.

Kang, H.G., Costa, M.D., Priplata, A.A., Starobinets, O.V., Goldberger, A.L., Peng, C.K., Kiely, D.K., Cupples, L.A., and Lipsitz, L.A. (2009). Frailty and the degradation of complex balance dynamics during a dual-task protocol. *Journal of Gerontology, Series A: Biological Sciences and Medical Sciences, 64*(12), 1304–1311.

Karamanos, K., Dakopoulos, D., Aloupis, K., Peratzakis, A., Athanasopoulou, L., Nikolopoulos, S., Kapiris, P., and Eftaxias, K. (2006). Preseismic electromagnetic signals in terms of complexity. *Physical Review E, 74,* 016104.

Katsavelis, D., Mukherjee, M., Decker, L., and Stergiou, N. (2010). The effect of virtual reality on gait variability. *Nonlinear Dynamics in Psychology and Life Sciences, 14*(3), 239–256.

Kleppe, I.C. and Robinson, H.P.C. (2006). Correlation entropy of synaptic input-output dynamics. *Physical Review E, 74*(4 pt 1), 041909.

Kolmogorov, A.N. (1958). New metric invariant of transitive dynamical systems and endomorphisms of Lebesgue spaces. *Doklady of Russian Academy of Sciences, 119*(N5), 861–864.

Kondepudi, D. and Progogine, I. (1998). *Modern Thermodynamics: From Heat Engines to Dissipative Structures.* New York: Wiley.

Kuczyński, M., Szymańska, M., and Bieć, E. (2011). Dual-task effect on postural control in high-level competitive dancers. *Journal of Sports Science, 29*(5), 539–545.

Kurz, M. and Hou, J.G. (2010). Levodopa influences the regularity of the ankle joint kinematics in individuals with Parkinson's disease. *Journal of Computational Neuroscience, 28*(1), 131–136.

Kurz, M. and Stergiou, N. (2003). The aging neuromuscular system expresses less certainty for selecting joint kinematics during gait in humans. *Neuroscience Letters, 348*(3), 155–158.

Lake, D.E., Richman, J.S., Griffin, M.P., and Moorman, J.R. (2002). Sample entropy analysis of neonatal heart rate variability. *American Journal of Physiology: Regulatory, Integrative and Comparative Physiology, 283*(3), R789–R797.

Lamoth, C.J., Ainsworth, E., Polomski, W., and Houdijk, H. (2010). Variability and stability analysis of walking of transfemoral amputees. *Medical Engineering and Physics, 32*(9), 1009–1014.

Lamoth, C.J., van Deudekom, F.J., van Campen, J.P., Appels, B.A., de Vries, O.J., and Pijnappels, M. (2011). Gait stability and variability measures show effects of impaired cognition and dual tasking in frail people. *Journal of Neuroengineering and Rehabilitation, 8,* 2.

Lamoth, C.J. and van Heuvelen, M.J. (2012). Sports activities are reflected in the local stability and regularity of body sway: Older ice-skaters have better postural control than inactive elderly. *Gait and Posture, 35*(3), 489–493.

Lamoth, C.J., van Lummel, R.C., and Beek, P.J. (2009). Athletic skill level is reflected in body sway: A test case for accelometry in combination with stochastic dynamics. *Gait and Posture, 29*(4), 546–551.

Lempel, A. and Ziv, J. (1976). On the complexity of finite sequences. *IEEE Transactions on Information Theory, 22*(1), 75–81.

Li, S.C., Zhou, Q.F., Wu, S.H., and Dai, E.F. (2006). Measurement of climate complexity using sample entropy. *International Journal of Climatology, 26(15)*, 2131–2139.

Li, Y., Qiu, J., Yan, R., Yang, Z., and Zhang, T. (2008a). Weakened long-range correlation of renal sympathetic nerve activity in Wistar rats after anaesthesia. *Neuroscience Letters, 433(1)*, 28–32.

Li, Y., Qiu, J., Yang, Z., Johns, E.J., and Zhang, T. (2008b). Long-range correlation of renal sympathetic nerve activity in both conscious and anesthetized rats. *Journal of Neuroscience Methods, 172(1)*, 131–136.

Liu, C., Li, K., Zhao, L, Liu, F., Zheng, D., Liu, C., and Liu, S. (2013). Analysis of heart rate variability using fuzzy measure entropy. *Computers in Biology and Medicine, 43(2)*, 100–108.

Liu, Y., Sun, L., Zhu, Y., and Beadle, P. (2005). Novel method for measuring the complexity of schizophrenic EEG based on symbolic entropy analysis. *Conference Proceedings of IEEE Engineering in Medicine and Biology Society*, Shanghai, *2005*, pp. 37–40.

Lu, S., Chen, X., Kanters, J., Solomon, I.C., and Chon, K.H. (2008). Automatic selection of the threshold value R for approximate entropy. *IEEE Transactions on Biomedical Engineering, 55*, 115–125.

Manor, B., Costa, M.D., Hu, K., Newton, E., Starobinets, O., Kang, H.G., Peng, C.K., Novak, V., and Lipsitz, L.A. (2010). Physiological complexity and system adaptability: Evidence from postural control dynamics of older adults. *Journal of Applied Physiology, 109(6)*, 1786–1791.

Mei, Z., Zhao, G., Ivanov, K., Guo, Y., Zhu, Q., Zhou, Y., and Wang, L. (2013). Sample entropy characteristics of movement for four foot types based on plantar centre of pressure during stance phase. *Biomedical Engineering Online, 12(1)*, 101.

Millar, P.J., Rakobowchuk, M., McCartney, N., and MacDonald, M.J. (2009). Heart rate variability and nonlinear analysis of heart rate dynamics following single and multiple Wingate bouts. *Applied Physiology, Nutrition, and Metabolism, 34(5)*, 875–883.

Mir, A.H. (2007). Fuzzy entropy based interactive enhancement of radiographic images. *Journal of Medical Engineering and Technology, 31(3)*, 220–231.

Misra, M., Miller, K.K., Almazan, C., Ramaswamy, K., Lapcharoensap, W., Worley, M., Neubauer, G., Herzog, D.B., and Klibanski, A. (2004). Alterations in cortisol secretory dynamics in adolescent girls with anorexia nervosa and effects on bone metabolism. *Journal of Clinical Endocrinology and Metabolism, 89(10)*, 4972–4980.

Misra, M., Miller, K.K., Bjornson, J., Hackman, A., Aggarwal, A., Chung, J., Ott, M., Herzog, D.B., Johnson, M.L., and Klibanski, A. (2003). Alterations in growth hormone secretory dynamics in adolescent girls with anorexia nervosa and effects on bone metabolism. *Journal of Clinical Endocrinology and Metabolism, 88(12)*, 5615–5623.

Molina-Picó, A., Cuesta-Frau, D., Aboy, M., Crespo, C., Miró-Martínez, P., and Oltra-Crespo, S. (2011). Comparative study of approximate entropy and sample entropy robustness to spikes. *Artificial Intelligence in Medicine, 53*, 97–106.

Myers, S.A., Stergiou, N., Pipinos, I.I., and Johanning, J.M. (2010). Gait variability patterns are altered in healthy young individuals during the acute reperfusion phase of ischemia-reperfusion. *Journal of Surgical Research, 164(1)*, 6–12.

Nagarajan, R. (2002). Quantifying physiological data with Lempel-Ziv complexity—Certain issues. *IEEE Transactions in Biomedical Engineering, 49(11)*, 1371–1373.

National Center for Biotechnology Information, U.S. National Library of Medicine. (2015). *pubmed.gov.* http://www.ncbi.nlm.nih.gov/pubmed, accessed August 27, 2015.

Norris, P.R., Anderson, S.M., Jenkins, J.M., Williams, A.E., and Morris, J.A. Jr. (2008). Heart rate multiscale entropy at three hours predicts hospital mortality in 3,154 trauma patients. *Shock, 30(1)*, 17–22.

Papaioannou, V.E., Chouvarda, I.G., Maglaveras, N.K., and Pneumatikos, I.A. (2011). Study of multiparameter respiratory pattern complexity in surgical critically ill patients during weaning trials. *BMC Physiology, 11*, 2.

Pau, M., Kim, S., and Nussbaum, M.A. (2012). Does load carriage differentially alter postural sway in overweight vs. normal-weight schoolchildren? *Gait and Posture, 35(3)*, 378–382.

Peev, M.P., Naraghi, L., Chang, Y., Demoya, M., Fagenholz, P., Yeh, D., Velmahos, G., and King, D.R. (2013). Real-time sample entropy predicts life-saving interventions after the Boston Marathon bombing. *Journal of Critical Care, 28(6)*, e1–e4.

Perlmutter, S., Lin, F., and Makhsous, M. (2010). Quantitative analysis of static sitting posture in chronic stroke. *Gait and Posture, 32(1)*, 53–56.

Pham, T.D. and Ichikawa, K. (2013). Spatial chaos and complexity in the intracellular space of cancer and normal cells. *Theoretical Biology & Medical Modelling, 10(1)*, 62.

Pincus, S. (1995). Approximate entropy (ApEn) as a complexity measure. *Chaos, 5(1)*, 110–117.

Pincus, S. and Huang, W. (1992). Approximate entropy—Statistical properties and applications. *Communications in Statistical Theory Methods, 21*, 3061–3077.

Pincus, S. and Kalman, R.E. (1997). Not all (possibly) "random" sequences are created equal. *Proceedings of the National Academy of Sciences, 94(8)*, 3513–3518.

Pincus, S. and Singer, B.H. (1995). Randomness and degrees of irregularity. *Proceedings of the National Academy of Sciences of the United States of America, 93*, 2083–2088.

Pincus, S.M. (1991). Approximate entropy as a measure of system complexity. *Proceedings of the National Academy of Sciences of the United States of America, 88*, 2297–2301.

Pincus, S.M. (1998). Approximate entropy (ApEn) as a regularity measure. In *Applications of Nonlinear Dynamics to Developmental Process Modeling*. Eds.: Newell, K.M. and Molenaar, P.C.M. Mahwah, NJ: Lawrence Erlbaum Associates.

Pincus, S.M., Gladstone, I.M., and Ehrenkranz, R.A. (1991). A regularity statistic for medical data analysis. *Journal of Clinical Monitoring, 7(4)*, 335–345.

Pincus, S.M. and Goldberger, A.L. (1994). Physiological time-series analysis: What does regularity quantify? *American Journal of Physiology—Heart and Circulatory Physiology, 266(4)*, H1643–H1656.

Pincus, S.M., Mulligan, T., Iranmanesh, A., Gheorghiu, S., Godschalk, M., and Vedlhuis, J.D. (1996). Older males secrete luteinizing hormone and testosterone more irregularly, and jointly more asynchronously, than younger males. *Proceedings of the National Academy of Sciences of the United States of America, 93*, 14100–14105.

Platisa, M.M., Mazic, S., Nestorovic, Z., and Gal, V. (2008). Complexity of heartbeat interval series in young healthy trained and untrained men. *Physiological Measures, 29(4)*, 439–450.

Platisa, M.M., Nestorovic, Z., Damjanovic, S., and Gal, V. (2006). Linear and non-linear heart rate variability measures in chronic and acute phase of anorexia nervosa. *Clinical Physiology and Functional Imaging, 26(1)*, 54–60.

Popivanov, D., Dushanova, J., and Sauleva, Z. (2001). Nonlinear EEG dynamics during imagined self-paced movements. *Acta Physiologica et Pharmacologica Bulgarica, 26(1–2)*, 119–122.

Porta, A., Baselli, G., Liberati, D., Montano, N., Cogliati, C., Gnecchi-Ruscone, T., Malliani, A., and Cerutti, S. (1998). Measuring regularity by means of a corrected conditional entropy in sympathetic outflow. *Biological Cybernetics, 78(1)*, 71–78.

Public database. (2011). Physionet.org. http://www.physionet.org/, accessed August 27, 2015.

Rényi, A. (1961). On measures of entropy and information. *Proceedings of the Fourth Berkeley Symposium on Mathematics, Statistics and Probability*, Vol. *1*. Berkeley, CA: University of California Press, pp. 547–561.

Richman, J.S. and Moorman, J.R. (2000). Physiological time series analysis using approximate entropy and sample entropy. *American Journal of Physiology: Heart and Circulatory Physiology, 278*, H2039–H2049.

Riedl, M., Muller, A., Wessel, N. (2013). Practical considerations of permutation entropy. *European Physical Journal-Special Topics, 222*(2), 249–262.

Riley, M.A., Balaubrahanian, R., and Turvey, M.T. (1999). Recurrence quantification analysis of postural fluctuations. *Gait and Posture, 9*, 65–78.

Rukhin, A.L. (2000). Approximate entropy for testing randomness. *Journal of Applied Probability, 37*, 88–100.

Sarà, M., Sebastiano, F., Sacco, S., Pistoia, F., Onorati, P., Albertini, G., and Carolei, A. (2008). Heart rate non linear dynamics in patients with persistent vegetative state: A preliminary report. *Brain Injury, 22*(1), 33–37.

Sarlabous, L., Torres, A., Fiz, J.A., Gea, J., Martinez-Llorens, J., Morera, J., and Jane, R. (2010). Interpretation of the approximate entropy using fixed tolerance values as a measure of amplitude variations in biomedical signals. *Conference Proceedings of IEEE Engineering in Medicine and Biology Society,* Buenos Aires, *2010,* pp. 5967–5970.

Schneider, G., Hollweck, R., Ningler, M., Stockmanns, G., and Kochs, E.F. (2005). Detection of consciousness by electroencephalogram and auditory evoked potentials. *Anesthesiology, 103*(5), 934–943.

Schniepp, R., Wuehr, M., Pradhan, C., Novozhilov, S., Krafczyk, S., Brandt, T., and Jahn, K. (2013). Nonlinear variability of body sway in patients with phobic postural vertigo. *Frontiers in Neurology, 4,* 115.

Shalbaf, R., Behnam, H., Sleigh, J.W., Steyn-Ross, A., and Voss, L.J. (2013). Monitoring the depth of anesthesia using entropy features and an artificial neural network. *Journal of Neuroscience Methods, 218*(1), 17–24.

Shannon, C.E. (1948a). A mathematical theory of communication. *Bell System Technical Journal, 27,* 379–423.

Shannon, C.E. (1948b). A mathematical theory of communication. *Bell System Technical Journal, 27,* 623–656.

Shin, D.G., Yoo, C.S., Yi, S.H., Bae, J.H., Kim, Y.J., Park, J.S., and Hong, G.R. (2006). Prediction of paroxysmal atrial fibrillation using nonlinear analysis of the R-R interval dynamics before the spontaneous onset of atrial fibrillation. *Circulation Journal, 70*(1), 94–99.

Signorini, M.G., Ferrario, M., Marchetti, M., and Marseglia, A. (2006). Nonlinear analysis of heart rate variability signal for the characterization of cardiac heart failure patients. *Conference Proceedings of IEEE Engineering in Medicine and Biology Society,* New York, NY, Vol. *1,* pp. 3431–3434.

Sleigh, J.W. (1999). Postoperative respiratory arrhythmias: Incidence and measurement. *Acta Anaesthesiologica Scandinavica, 43*(7), 708–714.

Sokunbi, M.O., Fung, W., Sawlani, V., Choppin, S., Linden, D.E., and Thome, J. (2013). Resting state fMRI entropy probes complexity of brain activity in adults with ADHD. *Psychiatry Research, 214*(3), 341–348.

Song, Y., Crowcroft, J., and Zhang, J. (2012). Automatic epileptic seizure detection in EEGs based on optimized sample entropy and extreme learning machine. *Journal of Neuroscience Methods, 210*(2), 132–146.

Sosnoff, J.J., Broglio, S.P., Shin, S., and Ferrara, M.S. (2011). Previous mild traumatic brain injury and postural-control dynamics. *Journal of Athletic Training, 46*(1), 85–91.

Stam, C.J., Jelles, B., Achtereekte, H.A., Rombouts, S.A., Slaets, J.P., and Keunen, R.W. (1995). Investigation of EEG non-linearity in dementia and Parkinson's disease. *Electroencephalography and Clinical Neurophysiology, 95*(5), 309–317.

Stergiou, N. and Decker, L.M. (2011). Human movement variability, nonlinear dynamics, and pathology: Is there a connection? *Human Movement Science, 30*(5), 869–888.

Stergiou, N., Harbourne, R.T., and Cavanaugh, J.T. (2006). Optimal movement variability: A new theoretical perspective for neurologic physical therapy. *Journal of Neurologic Physical Therapy, 30*(3), 120–129.

Stewart, I. (2002). *Does God Play Dice: The New Mathematics of Chaos*. Malden, MA: Blackwell.

Stins, J.F., Michielsen, M.E., Roerdink, M., and Beek, P.J. (2009). Sway regularity reflects attentional involvement in postural control: Effects of expertise, vision and cognition. *Gait and Posture, 30(1)*, 106–109.

Svensson, J., Johannsson, G., Iranmanesh, A., Albertsson-Wikland, K., Veldhuis, J.D., and Bengtsson, B.A. (2006). GH secretory pattern in young adults who discontinued GH treatment for GH deficiency and decreased longitudinal growth in childhood. *European Journal of Endocrinology, 155(1)*, 91–99.

Talebi, N., Nasrabadi, A.M., and Curran, T. (2012). Investigation of changes in EEG complexity during memory retrieval: The effect of midazolam. *Cognitive Neurodynamics, 6(6)*, 537–546.

Tobaldini, E., Porta, A., Bulgheroni, M., Pecis, M., Muratori, M, Bevilacqua, M, and Montano, N. (2008). Increased complexity of short-term heart rate variability in hyperthyroid patients during orthostatic challenge. *Conference Proceedings of IEEE Engineering in Medicine and Biology Society,* Vancouver, BC, *2008*, pp. 1988–1991.

Tran, Y., Wijesuryia, N., Thuraisingham, R.A., Craig, A., and Nguyen, H.T. (2008). Increase in regularity and decrease in variability seen in electroencephalography (EEG) signals from alert to fatigue during a driving simulated task. *Conference Proceedings of IEEE Engineering in Medicine and Biology Society,* Vancouver, BC, *2008*, pp. 1096–1099.

Trunkvalterova, Z., Javorka, M., Tonhajzerova, I., Javorkova, J., Lazarova, Z., Javorka, K., and Baumert, M. (2008). Reduced short-term complexity of heart rate and blood pressure dynamics in patients with diabetes mellitus type 1: Multiscale entropy analysis. *Physiological Measurement, 29(7)*, 817–828.

Vaillancourt, D.E. and Newell, K.M. (2002a). Changing complexity in human behavior and physiology through aging and disease. *Neurobiology of Aging, 23(1)*, 1–11.

Vaillancourt, D.E. and Newell, K.M. (2002b). Complexity in aging and disease: Response to commentaries. *Neurobiology of Aging, 23(1)*, 27–29.

Van Drongelen, W., Nayak, S., Frim, D.M., Kohrman, M.H., Towle, V.L., Lee, H.C., McGee, A.B., Chico, M.S., and Hecox, K.E. (2003). Seizure anticipation in pediatric epilepsy: Use of Kolmogorov entropy. *Pediatric Neurology, 29(3)*, 207–213.

Van Leeuwen, P., Cysarz, D., Lange, S., and Grönemeyer, D. (2006). Increase in regularity of fetal heart rate variability with age. *Biomedizinische Technik (Berlin), 51(4)*, 244–247.

Van Leeuwen, P., Cysarz, D., Lange, S., Geue, D., and Groenemeyer, D. (2007). Quantification of fetal heart rate regularity using symbolic dynamics. *Chaos, 17(1)*, 015119.

Varela, M., Calvo, M., Chana, M., Gomez-Mestre, I., Asensio, R., and Galdos, P. (2005). Clinical implications of temperature curve complexity in critically ill patients. *Critical Care Medicine, 33(12)*, 2764–2771.

Varela, M., Churruca, J., Gonzalez, A., Martin, A., Ode, J., and Galdos, P. (2006). Temperature curve complexity predicts survival in critically ill patients. *American Journal of Respiratory and Critical Care Medicine, 174(3)*, 290–298.

Varela, M., Jimenez, L., and Fariña, R. (2003). Complexity analysis of the temperature curve: New information from body temperature. *European Journal of Applied Physiology, 89(3–4)*, 230–237.

Veiga, J., Lopes, A.J., Jansen, J.M., and Melo, P.L. (2011). Airflow pattern complexity and airway obstruction in asthma. *Journal of Applied Physiology, 111*, 412–419.

Veldhuis, J.D. and Pincus, S.M. (1998). Orderliness of hormone release patterns: A complementary measure to conventional pulsatile and circadian analyses. *European Journal of Endocrinology, 138*, 358–362.

Veldman, R.G., Frölich, M., Pincus, S.M., Veldhuis, J.D., and Roelfsema, F. (2000). Growth hormone and prolactin are secreted more irregularly in patients with Cushing's disease. *Clinical Endocrinology, 52(5)*, 625–632.

Von Neumann, J. (1996). *Mathematical Foundations of Quantum Mechanics*. Princeton, NJ: Princeton University Press.

Vuksanović, V. and Gal, V. (2005). Nonlinear and chaos characteristics of heart period time series: Healthy aging and postural change. *Autonomic Neuroscience: Basic & Clinical, 121(1–2)*, 94–100.

Waters, D.L., Qualls, C.R., Dorin, R.I., Veldhuis, J.D., and Baumgartner, R.N. (2008). Altered growth hormone, cortisol, and leptin secretion in healthy elderly persons with sarcopenia and mixed body composition phenotypes. *Journal of Gerontology A Biological Sciences and Medical Sciences, 63(5)*, 536–541.

Weinstein, M., Gorrindo, T., Riley, A., Mormino, J., Niedfeldt, J., Singer, B., Rodríguez, G., Simon, J., and Pincus, S. (2003). Timing of menopause and patterns of menstrual bleeding. *American Journal of Epidemiology, 158(8)*, 782–791.

White, C.E., Batchinsky, A.I., Necsoiu, C., Nguyen, R., Walker, K.P., Chung, K.K., Wolf, S.E., and Cancio, L.C. (2010). Lower interbreath interval complexity is associated with extubation failure in mechanically ventilated patients during spontaneous breathing trials. *Journal of Trauma, 68(6)*, 1310–1316.

Yamauchi, M., Tamaki, S., Yoshikawa, M., Ohnishi, Y., Nakano, H., Jacono, F.J., Loparo, K.A., Strohl, K.P., and Kimura, H. (2011). Differences in breathing patterning during wakefulness in patients with mixed apnea-dominant vs obstructive-dominant sleep apnea. *Chest, 140(1)*, 54–61.

Yentes, J.M., Hunt, N., Schmid, K.K., Kaipust, J.P., McGrath, D., and Stergiou, N. (2013). The appropriate use of approximate entropy and sample entropy with short data sets. *Annals of Biomedical Engineering, 41(2)*, 349–365.

Yeragani, V.K., Pohl, R., Mallavarapu, M., and Balon, R. (2003). Approximate entropy of symptoms of mood: An effective technique to quantify regularity of mood. *Bipolar Disorders, 5(4)*, 279–286.

Zhang, X.S. and Roy, R.J. (1999). Predicting movement during anaesthesia by complexity analysis of electroencephalograms. *Medical & Biological Engineering & Computing, 37(3)*, 327–334.

Zyczkowski, K. (2003). Renyi extrapolation of Shannon entropy. *Open Systems and Information Dynamics, 10*, 297–310.

READING LIST: CARDIOLOGY

Acharya, U.R., Kannathal, N., Sing, O.W., Ping, L.Y., and Chua, T. (2004). Heart rate analysis in normal subjects of various age groups. *Biomedical Engineering Online, 3(1)*, 24.

Bajaj, N., Joshua Leon, L., Kimber, S., and Vigmond, E. (2005a). Fibrillation complexity as a predictor of successful defibrillation. *Conference Proceedings: Annual International Conference of the IEEE Engineering in Medicine and Biology Society*, Shanghai, Vol. 7, pp. 7208–7211.

Bajaj, N., Joshua Leon, L., Vigmond, E., and Kimber, S. (2005b). Fibrillation complexity as a predictor of successful defibrillation. *Conference Proceedings: Annual International Conference of the IEEE Engineering in Medicine and Biology Society*, Shanghai, Vol. 1, pp. 768–771.

Batchinsky, A.I., Cancio, L.C., Salinas, J., Kuusela, T., Cooke, W.H., Wang, J.J., Boehme, M., Convertino, V.A., and Holcomb, J.B. (2007a). Prehospital loss of R-to-R interval complexity is associated with mortality in trauma patients. *Journal of Trauma, 63(3)*, 512–518.

Batchinsky, A.I., Cooke, W.H., Kuusela, T., and Cancio, L.C. (2007b). Loss of complexity characterizes the heart rate response to experimental hemorrhagic shock in swine. *Critical Care Medicine, 35(2)*, 519–525.

Batchinsky, A.I., Wolf, S.E., Molter, N., Kuusela, T., Jones, J.A., Moraru, C., Boehme, M. et al. (2008). Assessment of cardiovascular regulation after burns by nonlinear analysis of the electrocardiogram. *Journal of Burn Care & Research, 29(1)*, 56–63.

Beckers, F., Verheyden, B., and Aubert, A.E. (2006a). Aging and nonlinear heart rate control in a healthy population. *American Journal of Physiology Heart and Circulatory Physiology, 290(6)*, H2560– H2570.

Beckers, F., Verheyden, B., Ramaekers, D., Swynghedauw, B., and Aubert, A.E. (2006b). Effects of autonomic blockade on non-linear cardiovascular variability indices in rats. *Clinical and Experimental Pharmacology and Physiology, 33(5–6)*, 431–439.

Bien, H., Yin, L., and Entcheva, E. (2006). Calcium instabilities in mammalian cardiomyocyte networks. *Biophysical Journal, 90(7)*, 2628–2640.

Bolanos, M., Nazeran, H., and Haltiwanger, E. (2006). Comparison of heart rate variability signal features derived from electrocardiography and photoplethysmography in healthy individuals. *Conference Proceedings: Annual International Conference of the IEEE Engineering in Medicine and Biology Society*, New York, NY, Vol. *1*, pp. 4289–4294.

Chaffin, D.G. Jr., Barnard, J.M., Phernetton, T., and Reed, K.L. (1998). Decreased approximate entropy of heart rate variability in the hypoxic ovine fetus. *Journal of Maternal-Fetal Investigation, 8(1)*, 23–26.

Chan, H.L., Lin, L.Y., Lin, M.A., Fang, S.C., and Lin, C.H. (2007). Nonlinear characteristics of heart rate variability during unsupervised and steady physical activities. *Physiological Measurement, 28(3)*, 277–286.

Chatlapalli, S., Nazeran, H., Melarkod, V., Krishnam, R., Estrada, E., Pamula, Y., and Cabrera, S. (2004). Accurate derivation of heart rate variability signal for detection of sleep disordered breathing in children. *Conference Proceedings: Annual International Conference of the IEEE Engineering in Medicine and Biology Society*, San Francisco, CA, Vol. *1*, pp. 538–541.

Comani, S., Srinivasan, V., Alleva, G., and Romani, G.L. (2007). Entropy-based automated classification of independent components separated from fMCG. *Physics in Medicine and Biology, 52(5)*, N87–N97.

Cysarz, D., Bettermann, H., and van Leeuwen, P. (2000). Entropies of short binary sequences in heart period dynamics. *American Journal of Physiology Heart and Circulatory Physiology, 278(6)*, H2163–H2172.

Cysarz, D., Lange, S., Matthiessen, P.F., and Leeuwen, P. (2007). Regular heartbeat dynamics are associated with cardiac health. *American Journal of Physiology: Regulatory, Integrative and Comparative Physiology, 292(1)*, R368–R372.

Dawes, G.S., Moulden, M., Sheil, O., and Redman, C.W. (1992). Approximate entropy, a statistic of regularity, applied to fetal heart rate data before and during labor. *Obstetrics and Gynecology, 80(5)*, 763–768.

Ferrario, M., Signorini, M.G., and Magenes, G. (2007). Comparison between fetal heart rate standard parameters and complexity indexes for the identification of severe intrauterine growth restriction. *Methods of Information in Medicine, 46(2)*, 186–190.

Ferrario, M., Signorini, M.G., Magenes, G., and Cerutti, S. (2006). Comparison of entropy-based regularity estimators: Application to the fetal heart rate signal for the identification of fetal distress. *IEEE Transactions on Biomedical Engineering, 53(1)*, 119–125.

Fleisher, L.A., Dipietro, J.A., Johnson, T.R., and Pincus, S. (1997). Complementary and non-coincident increases in heart rate variability and irregularity during fetal development. *Clinical Science, 92(4)*, 345–349.

Fleisher, L.A., Fleckenstein, J.F., Frank, S.M., and Thuluvath, P.J. (2000). Heart rate variability as a predictor of autonomic dysfunction in patients awaiting liver transplantation. *Digestive Diseases and Sciences, 45(2)*, 340–344.

Fleisher, L.A., Pincus, S.M., and Rosenbaum, S.H. (1993). Approximate entropy of heart rate as a correlate of postoperative ventricular dysfunction. *Anesthesiology, 78(4)*, 683–692.

Fukuta, H., Hayano, J., Ishihara, S., Sakata, S., Ohte, N., Takahashi, H., Yokoya, M. et al. (2003). Prognostic value of nonlinear heart rate dynamics in hemodialysis patients with coronary artery disease. *Kidney International, 64*(2), 641–648.

Garde, S., Regalado, M.G., Schechtman, V.L., and Khoo, M.C. (2001). Nonlinear dynamics of heart rate variability in cocaine-exposed neonates during sleep. *American Journal of Physiology Heart and Circulatory Physiology, 280*(6), H2920–H2928.

Godin, P.J., Fleisher, L.A., Eidsath, A., Vandivier, R.W., Preas, H.L., Banks, S.M., Buchman, T.G., and Suffredini, A.F. (1996). Experimental human endotoxemia increases cardiac regularity: Results from a prospective, randomized, crossover trial. *Critical Care Medicine, 24*(7), 1117–1124.

Goldberger, A.L., Mietus, J.E., Rigney, D.R., Wood, M.L., and Fortney, S.M. (1994). Effects of head-down bed rest on complex heart rate variability: Response to LBNP testing. *Journal of Applied Physiology, 77*(6), 2863–2869.

Gonçalves, H., Bernardes, J., Rocha, A.P., and Ayres-de-Campos, D. (2007). Linear and nonlinear analysis of heart rate patterns associated with fetal behavioral states in the antepartum period. *Early Human Development, 83*(9), 585–591.

Gonçalves, H., Rocha, A.P., Ayres-de-Campos, D., and Bernardes, J. (2006). Internal versus external intrapartum foetal heart rate monitoring: The effect on linear and nonlinear parameters. *Physiological Measurement, 27*(3), 307–319.

Groome, L.J., Mooney, D.M., Holland, S.B., Smith, L.A., Atterbury, J.L., and Loizou, P.C. (1999). Human fetuses have nonlinear cardiac dynamics. *Journal of Applied Physiology, 87*(2), 530–537.

Hamzei, A., Ohara, T., Kim, Y.H., Lee, M.H., Voroshilovski, O., Lin, S.F., Weiss, J.N., Chen, P.S., and Karagueuzian, H.S. (2002). The role of approximate entropy in predicting ventricular defibrillation threshold. *Journal of Cardiovascular Pharmacology and Therapeutics, 7*(1), 45–52.

Ho, K.K., Moody, G.B., Peng, C.K., Mietus, J.E., Larson, M.G., Levy, D., and Goldberger, A.L. (1997). Predicting survival in heart failure case and control subjects by use of fully automated methods for deriving nonlinear and conventional indices of heart rate dynamics. *Circulation, 96*(3), 842–848.

Hogue, C.W. Jr., Domitrovich, P.P., Stein, P.K., Despotis, G.D., Re, L., Schuessler, R.B., Kleiger, R.E., and Rottman, J.N. (1998). RR interval dynamics before atrial fibrillation in patients after coronary artery bypass graft surgery. *Circulation, 98*(5), 429–434.

Hoh, J.K., Park, Y.S., Cha, K.J., Oh, J.E., Lee, H.J., Lee, G.T., and Park, M.I. (2007). Chaotic indices and canonical ensemble of heart rate patterns in small-for-gestational age fetuses. *Journal of Perinatal Medicine, 35*(3), 210–216.

Hoyer, D., Pompe, B., Chon, K.H., Hardraht, H., Wicher, C., and Zwiener, U. (2005). Mutual information function assesses autonomic information flow of heart rate dynamics at different time scales. *IEEE Transactions on Biomedical Engineering, 52*(4), 584–592.

Huikuri, H.V., Mäkikallio, T.H., and Perkiömäki, J. (2003). Measurement of heart rate variability by methods based on nonlinear dynamics. *Journal of Electrocardiology, 36*(Suppl), 95–99.

Huikuri, H.V., Poutiainen, A.M., Mäkikallio, T.H., Koistinen, M.J., Airaksinen, K.E., Mitrani, R.D., Myerburg, R.J., and Castellanos, A. (1999). Dynamic behavior and autonomic regulation of ectopic atrial pacemakers. *Circulation, 100*(13), 1416–1422.

Jartti, T.T., Kuusela, T.A., Kaila, T.J., Tahvanainen, K.U., and Välimäki, I.A. (1998). The dose-response effects of terbutaline on the variability, approximate entropy and fractal dimension of heart rate and blood pressure. *British Journal of Clinical Pharmacology, 45*(3), 277–285.

Jokinen, V., Sourander, L.B., Karanko, H., Mäkikallio, T.H., and Huikuri, H.V. (2005). Changes in cardiovascular autonomic regulation among elderly subjects: Follow-up of sixteen years. *Annals of Medicine, 37*(3), 206–212.

Jokinen, V., Syvänne, M., Mäkikallio, T.H., Airaksinen, K.E., and Huikuri, H.V. (2001). Temporal age-related changes in spectral, fractal and complexity characteristics of heart rate variability. *Clinical Physiology, 21(3)*, 273–281.

Kim, H.S., Kim, C.S., and Yum, M.K. (1999). Abnormal cardiac autonomic activity and complexity in newly diagnosed and untreated hypertensive patients after general anesthesia. *Clinical and Experimental Hypertension, 21(8)*, 1357–1372.

Kim, J.S., Park, J.E., Seo, J.D., Lee, W.R., Kim, H.S., Noh, J.I., Kim, N.S., and Yum, M.K. (2000). Decreased entropy of symbolic heart rate dynamics during daily activity as a predictor of positive head-up tilt test in patients with alleged neurocardiogenic syncope. *Physics in Medicine and Biology, 45(11)*, 3403–3412.

Kim, W.S., Yoon, Y.Z., Bae, J.H., and Soh, K.S. (2005). Nonlinear characteristics of heart rate time series: Influence of three recumbent positions in patients with mild or severe coronary artery disease. *Physiological Measurement, 26(4)*, 517–529.

Korpelainen, J.T., Sotaniemi, K.A., Mäkikallio, A., Huikuri, H.V., and Myllylä, V.V. (1999). Dynamic behavior of heart rate in ischemic stroke. *Stroke, 30(5)*, 1008–1013.

Krstacic, G., Krstacic, A., Smalcelj, A., Milicic, D., and Jembrek-Gostovic, M. (2007). The "Chaos Theory" and nonlinear dynamics in heart rate variability analysis: Does it work in short-time series in patients with coronary heart disease? *Annals of Noninvasive Electrocardiology, 12(2)*, 130–136.

Kubo, Y., Murakami, S., Matsuoka, O., Hotta, N., Oinuma, S., Shinagawa, M., Omori, K. et al. (2003). Toward chronocardiologic and chronomic insights: Dynamics of heart rate associated with head-up tilting. *Biomedicine & Pharmacotherapy, 57(Suppl 1)*, 110s–115s.

Kul Yum, M. and Su Kim, N. (1997). Change of complex and periodic heart rate dynamics with change of pulmonary artery pressure in infants with left-to-right shunt lesion. *International Journal of Cardiology, 60(2)*, 143–150.

Kuo, T.B. and Yang, C.C. (2002). Sexual dimorphism in the complexity of cardiac pacemaker activity. *American Journal of Physiology Heart and Circulatory Physiology, 283(4)*, H1695–H1702.

Laitio, T.T., Huikuri, H.V., Kentala, E.S., Mäkikallio, T.H., Jalonen, J.R., Helenius, H., Sariola-Heinonen, K., Yli-Mäyry, S., and Scheinin, H. (2000). Correlation properties and complexity of perioperative RR-interval dynamics in coronary artery bypass surgery patients. *Anesthesiology, 93(1)*, 69–80.

Laitio, T.T., Huikuri, H.V., Koskenvuo, J., Jalonen, J., Mäkikallio, T.H., Helenius, H., Kentala, E.S., Hartiala, J., and Scheinin, H. (2006). Long-term alterations of heart rate dynamics after coronary artery bypass graft surgery. *Anesthesia and Analgesia, 102(4)*, 1026–1031.

Lake, D.E. (2006). Renyi entropy measures of heart rate Gaussianity. *IEEE Transactions on Biomedical Engineering, 53(1)*, 21–27.

Lake, D.E., Richman, J.S., Griffin, M.P., and Moorman, J.R. (2002). Sample entropy analysis of neonatal heart rate variability. *American Journal of Physiology: Regulatory, Integrative and Comparative Physiology, 283(3)*, R789–R797.

Landry, D.P., Bennett, F.M., and Oriol, N.E. (1994). Analysis of heart rate dynamics as a measure of autonomic tone in obstetrical patients undergoing epidural or spinal anesthesia. *Regional Anesthesia, 19(3)*, 189–195.

Lange, S., Van Leeuwen, P., Geue, D., Hatzmann, W., and Grönemeyer, D. (2005). Influence of gestational age, heart rate, gender and time of day on fetal heart rate variability. *Medical and Biological Engineering and Computing, 43(4)*, 481–486.

Larsen, P.D. and Galletly, D.C. (2001). Cardioventilatory coupling in heart rate variability: The value of standard analytical techniques. *British Journal of Anaesthesia, 87(6)*, 819–826.

Lee, J., Lee, Y.W., and Warwick, W.J. (2007). High frequency chest compression effects heart rate variability. *Conference Proceedings: Annual International Conference of the IEEE Engineering in Medicine and Biology Society, Lyon, 2007*, pp. 1066–1069.

Lee, M.S., Rim, Y.H., Jeong, D.M., Kim, M.K., Joo, M.C., and Shin, S.H. (2005a). Nonlinear analysis of heart rate variability during Qi therapy (external Qigong). *American Journal of Chinese Medicine, 33*(4), 579–588.

Lee, M.S., Shin, B.C., Rim, Y.H., and Woo, W.H. (2005b). Effects of Korean traditional herbal remedy on heart rate variability: Linear and nonlinear analysis. *International Journal of Neuroscience, 115*(3), 393–403.

Li, X., Zheng, D., Zhou, S., Tang, D., Wang, C., and Wu, G. (2005). Approximate entropy of fetal heart rate variability as a predictor of fetal distress in women at term pregnancy. *Acta Obstetricia et Gynecologica Scandinavica, 84*(9), 837–843.

Lin, L.Y., Lin, J.L., Du, C.C., Lai, L.P., Tseng, Y.Z., and Huang, S.K. (2001). Reversal of deteriorated fractal behavior of heart rate variability by beta-blocker therapy in patients with advanced congestive heart failure. *Journal of Cardiovascular Electrophysiology, 12*(1), 26–32.

Lipsitz, L.A. (1995). Age-related changes in the "complexity" of cardiovascular dynamics: A potential marker of vulnerability to disease. *Chaos, 5*(1), 102–109.

Lipsitz, L.A., Pincus, S.M., Morin, R.J., Tong, S., Eberle, L.P., and Gootman, P.M. (1997). Preliminary evidence for the evolution in complexity of heart rate dynamics during autonomic maturation in neonatal swine. *Journal of the Autonomic Nervous System, 65*(1), 1–9.

Lopera, G., Castellanos, A., Moleiro, F., Huikuri, H.V., and Myerburg, R.J. (2003). Chronic inappropriate sinus tachycardia in elderly females. *Annals of Noninvasive Electrocardiology, 8*(2), 139–143.

Lu, S., Zhao, H., Ju, K., Shin, K., Lee, M., Shelley, K., and Chon, K.H. (2008). Can photoplethysmography variability serve as an alternative approach to obtain heart rate variability information? *Journal of Clinical Monitoring and Computing, 22*(1), 23–29.

Mäenpää, M., Penttilä, J., Laitio, T., Kaisti, K., Kuusela, T., Hinkka, S., and Scheinin, H. (2007). The effects of surgical levels of sevoflurane and propofol anaesthesia on heart rate variability. *European Journal of Anaesthesiology, 24*(7), 626–633.

Magenes, G., Signorini, M.G., Arduini, D., and Cerutti, S. (2004). Fetal heart rate variability due to vibroacoustic stimulation: Linear and nonlinear contribution. *Methods of Information in Medicine, 43*(1), 47–51.

Mäkikallio, T.H., Ristimäe, T., Airaksinen, K.E., Peng, C.K., Goldberger, A.L., and Huikuri, H.V. (1998). Heart rate dynamics in patients with stable angina pectoris and utility of fractal and complexity measures. *American Journal of Cardiology, 81*(1), 27–31.

Mäkikallio, T.H., Seppänen, T., Niemelä, M., Airaksinen, K.E., Tulppo, M., and Huikuri, H.V. (1996). Abnormalities in beat to beat complexity of heart rate dynamics in patients with a previous myocardial infarction. *Journal of the American College of Cardiology, 28*(4), 1005–1011.

Moraru, L., Cimponeriu, L., Tong, S., Thakor, N., and Bezerianos, A. (2004). Characterization of heart rate variability changes following asphyxia in rats. *Methods of Information in Medicine, 43*(1), 118–121.

Moraru, L., Tong, S., Malhotra, A., Geocadin, R., Thakor, N., and Bezerianos, A. (2005). Investigation of the effects of ischemic preconditioning on the HRV response to transient global ischemia using linear and nonlinear methods. *Medical Engineering & Physics, 27*(6), 465–473.

Nazeran, H., Chatlapalli, S., and Krishnam, R. (2005). Effect of novel nanoscale energy patches on spectral and nonlinear dynamic features of heart rate variability signals in healthy individuals during rest and exercise. *Conference Proceedings: Annual International Conference of the IEEE Engineering in Medicine and Biology Society*, Shanghai, Vol. 5, pp. 5563–5567.

Nazeran, H., Krishnam, R., Chatlapalli, S., Pamula, Y., Haltiwanger, E., and Cabrera, S. (2006). Nonlinear dynamics analysis of heart rate variability signals to detect sleep disordered breathing in children. *Conference Proceedings: Annual International Conference of the IEEE Engineering in Medicine and Biology Society*, New York, NY, Vol. 1, pp. 3873–3878.

Nelson, J.C., Rizwan-uddin, Griffin, M.P., and Moorman, J.R. (1998). Probing the order within neonatal heart rate variability. *Pediatric Research, 43*(6), 823–831.

Newlin, D.B., Wong, C.J., Stapleton, J.M., and London, E.D. (2000). Intravenous cocaine decreases cardiac vagal tone, vagal index (derived in Lorenz space), and heart period complexity (approximate entropy) in cocaine abusers. *Neuropsychopharmacology, 23*(5), 560–568.

Nikolopoulos, S., Alexandridi, A., Nikolakeas, S., and Manis, G. (2003). Experimental analysis of heart rate variability of long-recording electrocardiograms in normal subjects and patients with coronary artery disease and normal left ventricular function. *Journal of Biomedical Informatics, 36*(3), 202–217.

Ohara, T., Yashima, M., Hamzei, A., Favelyukis, M., Park, A., Kim, Y.H., Mandel, W.J., Chen, P.S., and Karagueuzian, H.S. (1999). Nicotine increases spatiotemporal complexity of ventricular fibrillation wavefront on the epicardial border zone of healed canine infarcts. *Journal of Cardiovascular Pharmacology and Therapeutics, 4*(2), 121–127.

Palazzolo, J.A., Estafanous, F.G., and Murray, P.A. (1998). Entropy measures of heart rate variation in conscious dogs. *American Journal of Physiology, 274*(4 Pt 2), H1099–H1105.

Papaioannou, T.G., Vlachopoulos, C., Ioakeimidis, N., Alexopoulos, N., and Stefanadis, C. (2006a). Nonlinear dynamics of blood pressure variability after caffeine consumption. *Clinical Medicine & Research, 4*(2), 114–118.

Papaioannou, V.E., Maglaveras, N., Houvarda, I., Antoniadou, E., and Vretzakis, G. (2006b). Investigation of altered heart rate variability, nonlinear properties of heart rate signals, and organ dysfunction longitudinally over time in intensive care unit patients. *Journal of Critical Care, 21*(1), 95–103; discussion 103–104.

Penttilä, J., Helminen, A., Jartti, T., Kuusela, T., Huikuri, H.V., Tulppo, M.P., and Scheinin, H. (2003). Effect of cardiac vagal outflow on complexity and fractal correlation properties of heart rate dynamics. *Autonomic and Autacoid Pharmacology, 23*(3), 173–179.

Perkiomaki, J.S., Couderc, J.P., Daubert, J.P., and Zareba, W. (2003). Temporal complexity of repolarization and mortality in patients with implantable cardioverter defibrillators. *Pacing and Clinical Electrophysiology, 26*(10), 1931–1936.

Perkiömäki, J.S., Mäkikallio, T.H., and Huikuri, H.V. (2005). Fractal and complexity measures of heart rate variability. *Clinical and Experimental Hypertension, 27*(2–3), 149–158.

Perkiomaki, J.S., Zareba, W., Badilini, F., and Moss, A.J. (2002). Influence of atropine on fractal and complexity measures of heart rate variability. *Annals of Noninvasive Electrocardiology, 7*(4), 326–331.

Perkiömäki, J.S., Zareba, W., Daubert, J.P., Couderc, J.P., Corsello, A., and Kremer, K. (2001). Fractal correlation properties of heart rate dynamics and adverse events in patients with implantable cardioverter-defibrillators. *American Journal of Cardiology, 88*(1), 17–22.

Pikkujämsä, S.M., Mäkikallio, T.H., Airaksinen, K.E., and Huikuri, H.V. (2001). Determinants and interindividual variation of R-R interval dynamics in healthy middle-aged subjects. *American Journal of Physiology Heart and Circulatory Physiology, 280*(3), H1400–H1406.

Pikkujämsä, S.M., Mäkikallio, T.H., Sourander, L.B., Räihä, I.J., Puukka, P., Skyttä, J., Peng, C.K., Goldberger, A.L., and Huikuri, H.V. (1999). Cardiac interbeat interval dynamics from childhood to senescence: Comparison of conventional and new measures based on fractals and chaos theory. *Circulation, 100*(4), 393–399.

Pincus, S.M., Cummins, T.R., and Haddad, G.G. (1993). Heart rate control in normal and aborted-SIDS infants. *American Journal of Physiology, 264*(3 Pt 2), R638–R646.

Pincus, S.M. and Minkin, M.J. (1998). Assessing sequential irregularity of both endocrine and heart rate rhythms. *Current Opinion in Obstetrics & Gynecology, 10*(4), 281–291.

Pincus, S.M. and Viscarello, R.R. (1992). Approximate entropy: A regularity measure for fetal heart rate analysis. *Obstetrics and Gynecology, 79(2)*, 249–255.

Podgoreanu, M.V., Stout, R.G., El-Moalem, H.E., and Silverman, D.G. (2002). Synchronous rhythmical vasomotion in the human cutaneous microvasculature during nonpulsatile cardiopulmonary bypass. *Anesthesiology, 97(5)*, 1110–1117.

Porta, A., Gnecchi-Ruscone, T., Tobaldini, E., Guzzetti, S., Furlan, R., and Montano, N. (2007). Progressive decrease of heart period variability entropy-based complexity during graded head-up tilt. *Journal of Applied Physiology, 103(4)*, 1143–1149.

Rassias, A.J., Holzberger, P.T., Givan, A.L., Fahrner, S.L., and Yeager, M.P. (2005). Decreased physiologic variability as a generalized response to human endotoxemia. *Critical Care Medicine, 33(3)*, 512–519.

Richman, J.S. and Moorman, J.R. (2000). Physiological time-series analysis using approximate entropy and sample entropy. *American Journal of Physiology Heart and Circulatory Physiology, 278(6)*, H2039–H2049.

Ryan, S.M., Goldberger, A.L., Pincus, S.M., Mietus, J., and Lipsitz, L.A. (1994). Gender- and age-related differences in heart rate dynamics: Are women more complex than men? *Journal of the American College of Cardiology, 24(7)*, 1700–1707.

Sapoznikov, D., Luria, M.H., and Gotsman, M.S. (1995). Detection of regularities in heart rate variations by linear and non-linear analysis: Power spectrum versus approximate entropy. *Computer Methods and Programs in Biomedicine, 48(3)*, 201–209.

Sarà, M., Sebastiano, F., Sacco, S., Pistoia, F., Onorati, P., Albertini, G., and Carolei, A. (2008). Heart rate non linear dynamics in patients with persistent vegetative state: A preliminary report. *Brain Injury, 22(1)*, 33–37.

Schuckers, S.A. (1998). Use of approximate entropy measurements to classify ventricular tachycardia and fibrillation. *Journal of Electrocardiology, 31(Suppl)*, 101–105.

Schoenenberger, A.W., Erne, P., Ammann, S., Perrig, M., Bürgi, U., and Stuck, A.E. (2008). Prediction of hypertensive crisis based on average, variability and approximate entropy of 24-h ambulatory blood pressure monitoring. *Journal of Human Hypertension, 22(1)*, 32–37.

Shin, D.G., Yoo, C.S., Yi, S.H., Bae, J.H., Kim, Y.J., Park, J.S., and Hong, G.R. (2006). Prediction of paroxysmal atrial fibrillation using nonlinear analysis of the R-R interval dynamics before the spontaneous onset of atrial fibrillation. *Circulation Journal, 70(1)*, 94–99.

Signorini, M.G. (2004). Nonlinear analysis of heart rate variability signal: Physiological knowledge and diagnostic indications. *Conference Proceedings: Annual International Conference of the IEEE Engineering in Medicine and Biology Society*, San Francisco, CA, Vol. 7, pp. 5407–5410.

Signorini, M.G., Ferrario, M., Marchetti, M., and Marseglia, A. (2006). Nonlinear analysis of heart rate variability signal for the characterization of cardiac heart failure patients. *Conference Proceedings: Annual International Conference of the IEEE Engineering in Medicine and Biology Society*, New York, NY, Vol. 1, pp. 3431–3434.

Signorini, M.G., Magenes, G., Cerutti, S., and Arduini, D. (2003). Linear and nonlinear parameters for the analysis of fetal heart rate signal from cardiotocographic recordings. *IEEE Transactions on Biomedical Engineering, 50(3)*, 365–374.

Sipinková, I., Hahn, G., Meyer, M., Tadlánek, M., and Hájek, J. (1997). Effect of respiration and posture on heart rate variability. *Physiological Research, 46(3)*, 173–179.

Snieder, H., van Doornen, L.J., Boomsma, D.I., and Thayer, J.F. (2007). Sex differences and heritability of two indices of heart rate dynamics: A twin study. *Twin Research and Human Genetics, 10(2)*, 364–372.

Srinivasan, K., Ashok, M.V., Vaz, M., and Yeragani, V.K. (2004). Effect of imipramine on linear and nonlinear measures of heart rate variability in children. *Pediatric Cardiology, 25(1)*, 20–25.

Storella, R.J., Horrow, J.C., and Polansky, M. (1999). Differences among heart rate variability measures after anesthesia and cardiac surgery. *Journal of Cardiothoracic and Vascular Anesthesia, 13*(4), 451–453.

Storella, R.J., Wood, H.W., Mills, K.M., Kanters, J.K., Højgaard, M.V., and Holstein-Rathlou, N.H. (1998). Approximate entropy and point correlation dimension of heart rate variability in healthy subjects. *Integrative Physiological and Behavioral Science, 33*(4), 315–320.

Tabor, Z., Michalski, J., and Rokita, E. (2004). Influence of 50 Hz magnetic field on human heart rate variability: Linear and nonlinear analysis. *Bioelectromagnetics, 25*(6), 474–480.

Tarkiainen, T.H., Kuusela, T.A., Tahvanainen, K.U., Hartikainen, J.E., Tiittanen, P., Timonen, K.L., and Vanninen, E.J. (2007). Comparison of methods for editing of ectopic beats in measurements of short-term non-linear heart rate dynamics. *Clinical Physiology and Functional Imaging, 27*(2), 126–133.

Thayer, J.F., Yonezawa, Y., and Sollers, J.J. 3rd (2000). A system for the ambulatory recording and analysis of nonlinear heart rate dynamics. *Biomedical Sciences Instrumentation, 36,* 295–299.

Toweill, D.L., Kovarik, W.D., Carr, R., Kaplan, D., Lai, S., Bratton, S., and Goldstein, B. (2003). Linear and nonlinear analysis of heart rate variability during propofol anesthesia for short-duration procedures in children. *Pediatric Critical Care Medicine, 4*(3), 308–314.

Tulppo, M.P., Hughson, R.L., Mäkikallio, T.H., Airaksinen, K.E., Seppänen, T., and Huikuri, H.V. (2001). Effects of exercise and passive head-up tilt on fractal and complexity properties of heart rate dynamics. *American Journal of Physiology Heart and Circulatory Physiology, 280*(3), H1081–H1087.

Tulppo, M.P., Mäkikallio, T.H., Takala, T.E., Seppänen, T., and Huikuri, H.V. (1996). Quantitative beat-to-beat analysis of heart rate dynamics during exercise. *American Journal of Physiology, 271*(1 Pt 2), H244–H252.

Van Leeuwen, P., Cysarz, D., Lange, S., Geue, D., and Groenemeyer, D. (2007a). Quantification of fetal heart rate regularity using symbolic dynamics. *Chaos, 17*(1), 015119.

Van Leeuwen, P., Cysarz, D., Lange, S., and Grönemeyer, D. (2006). Increase in regularity of fetal heart rate variability with age. *Biomedizinische Technik/Biomedical Engineering, 51*(4), 244–247.

Van Leeuwen, P., Lange, S., Geue, D., and Grönemeyer, D. (2007b). Heart rate variability in the fetus: A comparison of measures. *Biomedizinische Technik/Biomedical Engineering, 52*(1), 61–65.

Vigo, D.E., Castro, M.N., Dörpinghaus, A., Weidema, H., Cardinali, D.P., Siri, L.N., Rovira, B., Fahrer, R.D., Nogués, M., Leiguarda, R.C., and Guinjoan, S.M. (2007). Nonlinear analysis of heart rate variability in patients with eating disorders. *World Journal of Biological Psychiatry, 11,* 1–7.

Vigo, D.E., Nicola Siri, L., Ladrón De Guevara, M.S., Martínez-Martínez, J.A., Fahrer, R.D., Cardinali, D.P., Masoli, O., and Guinjoan, S.M. (2004). Relation of depression to heart rate nonlinear dynamics in patients > or =60 years of age with recent unstable angina pectoris or acute myocardial infarction. *American Journal of Cardiology, 93*(6), 756–760.

Vikman, S., Lindgren, K., Mäkikallio, T.H., Yli-Mäyry, S., Airaksinen, K.E., and Huikuri, H.V. (2005). Heart rate turbulence after atrial premature beats before spontaneous onset of atrial fibrillation. *Journal of the American College of Cardiology, 45*(2), 278–284.

Vikman, S., Mäkikallio, T.H., Yli-Mäyry, S., Nurmi, M., Airaksinen, K.E., and Huikuri, H.V. (2003). Heart rate variability and recurrence of atrial fibrillation after electrical cardioversion. *Annals of Medicine, 35*(1), 36–42.

Vikman, S., Mäkikallio, T.H., Yli-Mäyry, S., Pikkujämsä, S., Koivisto, A.M., Reinikainen, P., Airaksinen, K.E., and Huikuri, H.V. (1999). Altered complexity and correlation properties of R-R interval dynamics before the spontaneous onset of paroxysmal atrial fibrillation. *Circulation, 100(20)*, 2079–2084.

Vikman, S., Yli-Mäyry, S., Mäkikallio, T.H., Airaksinen, K.E., and Huikuri, H.V. (2001). Differences in heart rate dynamics before the spontaneous onset of long and short episodes of paroxysmal atrial fibrillation. *Annals of Noninvasive Electrocardiology, 6(2)*, 134–142.

Virtanen, I., Ekholm, E., Polo-Kantola, P., and Huikuri, H. (2007). Sleep stage dependent patterns of nonlinear heart rate dynamics in postmenopausal women. *Autonomic Neuroscience, 134(1–2)*, 74–80.

Wang, S.Y., Zhang, L.F., Wang, X.B., and Cheng, J.H. (2000). Age dependency and correlation of heart rate variability, blood pressure variability and baroreflex sensitivity. *Journal of Gravitational Physiology, 7(2)*, P145–P146.

Wilhelm, F.H., Grossman, P., and Roth, W.T. (1999). Analysis of cardiovascular regulation. *Biomedical Sciences Instrumentation, 35*, 135–140.

Yamada, A., Hayano, J., Sakata, S., Okada, A., Mukai, S., Ohte, N., and Kimura, G. (2000). Reduced ventricular response irregularity is associated with increased mortality in patients with chronic atrial fibrillation. *Circulation, 102(3)*, 300–306.

Yeragani, V.K., Krishnan, S., Engels, H.J., and Gretebeck, R. (2005). Effects of caffeine on linear and nonlinear measures of heart rate variability before and after exercise. *Depression and Anxiety, 21(3)*, 130–134.

Yeragani, V.K., Sobolewski, E., Jampala, V.C., Kay, J., Yeragani, S., and Igel, G. (1998). Fractal dimension and approximate entropy of heart period and heart rate: Awake versus sleep differences and methodological issues. *Clinical Science, 95(3)*, 295–301.

Yeragani, V.K., Srinivasan, K., Vempati, S., Pohl, R., and Balon, R. (1993). Fractal dimension of heart rate time series: An effective measure of autonomic function. *Journal of Applied Physiology, 75(6)*, 2429–2438.

Yum, M.K., Kim, N.S., Oh, J.W., Kim, C.R., Lee, J.W., Kim, S.K., Noh, C.I., Choi, J.Y., and Yun, Y.S. (1999). Non-linear cardiac dynamics and morning dip: An unsound circadian rhythm. *Clinical Physiology, 19(1)*, 56–67.

Yum, M.K., Oh, A.Y., Lee, H.M., Kim, C.S., Kim, S.D., Lee, Y.S., Wang, K.C., Chung, Y.N., and Kim, H.S. (2006). Identification of patients with childhood moyamoya diseases showing temporary hypertension after anesthesia by preoperative multifractal Hurst analysis of heart rate variability. *Journal of Neurosurgical Anesthesiology, 18(4)*, 223–229.

Yum, M.K., Park, E.Y., Kim, C.R., and Hwang, J.H. (2001). Alterations in irregular and fractal heart rate behavior in growth restricted fetuses. *European Journal of Obstetrics, Gynecology, and Reproductive Biology, 94(1)*, 51–58.

Zamarrón, C., Hornero, R., del Campo, F., Abásolo, D., and Alvarez, D. (2006). Heart rate regularity analysis obtained from pulse oximetric recordings in the diagnosis of obstructive sleep apnea. *Sleep and Breathing, 10(2)*, 83–89.

Zhang, L.F., Zhang, Z.Y., Wang, S.Y., and Zheng, J. (1997). Change in heart rate dynamics after aerobic training detected by approximate entropy and its association with orthostasis. *Journal of Gravitational Physiology, 4(2)*, P47–P48.

Zhang, L.F., Zheng, J., Wang, S.Y., Zhang, Z.Y., and Liu, C. (1999). Effect of aerobic training on orthostatic tolerance, circulatory response, and heart rate dynamics. *Aviation, Space, and Environmental Medicine, 70(10)*, 975–982.

Zohar, P., Kovacic, M., Brezocnik, M., and Podbregar, M. (2005). Prediction of maintenance of sinus rhythm after electrical cardioversion of atrial fibrillation by non-deterministic modelling. *Europace, 7(5)*, 500–507.

READING LIST: RESPIRATION

Akay, M. (2005a). Influence of peripheral chemodenervation on the complexity of respiratory patterns during early maturation. *Medical and Biological Engineering and Computing, 43(6)*, 793–799.

Akay, M. (2005b). Influence of the vagus nerve on respiratory patterns during early maturation. *IEEE Transactions on Biomedical Engineering, 52(11)*, 1863–1868.

Akay, M., Lipping, T., Moodie, K., and Hoopes, P.J. (2002). Effects of hypoxia on the complexity of respiratory patterns during maturation. *Early Human Development, 70(1–2)*, 55–71.

Akay, M., Moodie, K.L., and Hoopes, P.J. (2003). Age related alterations in the complexity of respiratory patterns. *Journal of Integrative Neuroscience, 2(2)*, 165–178.

Akay, M. and Sekine, N. (2004). Investigating the complexity of respiratory patterns during recovery from severe hypoxia. *Journal of Neural Engineering, 1(1)*, 16–20.

Alvarez, D., Hornero, R., García, M., del Campo, F., and Zamarrón, C. (2007a). Improving diagnostic ability of blood oxygen saturation from overnight pulse oximetry in obstructive sleep apnea detection by means of central tendency measure. *Artificial Intelligence in Medicine, 41(1)*, 13–24.

Alvarez, D., Hornero, R., Marcos, J.V., del Campo, F., and López, M. (2007b). Obstructive sleep apnea detection using clustering classification of nonlinear features from nocturnal oximetry. *Conference Proceedings: Annual International Conference of the IEEE Engineering in Medicine and Biology Society*, Lyon, *2007*, pp. 1937–1940.

Burioka, N., Cornélissen, G., Halberg, F., Kaplan, D.T., Suyama, H., Sako, T., and Shimizu, E. (2003). Approximate entropy of human respiratory movement during eye-closed waking and different sleep stages. *Chest, 123(1)*, 80–86.

Burioka, N., Suyama, H., Sako, T., Miyata, M., Takeshima, T., Endo, M., Kurai, J., Fukuoka, Y., Takata, M., Nomura, T., Nakashima, K., and Shimizu, E. (2002). Non-linear dynamics applied to human respiratory movement during sleep. *Biomedicine & Pharmacotherapy, 56(Suppl 2)*, 370s–373s.

BuSha, B.F. and Stella, M.H. (2002). State and chemical drive modulate respiratory variability. *Journal of Applied Physiology, 93(2)*, 685–696.

Butler, J.P. and Tsuda, A. (1997). Effect of convective stretching and folding on aerosol mixing deep in the lung, assessed by approximate entropy. *Journal of Applied Physiology, 83(3)*, 800–809.

Caldirola, D., Bellodi, L., Cammino, S., and Perna, G. (2004a). Smoking and respiratory irregularity in panic disorder. *Biological Psychiatry, 56(6)*, 393–398.

Caldirola, D., Bellodi, L., Caumo, A., Migliarese, G., and Perna, G. (2004b). Approximate entropy of respiratory patterns in panic disorder. *American Journal of Psychiatry, 161(1)*, 79–87.

Chen, X., Chon, K.H., and Solomon, I.C. (2005a). Chemical activation of pre-Bötzinger complex in vivo reduces respiratory network complexity. *American Journal of Physiology: Regulatory, Integrative and Comparative Physiology, 288(5)*, R1237–R1247.

Chen, X., Solomon, I., and Chon, K. (2005b). Comparison of the use of approximate entropy and sample entropy: Applications to neural respiratory signal. *Conference Proceedings: Annual International Conference of the IEEE Engineering in Medicine and Biology Society*, Shanghai, Vol. *4*, pp. 4212–4215.

del Campo, F., Hornero, R., Zamarrón, C., Abasolo, D.E., and Alvarez, D. (2006). Oxygen saturation regularity analysis in the diagnosis of obstructive sleep apnea. *Artificial Intelligence in Medicine, 37(2)*, 111–118.

Dragomir, A., Akay, Y., Curran, A.K., Akay, M. (2008). Complexity measures of the central respiratory networks during wakefulness and sleep. *Journal of Neural Engineering, 5(2)*, 254–261.

El-Khatib, M.F. (2007). A diagnostic software tool for determination of complexity in respiratory pattern parameters. *Computers in Biology and Medicine, 37(10)*, 1522–1527.

Engoren, M. (1998). Approximate entropy of respiratory rate and tidal volume during weaning from mechanical ventilation. *Critical Care Medicine, 26(11)*, 1817–1823.

Hornero, R., Alvarez, D., Abásolo, D., del Campo, F., and Zamarrón, C. (2007). Utility of approximate entropy from overnight pulse oximetry data in the diagnosis of the obstructive sleep apnea syndrome. *IEEE Transactions on Biomedical Engineering, 54(1)*, 107–113.

Hornero, R., Alvarez, D., Abasolo, D., Gomez, C., Del Campo, F., and Zamarron, C. (2005). Approximate entropy from overnight pulse oximetry for the obstructive sleep apnea syndrome. *Conference Proceedings: Annual International Conference of the IEEE Engineering in Medicine and Biology Society*, Shanghai, Vol. 6, pp. 6157–6160.

Nazeran, H., Krishnam, R., Chatlapalli, S., Pamula, Y., Haltiwanger, E., and Cabrera, S. (2006). Nonlinear dynamics analysis of heart rate variability signals to detect sleep disordered breathing in children. *Conference Proceedings: Annual International Conference of the IEEE Engineering in Medicine and Biology Society*, New York, NY, Vol. 1, pp. 3873–3878.

Sipinková, I., Hahn, G., Meyer, M., Tadlánek, M., and Hájek, J. (1997). Effect of respiration and posture on heart rate variability. *Physiological Research, 46(3)*, 173–179.

Sleigh, J.W. (1999). Postoperative respiratory arrhythmias: Incidence and measurement. *Acta Anaesthesiologica Scandinavica, 43(7)*, 708–714.

Yeragani, V.K., Radhakrishna, R.K., Tancer, M., and Uhde, T. (2002). Nonlinear measures of respiration: Respiratory irregularity and increased chaos of respiration in patients with panic disorder. *Neuropsychobiology, 46(3)*, 111–120.

Yeragani, V.K., Rao, R., Tancer, M., and Uhde, T. (2004). Paroxetine decreases respiratory irregularity of linear and nonlinear measures of respiration in patients with panic disorder: A preliminary report. *Neuropsychobiology, 49(2)*, 53–57.

Yu, H.J., Chen, X., Foglyano, R.M., Wilson, C.G., and Solomon, I.C. (2008). Respiratory network complexity in neonatal rat in vivo and in vitro. *Advances in Experimental Medicine and Biology, 605*, 393–398.

Zhang, T. and Turner, D. (2001). A visuomotor reaction time task increases the irregularity and complexity of inspiratory airflow pattern in man. *Neuroscience Letters, 297(1)*, 41–44.

READING LIST: ENDOCRINOLOGY

Alesci, S., Martinez, P.E., Kelkar, S., Ilias, I., Ronsaville, D.S., Listwak, S.J., Ayala, A.R. et al. (2005). Major depression is associated with significant diurnal elevations in plasma interleukin-6 levels, a shift of its circadian rhythm, and loss of physiological complexity in its secretion: Clinical implications. *Journal of Clinical Endocrinology and Metabolism, 90(5)*, 2522–2530.

Alexander, S.L., Irvine, C.H., and Evans, M.J. (2004). Inter-relationships between the secretory dynamics of thyrotrophin-releasing hormone, thyrotrophin and prolactin in periovulatory mares: Effect of hypothyroidism. *Journal of Neuroendocrinology, 16(11)*, 906–915.

Aloi, J.A., Bergendahl, M., Iranmanesh, A., and Veldhuis, J.D. (1997). Pulsatile intravenous gonadotropin-releasing hormone administration averts fasting-induced hypogonadotropism and hypoandrogenemia in healthy, normal weight men. *Journal of Clinical Endocrinology and Metabolism, 82(5)*, 1543–1548.

Bergendahl, M., Aloi, J.A., Iranmanesh, A., Mulligan, T.M., and Veldhuis, J.D. (1998). Fasting suppresses pulsatile luteinizing hormone (LH) secretion and enhances orderliness of LH release in young but not older men. *Journal of Clinical Endocrinology and Metabolism, 83(6)*, 1967–1975.

Bergendahl, M., Evans, W.S., Pastor, C., Patel, A., Iranmanesh, A., and Veldhuis, J.D. (1999). Short-term fasting suppresses leptin and (conversely) activates disorderly growth hormone secretion in midluteal phase women—A clinical research center study. *Journal of Clinical Endocrinology and Metabolism, 84(3)*, 883–894.

Bergendahl, M., Iranmanesh, A., Evans, W.S., and Veldhuis, J.D. (2000a). Short-term fasting selectively suppresses leptin pulse mass and 24-hour rhythmic leptin release in healthy midluteal phase women without disturbing leptin pulse frequency or its entropy control (pattern orderliness). *Journal of Clinical Endocrinology and Metabolism, 85(1)*, 207–213.

Bergendahl, M., Iranmanesh, A., Mulligan, T., and Veldhuis, J.D. (2000b). Impact of age on cortisol secretory dynamics basally and as driven by nutrient-withdrawal stress. *Journal of Clinical Endocrinology and Metabolism, 85(6)*, 2203–2214.

Biermasz, N.R., Pereira, A.M., Frölich, M., Romijn, J.A., Veldhuis, J.D., and Roelfsema, F. (2004). Octreotide represses secretory-burst mass and nonpulsatile secretion but does not restore event frequency or orderly GH secretion in acromegaly. *American Journal of Physiology: Endocrinology and Metabolism, 286(1)*, E25–E30.

Blackman, M.R., Muniyappa, R., Wilson, M., Moquin, B.E., Baldwin, H.L., Wong, K.A., Snyder, C. et al. (2007). Diurnal secretion of growth hormone, cortisol, and dehydroepiandrosterone in pre- and perimenopausal women with active rheumatoid arthritis: A pilot case-control study. *Arthritis Research and Therapy, 9(4)*, R73.

Bonadonna, S., Burattin, A., Nuzzo, M., Bugari, G., Rosei, E.A., Valle, D., Iori, N., Bilezikian, J.P., Veldhuis, J.D., and Giustina, A. (2005). Chronic glucocorticoid treatment alters spontaneous pulsatile parathyroid hormone secretory dynamics in human subjects. *European Journal of Endocrinology, 152(2)*, 199–205.

Brabant, G. and Prank, K. (2000). Prediction and significance of the temporal pattern of hormone secretion in disease states. *Novartis Foundation Symposium, 227*, 105–114; discussion 114–118.

Bray, M.J., Vick, T.M., Shah, N., Anderson, S.M., Rice, L.W., Iranmanesh, A., Evans, W.S., and Veldhuis, J.D. (2001). Short-term estradiol replacement in postmenopausal women selectively mutes somatostatin's dose-dependent inhibition of fasting growth hormone secretion. *Journal of Clinical Endocrinology and Metabolism, 86(7)*, 3143–3149.

Carroll, B.J., Cassidy, F., Naftolowitz, D., Tatham, N.E., Wilson, W.H., Iranmanesh, A., Liu, P.Y., and Veldhuis, J.D. (2007). Pathophysiology of hypercortisolism in depression. *Acta Psychiatrica Scandinavica Supplementum, 433*, 90–103.

Charmandari, E., Pincus, S.M., Matthews, D.R., Dennison, E., Fall, C.H., and Hindmarsh, P.C. (2001). Joint growth hormone and cortisol spontaneous secretion is more asynchronous in older females than in their male counterparts. *Journal of Clinical Endocrinology and Metabolism, 86(7)*, 3393–3399.

Charmandari, E., Pincus, S.M., Matthews, D.R., Johnston, A., Brook, C.G., and Hindmarsh, P.C. (2002). Oral hydrocortisone administration in children with classic 21-hydroxylase deficiency leads to more synchronous joint GH and cortisol secretion. *Journal of Clinical Endocrinology and Metabolism, 87(5)*, 2238–2244.

Charmandari, E., Pincus, S.M., Matthews, D.R., Johnston, A., Brook, C.G., and Hindmarsh, P.C. (2003). Sexual dimorphism in the synchrony of joint growth hormone and cortisol dynamics in children with classic 21-hydroxylase deficiency. *Journal of Pediatric Endocrinology and Metabolism, 16(8)*, 1119–1130.

Clark, P.A., Iranmanesh, A., Veldhuis, J.D., and Rogol, A.D. (1997). Comparison of pulsatile luteinizing hormone secretion between prepubertal children and young adults: Evidence for a mass/amplitude-dependent difference without gender or day/night contrasts. *Journal of Clinical Endocrinology and Metabolism, 82(9)*, 2950–2955.

Clarke, I., Moore, L., and Veldhuis, J. (2002). Intensive direct cavernous sinus sampling identifies high-frequency, nearly random patterns of FSH secretion in ovariectomized ewes: Combined appraisal by RIA and bioassay. *Endocrinology, 143(1)*, 117–129.

Darzy, K.H., Murray, R.D., Gleeson, H.K., Pezzoli, S.S., Thorner, M.O., and Shalet, S.M. (2006). The impact of short-term fasting on the dynamics of 24-hour growth hormone (GH) secretion in patients with severe radiation-induced GH deficiency. *Journal of Clinical Endocrinology and Metabolism, 91(3)*, 987–994.

Darzy, K.H., Pezzoli, S.S., Thorner, M.O., and Shalet, S.M. (2005). The dynamics of growth hormone (GH) secretion in adult cancer survivors with severe GH deficiency acquired after brain irradiation in childhood for nonpituitary brain tumors: Evidence for preserved pulsatility and diurnal variation with increased secretory disorderliness. *Journal of Clinical Endocrinology and Metabolism, 90(5)*, 2794–2803.

Evans, W.S., Anderson, S.M., Hull, L.T., Azimi, P.P., Bowers, C.Y., and Veldhuis, J.D. (2001). Continuous 24-hour intravenous infusion of recombinant human growth hormone (GH)-releasing hormone-(1-44)-amide augments pulsatile, entropic, and daily rhythmic GH secretion in postmenopausal women equally in the estrogen-withdrawn and estrogen-supplemented states. *Journal of Clinical Endocrinology and Metabolism, 86(2)*, 700–712.

Evans, W.S., Taylor, A.E., Boyd, D.G., Johnson, M.L., Matt, D.W., Jimenez, Y., and Nestler, J.E. (2007). Lack of effect of short-term diazoxide administration on luteinizing hormone secretion in women with polycystic ovary syndrome. *Fertility and Sterility, 88(1)*, 118–124.

Fall, C.H., Dennison, E., Cooper, C., Pringle, J., Kellingray, S.D., and Hindmarsh, P. (2002). Does birth weight predict adult serum cortisol concentrations? Twenty-four-hour profiles in the United Kingdom 1920–1930 Hertfordshire Birth Cohort. *Journal of Clinical Endocrinology and Metabolism, 87(5)*, 2001–2007.

Feneberg, R., Sparber, M., Veldhuis, J.D., Mehls, O., Ritz, E., and Schaefer, F. (2002). Altered temporal organization of plasma insulin oscillations in chronic renal failure. *Journal of Clinical Endocrinology and Metabolism, 87(5)*, 1965–1973.

Fliser, D., Schaefer, F., Schmid, D., Veldhuis, J.D., and Ritz, E. (1997). Angiotensin II affects basal, pulsatile, and glucose-stimulated insulin secretion in humans. *Hypertension, 30(5)*, 1156–1161.

Fliser, D., Veldhuis, J.D., Dikow, R., Schmidt-Gayk, H., and Ritz, E. (1998). Effects of acute ACE inhibition on pulsatile renin and aldosterone secretion and their synchrony. *Hypertension, 32(5)*, 929–934.

Franco, C., Veldhuis, J.D., Iranmanesh, A., Brandberg, J., Lönn, L., Andersson, B., Bengtsson, B.A., Svensson, J., and Johannsson, G. (2006). Thigh intermuscular fat is inversely associated with spontaneous GH release in post-menopausal women with abdominal obesity. *European Journal of Endocrinology, 155(2)*, 261–268.

Friend, K., Iranmanesh, A., Login, I.S., and Veldhuis, J.D. (1997). Pyridostigmine treatment selectively amplifies the mass of GH secreted per burst without altering GH burst frequency, half-life, basal GH secretion or the orderliness of GH release. *European Journal of Endocrinology, 137(4)*, 377–386.

Friend, K., Iranmanesh, A., and Veldhuis, J.D. (1996). The orderliness of the growth hormone (GH) release process and the mean mass of GH secreted per burst are highly conserved in individual men on successive days. *Journal of Clinical Endocrinology and Metabolism, 81(10)*, 3746–3753.

García-Rudaz, M.C., Ropelato, M.G., Escobar, M.E., Veldhuis, J.D., and Barontini, M. (1998). Augmented frequency and mass of LH discharged per burst are accompanied by marked disorderliness of LH secretion in adolescents with polycystic ovary syndrome. *European Journal of Endocrinology, 139(6)*, 621–630.

Garcia-Rudaz, M.C., Ropelato, M.G., Escobar, M.E., Veldhuis, J.D., and Barontini, M. (2002). Amplified and orderly growth hormone secretion characterizes lean adolescents with polycystic ovary syndrome. *European Journal of Endocrinology, 147(2)*, 207–216.

Gasperi, M., Cecconi, E., Grasso, L., Bartalena, L., Centoni, R., Aimaretti, G., Broglio, F., Miccoli, P., Marcocci, C., Ghigo, E., and Martino, E. (2002). GH secretion is impaired in patients with primary hyperparathyroidism. *Journal of Clinical Endocrinology and Metabolism, 87(5)*, 1961–1964.

Gentili, A., Mulligan, T., Godschalk, M., Clore, J., Patrie, J., Iranmanesh, A., and Veldhuis, J.D. (2002). Unequal impact of short-term testosterone repletion on the somatotropic axis of young and older men. *Journal of Clinical Endocrinology and Metabolism, 87(2)*, 825–834.

Getty, L., Panteleon, A.E., Mittelman, S.D., Dea, M.K., and Bergman, R.N. (2000). Rapid oscillations in omental lipolysis are independent of changing insulin levels in vivo. *Journal of Clinical Investigation, 106(3)*, 421–430.

Gevers, E., Pincus, S.M., Robinson, I.C., and Veldhuis, J.D. (1998). Differential orderliness of the GH release process in castrate male and female rats. *American Journal of Physiology, 274(2 Pt 2)*, R437–R444.

Gianotti, L., Veldhuis, J.D., Destefanis, S., Lanfranco, F., Ramunni, J., Arvat, E., Marzetto, M., Boutignon, F., Deghenghi, R., and Ghigo, E. (2003). Suppression and recovery of LH secretion by a potent and selective GnRH-receptor antagonist peptide in healthy early follicular-phase women are mediated via selective control of LH secretory burst mass. *Clinical Endocrinology, 59(4)*, 526–532.

Gill, M.S., Tillmann, V., Veldhuis, J.D., and Clayton, P.E. (2001). Patterns of GH output and their synchrony with short-term height increments influence stature and growth performance in normal children. *Journal of Clinical Endocrinology and Metabolism, 86(12)*, 5860–5863.

Glintborg, D., Støving, R.K., Hagen, C., Hermann, A.P., Frystyk, J., Veldhuis, J.D., Flyvbjerg, A., and Andersen, M. (2005). Pioglitazone treatment increases spontaneous growth hormone (GH) secretion and stimulated GH levels in polycystic ovary syndrome. *Journal of Clinical Endocrinology and Metabolism, 90(10)*, 5605–5612.

Goodman, W.G., Misra, S., Veldhuis, J.D., Portale, A.A., Wang, H.J., Ament, M.E., and Salusky, I.B. (2000). Altered diurnal regulation of blood ionized calcium and serum parathyroid hormone concentrations during parenteral nutrition. *American Journal of Clinical Nutrition, 71(2)*, 560–568.

Gravholt, C.H., Veldhuis, J.D., and Christiansen, J.S. (1998). Increased disorderliness and decreased mass and daily rate of endogenous growth hormone secretion in adult Turner syndrome: The impact of body composition, maximal oxygen uptake and treatment with sex hormones. *Growth Hormone and IGF Research, 8(4)*, 289–298.

Grimmichová, T., Vrbíková, J., Matucha, P., Vondra, K., Veldhuis, P.P., and Johnson, M.L. (2008). Fasting insulin pulsatile secretion in lean women with polycystic ovary syndrome. *Physiological Research, 57*, S91–S98.

Groote Veldman, R., van den Berg, G., Pincus, S.M., Frölich, M., Veldhuis, J.D., and Roelfsema, F. (1999). Increased episodic release and disorderliness of prolactin secretion in both micro- and macroprolactinomas. *European Journal of Endocrinology, 140(3)*, 192–200.

Gusenoff, J.A., Harman, S.M., Veldhuis, J.D., Jayme, J.J., St Clair, C., Münzer, T., Christmas, C. et al. (2001). Cortisol and GH secretory dynamics, and their interrelationships, in healthy aged women and men. *American Journal of Physiology: Endocrinology and Metabolism, 280(4)*, E616–E625.

Hartman, M.L., Pincus, S.M., Johnson, M.L., Matthews, D.H., Faunt, L.M., Vance, M.L., Thorner, M.O., and Veldhuis, J.D. (1994). Enhanced basal and disorderly growth hormone secretion distinguish acromegalic from normal pulsatile growth hormone release. *Journal of Clinical Investigation, 94(3)*, 1277–1288.

Hindmarsh, P.C., Dennison, E., Pincus, S.M., Cooper, C., Fall, C.H., Matthews, D.R., Pringle, P.J., and Brook, C.G. (1999). A sexually dimorphic pattern of growth hormone secretion in the elderly. *Journal of Clinical Endocrinology and Metabolism, 84(8)*, 2679–2685.

Hoeger, K.M., Kolp, L.A., Strobl, F.J., and Veldhuis, J.D. (1999). Evaluation of LH secretory dynamics during the rat proestrous LH surge. *American Journal of Physiology, 276(1 Pt 2)*, R219–R225.

Hollingdal, M., Juhl, C.B., Pincus, S.M., Sturis, J., Veldhuis, J.D., Polonsky, K.S., Pørksen, N., and Schmitz, O. (2000). Failure of physiological plasma glucose excursions to entrain high-frequency pulsatile insulin secretion in type 2 diabetes. *Diabetes, 49(8)*, 1334–1340.

Iranmanesh, A., Bowers, C.Y., and Veldhuis, J.D. (2004). Activation of somatostatin-receptor subtype-2/-5 suppresses the mass, frequency, and irregularity of growth hormone (GH)-releasing peptide-2-stimulated GH secretion in men. *Journal of Clinical Endocrinology and Metabolism, 89(9)*, 4581–4587.

Juhl, C.B., Pørksen, N., Hollingdal, M., Sturis, J., Pincus, S., Veldhuis, J.D., Dejgaard, A., and Schmitz, O. (2000a). Repaglinide acutely amplifies pulsatile insulin secretion by augmentation of burst mass with no effect on burst frequency. *Diabetes Care, 23(5)*, 675–681.

Juhl, C.B., Pørksen, N., Pincus, S.M., Hansen, A.P., Veldhuis, J.D., and Schmitz, O. (2001). Acute and short-term administration of a sulfonylurea (gliclazide) increases pulsatile insulin secretion in type 2 diabetes. *Diabetes, 50(8)*, 1778–1784.

Juhl, C.B., Pørksen, N., Sturis, J., Hansen, A.P., Veldhuis, J.D., Pincus, S., Fineman, M., and Schmitz, O. (2000b). High-frequency oscillations in circulating amylin concentrations in healthy humans. *American Journal of Physiology: Endocrinology and Metabolism, 278(3)*, E484–E490.

Juhl, C.B., Schmitz, O., Pincus, S., Holst, J.J., Veldhuis, J., and Pørksen, N. (2000c). Short-term treatment with GLP-1 increases pulsatile insulin secretion in Type II diabetes with no effect on orderliness. *Diabetologia, 43(5)*, 583–588.

Keenan, D.M., Evans, W.S., and Veldhuis, J.D. (2003). Control of LH secretory-burst frequency and interpulse-interval regularity in women. *American Journal of Physiology: Endocrinology and Metabolism, 285(5)*, E938–E948.

Keenan, D.M. and Veldhuis, J.D. (2001). Disruption of the hypothalamic luteinizing hormone pulsing mechanism in aging men. *American Journal of Physiology: Regulatory, Integrative and Comparative Physiology, 281(6)*, R1917–R1924.

Khoromi, S., Muniyappa, R., Nackers, L., Gray, N., Baldwin, H., Wong, K.A., Matheny, L.A. et al. (2006). Effects of chronic osteoarthritis pain on neuroendocrine function in men. *Journal of Clinical Endocrinology and Metabolism, 91(11)*, 4313–4318.

Kok, S.W., Roelfsema, F., Overeem, S., Lammers, G.J., Frölich, M., Meinders, A.E., and Pijl, H. (2004). Pulsatile LH release is diminished, whereas FSH secretion is normal, in hypocretin-deficient narcoleptic men. *American Journal of Physiology: Endocrinology and Metabolism, 287(4)*, E630–E636.

Kok, S.W., Roelfsema, F., Overeem, S., Lammers, G.J., Frölich, M., Meinders, A.E., and Pijl, H. (2005). Altered setting of the pituitary-thyroid ensemble in hypocretin-deficient narcoleptic men. *American Journal of Physiology: Endocrinology and Metabolism, 288(5)*, E892–E899.

Kok, S.W., Roelfsema, F., Overeem, S., Lammers, G.J., Strijers, R.L., Frölich, M., Meinders, A.E., and Pijl, H. (2002). Dynamics of the pituitary-adrenal ensemble in hypocretin-deficient narcoleptic humans: Blunted basal adrenocorticotropin release and evidence for normal time-keeping by the master pacemaker. *Journal of Clinical Endocrinology and Metabolism, 87(11)*, 5085–5091.

Koutkia, P., Canavan, B., Breu, J., Johnson, M.L., and Grinspoon, S.K. (2004). Nocturnal ghrelin pulsatility and response to growth hormone secretagogues in healthy men. *American Journal of Physiology: Endocrinology and Metabolism, 287(3)*, E506–E512.

Koutkia, P., Canavan, B., Johnson, M.L., DePaoli, A., and Grinspoon, S. (2003). Characterization of leptin pulse dynamics and relationship to fat mass, growth hormone, cortisol, and insulin. *American Journal of Physiology: Endocrinology and Metabolism, 285(2)*, E372–E379.

Lado-Abeal, J., Hickox, J.R., Cheung, T.L., Veldhuis, J.D., Hardy, D.M., and Norman, R.L. (2000). Neuroendocrine consequences of fasting in adult male macaques: Effects of recombinant rhesus macaque leptin infusion. *Neuroendocrinology, 71(3)*, 196–208.

Lado-Abeal, J., Veldhuis, J.D., and Norman, R.L. (2002). Glucose relays information regarding nutritional status to the neural circuits that control the somatotropic, corticotropic, and gonadotropic axes in adult male rhesus macaques. *Endocrinology, 143(2)*, 403–410.

Larsen, M.O., Juhl, C.B., Pørksen, N., Gotfredsen, C.F., Carr, R.D., Ribel, U., Wilken, M., and Rolin, B. (2005). Beta-cell function and islet morphology in normal, obese, and obese beta-cell mass-reduced Göttingen minipigs. *American Journal of Physiology: Endocrinology and Metabolism, 288(2)*, E412–E421.

Licinio, J., Negrão, A.B., Mantzoros, C., Kaklamani, V., Wong, M.L., Bongiorno, P.B., Mulla, A. et al. (1998a). Synchronicity of frequently sampled, 24-h concentrations of circulating leptin, luteinizing hormone, and estradiol in healthy women. *Proceedings of the National Academy of Sciences, 95(5)*, 2541–2546.

Licinio, J., Negrão, A.B., Mantzoros, C., Kaklamani, V., Wong, M.L., Bongiorno, P.B., Negro, P.P. et al. (1998b). Sex differences in circulating human leptin pulse amplitude: Clinical implications. *Journal of Clinical Endocrinology and Metabolism, 83(11)*, 4140–4147.

Liu, P.Y., Iranmanesh, A., Keenan, D.M., Pincus, S.M., and Veldhuis, J.D. (2007). A noninvasive measure of negative-feedback strength, approximate entropy, unmasks strong diurnal variations in the regularity of LH secretion. *American Journal of Physiology: Endocrinology and Metabolism, 293(5)*, E1409–E1415.

Liu, P.Y., Pincus, S.M., Keenan, D.M., Roelfsema, F., and Veldhuis, J.D. (2005a). Joint synchrony of reciprocal hormonal signaling in human paradigms of both ACTH excess and cortisol depletion. *American Journal of Physiology: Endocrinology and Metabolism, 289(1)*, E160–E165.

Liu, P.Y., Pincus, S.M., Keenan, D.M., Roelfsema, F., and Veldhuis, J.D. (2005b). Analysis of bidirectional pattern synchrony of concentration-secretion pairs: Implementation in the human testicular and adrenal axes. *American Journal of Physiology: Regulatory, Integrative and Comparative Physiology, 288(2)*, R440–R446.

Liu, P.Y., Pincus, S.M., Takahashi, P.Y., Roebuck, P.D., Iranmanesh, A., Keenan, D.M., and Veldhuis, J.D. (2006). Aging attenuates both the regularity and joint synchrony of LH and testosterone secretion in normal men: Analyses via a model of graded GnRH receptor blockade. *American Journal of Physiology: Endocrinology and Metabolism, 290(1)*, E34–E41.

Maccario, M., Veldhuis, J.D., Broglio, F., Vito, L.D., Arvat, E., Deghenghi, R., and Ghigo, E. (2002). Impact of two or three daily subcutaneous injections of hexarelin, a synthetic growth hormone (GH) secretagogue, on 24-h GH, prolactin, adrenocorticotropin and cortisol secretion in humans. *European Journal of Endocrinology, 146(3)*, 310–318.

Maheshwari, H.G., Pezzoli, S.S., Rahim, A., Shalet, S.M., Thorner, M.O., and Baumann, G. (2002). Pulsatile growth hormone secretion persists in genetic growth hormone-releasing hormone resistance. *American Journal of Physiology: Endocrinology and Metabolism, 282(4)*, E943–E951.

Martha, P.M. Jr., Rogol, A.D., Veldhuis, J.D., and Blizzard, R.M. (1996). A longitudinal assessment of hormonal and physical alterations during normal puberty in boys. III. The neuroendocrine growth hormone axis during late prepuberty. *Journal of Clinical Endocrinology and Metabolism, 81(11)*, 4068–4074.

Marzullo, P., Caumo, A., Savia, G., Verti, B., Walker, G.E., Maestrini, S., Tagliaferri, A., Di Blasio, A.M., and Liuzzi, A. (2006). Predictors of postabsorptive ghrelin secretion after intake of different macronutrients. *Journal of Clinical Endocrinology and Metabolism, 91(10)*, 4124–4130.

Matt, D.W., Gilson, M.P., Sales, T.E., Krieg, R.J., Kerbeshian, M.C., Veldhuis, J.D., and Evans, W.S. (1998a). Characterization of attenuated proestrous luteinizing hormone surges in middle-aged rats by deconvolution analysis. *Biology of Reproduction, 59(6)*, 1477–1482.

Matt, D.W., Kauma, S.W., Pincus, S.M., Veldhuis, J.D., and Evans, W.S. (1998b). Characteristics of luteinizing hormone secretion in younger versus older premenopausal women. *American Journal of Obstetrics and Gynecology, 178(3)*, 504–510.

Mazziotti, G., Cimino, V., De Menis, E., Bonadonna, S., Bugari, G., De Marinis, L., Veldhuis, J.D., and Giustina, A. (2006). Active acromegaly enhances spontaneous parathyroid hormone pulsatility. *Metabolism, 55(6)*, 736–740.

McComb, J.J., Qian, X.P., Veldhuis, J.D., J. McGlone, J., and Norman, R.L. (2006). Neuroendocrine responses to psychological stress in eumenorrheic and oligomenorrheic women. *Stress, 9(1)*, 41–51.

Meier, J.J., Kjems, L.L., Veldhuis, J.D., Lefèbvre, P., and Butler, P.C. (2006). Postprandial suppression of glucagon secretion depends on intact pulsatile insulin secretion: Further evidence for the intraislet insulin hypothesis. *Diabetes, 55(4)*, 1051–1056.

Meneilly, G.S., Ryan, A.S., Veldhuis, J.D., and Elahi, D. (1997). Increased disorderliness of basal insulin release, attenuated insulin secretory burst mass, and reduced ultradian rhythmicity of insulin secretion in older individuals. *Journal of Clinical Endocrinology and Metabolism, 82(12)*, 4088–4093.

Meneilly, G.S., Veldhuis, J.D., and Elahi, D. (1999). Disruption of the pulsatile and entropic modes of insulin release during an unvarying glucose stimulus in elderly individuals. *Journal of Clinical Endocrinology and Metabolism, 84(6)*, 1938–1943.

Meneilly, G.S., Veldhuis, J.D., and Elahi, D. (2005). Deconvolution analysis of rapid insulin pulses before and after six weeks of continuous subcutaneous administration of glucagon-like peptide-1 in elderly patients with type 2 diabetes. *Journal of Clinical Endocrinology and Metabolism, 90(11)*, 6251–6256.

Misra, M., Miller, K.K., Almazan, C., Ramaswamy, K., Lapcharoensap, W., Worley, M., Neubauer, G., Herzog, D.B., and Klibanski, A. (2004). Alterations in cortisol secretory dynamics in adolescent girls with anorexia nervosa and effects on bone metabolism. *Journal of Clinical Endocrinology and Metabolism, 89(10)*, 4972–4980.

Misra, M., Miller, K.K., Bjornson, J., Hackman, A., Aggarwal, A., Chung, J., Ott, M., Herzog, D.B., Johnson, M.L., and Klibanski, A. (2003). Alterations in growth hormone secretory dynamics in adolescent girls with anorexia nervosa and effects on bone metabolism. *Journal of Clinical Endocrinology and Metabolism, 88(12)*, 5615–5623.

Moore, C., Shalet, S., Manickam, K., Willard, T., Maheshwari, H., and Baumann, G. (2005). Voice abnormality in adults with congenital and adult-acquired growth hormone deficiency. *Journal of Clinical Endocrinology and Metabolism, 90(7)*, 4128–4132.

Mulligan, T., Iranmanesh, A., Kerzner, R., Demers, L.W., and Veldhuis, J.D. (1999). Two-week pulsatile gonadotropin releasing hormone infusion unmasks dual (hypothalamic and Leydig cell) defects in the healthy aging male gonadotropic axis. *European Journal of Endocrinology, 141(3)*, 257–266.

Muniyappa, R., Sorkin, J.D., Veldhuis, J.D., Harman, S.M., Münzer, T., Bhasin, S., and Blackman, M.R. (2007). Long-term testosterone supplementation augments overnight growth hormone secretion in healthy older men. *American Journal of Physiology: Endocrinology and Metabolism, 293(3)*, E769–E775.

Muniyappa, R., Wong, K.A., Baldwin, H.L., Sorkin, J.D., Johnson, M.L., Bhasin, S., Harman, S.M., and Blackman, M.R. (2006). Dehydroepiandrosterone secretion in healthy older men and women: Effects of testosterone and growth hormone administration in older men. *Journal of Clinical Endocrinology and Metabolism, 91(11)*, 4445–4452.

Naguib, M., Schmid, P.G. 3rd, and Baker, M.T. (2003). The electroencephalographic effects of IV anesthetic doses of melatonin: Comparative studies with thiopental and propofol. *Anesthesia and Analgesia, 97(1)*, 238–243, table of contents.

Nyholm, B., Pørksen, N., Juhl, C.B., Gravholt, C.H., Butler, P.C., Weeke, J., Veldhuis, J.D., Pincus, S., and Schmitz, O. (2000). Assessment of insulin secretion in relatives of patients with type 2 (non-insulin-dependent) diabetes mellitus: Evidence of early beta-cell dysfunction. *Metabolism, 49(7),* 896–905.

Painson, J.C., Veldhuis, J.D., and Tannenbaum, G.S. (2000). Single exposure to testosterone in adulthood rapidly induces regularity in the growth hormone release process. *American Journal of Physiology: Endocrinology and Metabolism, 278(5),* E933–E940.

Parra, A., Reyes-Terán, G., Ramírez-Peredo, J., Jacquemin, B., Quiroz, V., Cárdenas, M., García-Sancho, M.C., and Larrea, F. (2004). Differences in nocturnal basal and rhythmic prolactin secretion in untreated compared to treated HIV-infected men are associated with CD4+ T-lymphocytes. *Immunology and Cell Biology, 82(1),* 24–31.

Peacey, S.R. and Shalet, S.M. (1999). Growth hormone pulsatility in acromegaly following radiotherapy. *Pituitary, 2(1),* 63–69.

Peacey, S.R., Toogood, A.A., Veldhuis, J.D., Thorner, M.O., and Shalet, S.M. (2001). The relationship between 24-hour growth hormone secretion and insulin-like growth factor I in patients with successfully treated acromegaly: Impact of surgery or radiotherapy. *Journal of Clinical Endocrinology and Metabolism, 86(1),* 259–266.

Pijl, H., Langendonk, J.G., Burggraaf, J., Frölich, M., Cohen, A.F., Veldhuis, J.D., and Meinders, A.E. (2001). Altered neuroregulation of GH secretion in viscerally obese premenopausal women. *Journal of Clinical Endocrinology and Metabolism, 86(11),* 5509–5515.

Pincus, S. (1995). Approximate entropy (ApEn) as a complexity measure. *Chaos, 5(1),* 110–117.

Pincus, S.M. (2000). Orderliness of hormone release. *Novartis Foundation Symposium, 227,* 82–96; discussion 96–104.

Pincus, S.M., Gevers, E.F., Robinson, I.C., van den Berg, G., Roelfsema, F., Hartman, M.L., and Veldhuis, J.D. (1996). Females secrete growth hormone with more process irregularity than males in both humans and rats. *American Journal of Physiology, 270(1 Pt 1),* E107–E115.

Pincus, S.M., Hartman, M.L., Roelfsema, F., Thorner, M.O., and Veldhuis, J.D. (1999). Hormone pulsatility discrimination via coarse and short time sampling. *American Journal of Physiology, 277(5 Pt 1),* E948–E957.

Pincus, S.M. and Keefe, D.L. (1992). Quantification of hormone pulsatility via an approximate entropy algorithm. *American Journal of Physiology, 262(5 Pt 1),* E741–E754.

Pincus, S.M. and Minkin, M.J. (1998). Assessing sequential irregularity of both endocrine and heart rate rhythms. *Current Opinion in Obstetrics & Gynecology, 10(4),* 281–291.

Pincus, S.M., Mulligan, T., Iranmanesh, A., Gheorghiu, S., Godschalk, M., and Veldhuis, J.D. (1996). Older males secrete luteinizing hormone and testosterone more irregularly, and jointly more asynchronously, than younger males. *Proceedings of the National Academy of Sciences, 93(24),* 14100–14105.

Pincus, S.M., Padmanabhan, V., Lemon, W., Randolph, J., and Rees Midgley, A. (1998). Follicle-stimulating hormone is secreted more irregularly than luteinizing hormone in both humans and sheep. *Journal of Clinical Investigation, 101(6),* 1318–1324.

Pincus, S.M., Veldhuis, J.D., Mulligan, T., Iranmanesh, A., and Evans, W.S. (1997). Effects of age on the irregularity of LH and FSH serum concentrations in women and men. *American Journal of Physiology, 273(5 Pt 1),* E989–E995.

Pincus, S.M., Veldhuis, J.D., and Rogol, A.D. (2000). Longitudinal changes in growth hormone secretory process irregularity assessed transpubertally in healthy boys. *American Journal of Physiology: Endocrinology and Metabolism, 279(2),* E417–E424.

Pørksen, N., Grøfte, B., Nyholm, B., Holst, J.J., Pincus, S.M., Veldhuis, J.D., Schmitz, O., and Butler, P.C. (1998). Glucagon-like peptide 1 increases mass but not frequency or orderliness of pulsatile insulin secretion. *Diabetes, 47(1),* 45–49.

Pørksen, N., Juhl, C., Hollingdal, M., Pincus, S.M., Sturis, J., Veldhuis, J.D., and Schmitz, O. (2000). Concordant induction of rapid in vivo pulsatile insulin secretion by recurrent punctuated glucose infusions. *American Journal of Physiology: Endocrinology and Metabolism, 278(1)*, E162–E170.

Posener, J.A., Charles DeBattista, Veldhuis, J.D., Province, M.A., Williams, G.H., and Schatzberg, A.F. (2004). Process irregularity of cortisol and adrenocorticotropin secretion in men with major depressive disorder. *Psychoneuroendocrinology, 29(9)*, 1129–1137.

Quigg, M., Kiely, J.M., Shneker, B., Veldhuis, J.D., and Bertram, E.H. 3rd (2002). Interictal and postictal alterations of pulsatile secretions of luteinizing hormone in temporal lobe epilepsy in men. *Annals of Neurology, 51(5)*, 559–566.

Ritzel, R., Schulte, M., Pørksen, N., Nauck, M.S., Holst, J.J., Juhl, C., März, W., Schmitz, O., Schmiegel, W.H., and Nauck, M.A. (2001). Glucagon-like peptide 1 increases secretory burst mass of pulsatile insulin secretion in patients with type 2 diabetes and impaired glucose tolerance. *Diabetes, 50(4)*, 776–784.

Roelfsema, F., Biermasz, N.R., and Veldhuis, J.D. (2002). Pulsatile, nyctohemeral and entropic characteristics of GH secretion in adult GH-deficient patients: Selectively decreased pulsatile release and increased secretory disorderliness with preservation of diurnal timing and gender distinctions. *Clinical Endocrinology, 56(1)*, 79–87.

Roelfsema, F., Biermasz, N.R., Veldman, R.G., Veldhuis, J.D., Frölich, M., Stokvis-Brantsma, W.H., and Wit, J.M. (2001). Growth hormone (GH) secretion in patients with an inactivating defect of the GH-releasing hormone (GHRH) receptor is pulsatile: Evidence for a role for non-GHRH inputs into the generation of GH pulses. *Journal of Clinical Endocrinology and Metabolism, 86(6)*, 2459–2464.

Roelfsema, F., Pincus, S.M., and Veldhuis, J.D. (1998a). Patients with Cushing's disease secrete adrenocorticotropin and cortisol jointly more asynchronously than healthy subjects. *Journal of Clinical Endocrinology and Metabolism, 83(2)*, 688–692.

Roelfsema, F., van den Berg, G., van Dulken, H., Veldhuis, J.D., and Pincus, S.M. (1998b). Pituitary apoplexy in acromegaly, a long-term follow-up study in two patients. *Journal of Endocrinological Investigation, 21(5)*, 298–303.

Rogol, A.D., Blethen, S.L., Sy, J.P., and Veldhuis, J.D. (2003). Do growth hormone (GH) serial sampling, insulin-like growth factor-I (IGF-I) or auxological measurements have an advantage over GH stimulation testing in predicting the linear growth response to GH therapy? *Clinical Endocrinology, 58(2)*, 229–237.

Samuels, M.H., Veldhuis, J.D., Kramer, P., Urban, R.J., Bauer, R., and Mundy, G.R. (1997). Episodic secretion of parathyroid hormone in postmenopausal women: Assessment by deconvolution analysis and approximate entropy. *Journal of Bone and Mineral Research, 12(4)*, 616–623.

Schmitt, C.P., Löcken, S., Mehls, O., Veldhuis, J.D., Lehnert, T., Ritz, E., and Schaefer, F. (2003a). PTH pulsatility but not calcium sensitivity is restored after total parathyroidectomy with heterotopic autotransplantation. *Journal of the American Society of Nephrology, 14(2)*, 407–414.

Schmitt, C.P., Obry, J., Feneberg, R., Veldhuis, J.D., Mehls, O., Ritz, E., and Schaefer, F. (2003b). Beta1-adrenergic blockade augments pulsatile PTH secretion in humans. *Journal of the American Society of Nephrology, 14(12)*, 3245–3250.

Schmitt, C.P., Schaefer, F., Bruch, A., Veldhuis, J.D., Schmidt-Gayk, H., Stein, G., Ritz, E., and Mehls, O. (1996). Control of pulsatile and tonic parathyroid hormone secretion by ionized calcium. *Journal of Clinical Endocrinology and Metabolism, 81(12)*, 4236–4243.

Schmitz, O., Juhl, C.B., Hollingdal, M., Veldhuis, J.D., Pørksen, N., and Pincus, S.M. (2001). Irregular circulating insulin concentrations in type 2 diabetes mellitus: An inverse relationship between circulating free fatty acid and the disorderliness of an insulin time series in diabetic and healthy individuals. *Metabolism, 50(1)*, 41–46.

Schmitz, O., Pørksen, N., Nyholm, B., Skjaerbaek, C., Butler, P.C., Veldhuis, J.D., and Pincus, S.M. (1997). Disorderly and nonstationary insulin secretion in relatives of patients with NIDDM. *American Journal of Physiology, 272(2 Pt 1)*, E218–E226.

Shah, N., Evans, W.S., and Veldhuis, J.D. (1999a). Actions of estrogen on pulsatile, nyctohemeral, and entropic modes of growth hormone secretion. *American Journal of Physiology, 276(5 Pt 2)*, R1351–R1358.

Shah, N., Evans, W.S., Bowers, C.Y., and Veldhuis, J.D. (1999b). Tripartite neuroendocrine activation of the human growth hormone (GH) axis in women by continuous 24-hour GH-releasing peptide infusion: Pulsatile, entropic, and nyctohemeral mechanisms. *Journal of Clinical Endocrinology and Metabolism, 84(6)*, 2140–2150.

Shah, N., Evans, W.S., Bowers, C.Y., and Veldhuis, J.D. (2000). Oral estradiol administration modulates continuous intravenous growth hormone (GH)-releasing peptide-2-driven GH secretion in postmenopausal women. *Journal of Clinical Endocrinology and Metabolism, 85(8)*, 2649–2659.

Siragy, H.M., Vieweg, W.V., Pincus, S., and Veldhuis, J.D. (1995). Increased disorderliness and amplified basal and pulsatile aldosterone secretion in patients with primary aldosteronism. *Journal of Clinical Endocrinology and Metabolism, 80(1)*, 28–33.

Soares-Welch, C., Mielke, K.L., Bowers, C.Y., and Veldhuis, J.D. (2005). Short-term testosterone supplementation does not activate GH and IGF-I production in postmenopausal women. *Clinical Endocrinology, 63(1)*, 32–38.

Sparacino, G., Bardi, F., and Cobelli, C. (2000). Approximate entropy studies of hormone pulsatility from plasma concentration time series: Influence of the kinetics assessed by simulation. *Annals of Biomedical Engineering, 28(6)*, 665–676.

Støving, R.K., Veldhuis, J.D., Flyvbjerg, A., Vinten, J., Hangaard, J., Koldkjaer, O.G., Kristiansen, J., and Hagen, C. (1999). Jointly amplified basal and pulsatile growth hormone (GH) secretion and increased process irregularity in women with anorexia nervosa: Indirect evidence for disruption of feedback regulation within the GH-insulin-like growth factor I axis. *Journal of Clinical Endocrinology and Metabolism, 84(6)*, 2056–2063.

Svensson, J., Johannsson, G., Iranmanesh, A., Albertsson-Wikland, K., Veldhuis, J.D., and Bengtsson, B.A. (2006). GH secretory pattern in young adults who discontinued GH treatment for GH deficiency and decreased longitudinal growth in childhood. *European Journal of Endocrinology, 155(1)*, 91–99.

Svensson, J., Veldhuis, J.D., Iranmanesh, A., Bengtsson, B.A., and Johannsson, G. (2002). Increased orderliness of growth hormone (GH) secretion in GH-deficient adults with low serum insulin-like growth factor I. *Journal of Clinical Endocrinology and Metabolism, 87(6)*, 2863–2869.

Tuckow, A.P., Rarick, K.R., Kraemer, W.J., Marx, J.O., Hymer, W.C., and Nindl, B.C. (2006). Nocturnal growth hormone secretory dynamics are altered after resistance exercise: Deconvolution analysis of 12-hour immunofunctional and immunoreactive isoforms. *American Journal of Physiology: Regulatory, Integrative and Comparative Physiology, 291(6)*, R1749–R1755.

Vahl, N., Jørgensen, J.O., Skjaerbaek, C., Veldhuis, J.D., Orskov, H., and Christiansen, J.S. (1997). Abdominal adiposity rather than age and sex predicts mass and regularity of GH secretion in healthy adults. *American Journal of Physiology, 272(6 Pt 1)*, E1108–E1116.

van Aken, M.O., Pereira, A.M., Frölich, M., Romijn, J.A., Pijl, H., Veldhuis, J.D., and Roelfsema, F. (2005a). Growth hormone secretion in primary adrenal Cushing's syndrome is disorderly and inversely correlated with body mass index. *American Journal of Physiology: Endocrinology and Metabolism, 288(1)*, E63–E70.

van Aken, M.O., Pereira, A.M., van den Berg, G., Romijn, J.A., Veldhuis, J.D., and Roelfsema, F. (2004). Profound amplification of secretory-burst mass and anomalous regularity of ACTH secretory process in patients with Nelson's syndrome compared with Cushing's disease. *Clinical Endocrinology, 60(6)*, 765–772.

van Aken, M.O., Pereira, A.M., van Thiel, S.W., van den Berg, G., Frölich, M., Veldhuis, J.D., Romijn, J.A., and Roelfsema, F. (2005b). Irregular and frequent cortisol secretory episodes with preserved diurnal rhythmicity in primary adrenal Cushing's syndrome. *Journal of Clinical Endocrinology and Metabolism, 90(3)*, 1570–1577.

Van Dam, E.W., Roelfsema, F., Helmerhorst, F.H., Frölich, M., Meinders, A.E., Veldhuis, J.D., and Pijl, H. (2002). Low amplitude and disorderly spontaneous growth hormone release in obese women with or without polycystic ovary syndrome. *Journal of Clinical Endocrinology and Metabolism, 87(9)*, 4225–4230.

van den Berg, G., Pincus, S.M., Frölich, M., Veldhuis, J.D., and Roelfsema, F. (1998). Reduced disorderliness of growth hormone release in biochemically inactive acromegaly after pituitary surgery. *European Journal of Endocrinology, 138(2)*, 164–169.

van den Berg, G., Pincus, S.M., Veldhuis, J.D., Frölich, M., and Roelfsema, F. (1997). Greater disorderliness of ACTH and cortisol release accompanies pituitary-dependent Cushing's disease. *European Journal of Endocrinology, 136(4)*, 394–400.

Van den Berghe, G., Baxter, R.C., Weekers, F., Wouters, P., Bowers, C.Y., and Veldhuis, J.D. (2000). A paradoxical gender dissociation within the growth hormone/insulin-like growth factor I axis during protracted critical illness. *Journal of Clinical Endocrinology and Metabolism, 85(1)*, 183–192.

van der Klaauw, A.A., Pereira, A.M., van Thiel, S.W., Frolich, M., Iranmanesh, A., Veldhuis, J.D., Roelfsema, F., and Romijn, J.A. (2007). Attenuated pulse size, disorderly growth hormone and prolactin secretion with preserved nyctohemeral rhythm distinguish irradiated from surgically treated acromegaly patients. *Clinical Endocrinology, 66(4)*, 489–498.

van der Klaauw, A.A., Pereira, A.M., van Thiel, S.W., Smit, J.W., Corssmit, E.P., Biermasz, N.R., Frolich, M., Iranmanesh, A., Veldhuis, J.D., Roelfsema, F., and Romijn, J.A. (2006). GH deficiency in patients irradiated for acromegaly: Significance of GH stimulatory tests in relation to the 24 h GH secretion. *European Journal of Endocrinology, 154(6)*, 851–858.

Veldhuis, J.D. (1996). New modalities for understanding dynamic regulation of the somatotropic (GH) axis: Explication of gender differences in GH neuroregulation in the human. *Journal of Pediatric Endocrinology and Metabolism, 9 Suppl 3*, 237–253.

Veldhuis, J.D. (1997a). Altered pulsatile and coordinate secretion of pituitary hormones in aging: Evidence of feedback disruption. *Aging, 9(4 Suppl)*, 19–20.

Veldhuis, J.D. (1997b). Novel modalities for appraising individual and coordinate pulsatile hormone secretion: The paradigm of luteinizing hormone and testosterone release in the aging male. *Molecular Psychiatry, 2(1)*, 70–80.

Veldhuis, J.D. (2000). Nature of altered pulsatile hormone release and neuroendocrine network signalling in human ageing: Clinical studies of the somatotropic, gonadotropic, corticotropic and insulin axes. *Novartis Foundation Symposium, 227*, 163–185; discussion 185–189.

Veldhuis, J.D., Evans, W.S., and Bowers, C.Y. (2002a). Impact of estradiol supplementation on dual peptidyl drive of GH secretion in postmenopausal women. *Journal of Clinical Endocrinology and Metabolism, 87(2)*, 859–866.

Veldhuis, J.D., Fletcher, T.P., Gatford, K.L., Egan, A.R., and Clarke, I.J. (2002b). Hypophyseal-portal somatostatin (SRIH) and jugular venous growth hormone secretion in the conscious unrestrained ewe. *Neuroendocrinology, 75(2)*, 83–91.

Veldhuis, J.D. and Iranmanesh, A. (2005). Short-term aromatase-enzyme blockade unmasks impaired feedback adaptations in luteinizing hormone and testosterone secretion in older men. *Journal of Clinical Endocrinology and Metabolism, 90(1)*, 211–218.

Veldhuis, J.D., Iranmanesh, A., Demers, L.M., and Mulligan, T. (1999a). Joint basal and pulsatile hypersecretory mechanisms drive the monotropic follicle-stimulating hormone (FSH) elevation in healthy older men: Concurrent preservation of the orderliness of the FSH release process: A general clinical research center study. *Journal of Clinical Endocrinology and Metabolism, 84(10)*, 3506–3514.

Veldhuis, J.D., Iranmanesh, A., and Mulligan, T. (2005). Age and testosterone feedback jointly control the dose-dependent actions of gonadotropin-releasing hormone in healthy men. *Journal of Clinical Endocrinology and Metabolism, 90(1)*, 302–309.

Veldhuis, J.D., Iranmanesh, A., Mulligan, T., and Pincus, S.M. (1999b). Disruption of the young-adult synchrony between luteinizing hormone release and oscillations in follicle-stimulating hormone, prolactin, and nocturnal penile tumescence (NPT) in healthy older men. *Journal of Clinical Endocrinology and Metabolism, 84(10)*, 3498–3505.

Veldhuis, J.D., Iranmanesh, A., Naftolowitz, D., Tatham, N., Cassidy, F., and Carroll, B.J. (2001a). Corticotropin secretory dynamics in humans under low glucocorticoid feedback. *Journal of Clinical Endocrinology and Metabolism, 86(11)*, 5554–5563.

Veldhuis, J.D., Iranmanesh, A., and Urban, R.J. (1997a). Primary gonadal failure in men selectively amplifies the mass of follicle stimulating hormone (FSH) secreted per burst and increases the disorderliness of FSH release patterns: Reversibility with testosterone replacement. *International Journal of Andrology, 20(5)*, 297–305.

Veldhuis, J.D., Iranmanesh, A., and Weltman, A. (1997b). Elements in the pathophysiology of diminished growth hormone (GH) secretion in aging humans. *Endocrine, 7(1)*, 41–48.

Veldhuis, J.D., Johnson, M.L., Veldhuis, O.L., Straume, M., and Pincus, S.M. (2001b). Impact of pulsatility on the ensemble orderliness (approximate entropy) of neurohormone secretion. *American Journal of Physiology: Regulatory, Integrative and Comparative Physiology, 281(6)*, R1975–R1985.

Veldhuis, J.D., Metzger, D.L., Martha, P.M. Jr., Mauras, N., Kerrigan, J.R., Keenan, B., Rogol, A.D., and Pincus, S.M. (1997c). Estrogen and testosterone, but not a nonaromatizable androgen, direct network integration of the hypothalamo-somatotrope (growth hormone)-insulin-like growth factor I axis in the human: Evidence from pubertal pathophysiology and sex-steroid hormone replacement. *Journal of Clinical Endocrinology and Metabolism, 82(10)*, 3414–3420.

Veldhuis, J.D. and Pincus, S.M. (1998). Orderliness of hormone release patterns: A complementary measure to conventional pulsatile and circadian analyses. *European Journal of Endocrinology, 138*, 358–362.

Veldhuis, J.D., Pincus, S.M., Garcia-Rudaz, M.C., Ropelato, M.G., Escobar, M.E., and Barontini, M. (2001c). Disruption of the synchronous secretion of leptin, LH, and ovarian androgens in nonobese adolescents with the polycystic ovarian syndrome. *Journal of Clinical Endocrinology and Metabolism, 86(8)*, 3772–3778.

Veldhuis, J.D., Pincus, S.M., Garcia-Rudaz, M.C., Ropelato, M.G., Escobar, M.E., and Barontini, M. (2001d). Disruption of the joint synchrony of luteinizing hormone, testosterone, and androstenedione secretion in adolescents with polycystic ovarian syndrome. *Journal of Clinical Endocrinology and Metabolism, 86(1)*, 72–79.

Veldhuis, J.D., Pincus, S.M., Mitamura, R., Yano, K., Suzuki, N., Ito, Y., Makita, Y., and Okuno, A. (2001e). Developmentally delimited emergence of more orderly luteinizing hormone and testosterone secretion during late prepuberty in boys. *Journal of Clinical Endocrinology and Metabolism, 86(1)*, 80–89.

Veldhuis, J.D., Roemmich, J.N., and Rogol, A.D. (2000). Gender and sexual maturation-dependent contrasts in the neuroregulation of growth hormone secretion in prepubertal and late adolescent males and females—A general clinical research center-based study. *Journal of Clinical Endocrinology and Metabolism, 85(7)*, 2385–2394.

Veldhuis, J.D., Straume, M., Iranmanesh, A., Mulligan, T., Jaffe, C., Barkan, A., Johnson, M.L., and Pincus, S. (2001f). Secretory process regularity monitors neuroendocrine feedback and feedforward signaling strength in humans. *American Journal of Physiology: Regulatory, Integrative and Comparative Physiology, 280(3)*, R721–R729.

Veldhuis, J.D., Zwart, A., Mulligan, T., and Iranmanesh, A. (2001g). Muting of androgen negative feedback unveils impoverished gonadotropin-releasing hormone/luteinizing hormone secretory reactivity in healthy older men. *Journal of Clinical Endocrinology and Metabolism, 86(2)*, 529–535.

Veldhuis, J.D., Zwart, A.D., and Iranmanesh, A. (1997d). Neuroendocrine mechanisms by which selective Leydig cell castration unleashes increased pulsatile LH release. *American Journal of Physiology, 272(2 Pt 2)*, R464–R474.

Veldman, R.G., Frölich, M., Pincus, S.M., Veldhuis, J.D., and Roelfsema, F. (2001a). Basal, pulsatile, entropic, and 24-hour rhythmic features of secondary hyperprolactinemia due to functional pituitary stalk disconnection mimic tumoral (primary) hyperprolactinemia. *Journal of Clinical Endocrinology and Metabolism, 86(4)*, 1562–1567.

Veldman, R.G., Frölich, M., Pincus, S.M., Veldhuis, J.D., and Roelfsema, F. (2001b). Hyperleptinemia in women with Cushing's disease is driven by high-amplitude pulsatile, but orderly and eurhythmic, leptin secretion. *European Journal of Endocrinology, 144(1)*, 21–27.

Veldman, R.G., Frölich, M., Pincus, S.M., Veldhuis, J.D., and Roelfsema, F. (2000a). Apparently complete restoration of normal daily adrenocorticotropin, cortisol, growth hormone, and prolactin secretory dynamics in adults with Cushing's disease after clinically successful transsphenoidal adenomectomy. *Journal of Clinical Endocrinology and Metabolism, 85(11)*, 4039–4046.

Veldman, R.G., Frölich, M., Pincus, S.M., Veldhuis, J.D., and Roelfsema, F. (2000b). Growth hormone and prolactin are secreted more irregularly in patients with Cushing's disease. *Clinical Endocrinology, 52(5)*, 625–632.

Wang, C., Berman, N.G., Veldhuis, J.D., Der, T., McDonald, V., Steiner, B., and Swerdloff, R.S. (1998). Graded testosterone infusions distinguish gonadotropin negative-feedback responsiveness in Asian and white men—A Clinical Research Center study. *Journal of Clinical Endocrinology and Metabolism, 83(3)*, 870–876.

Waters, D.L., Qualls, C.R., Dorin, R., Veldhuis, J.D., and Baumgartner, R.N. (2001). Increased pulsatility, process irregularity, and nocturnal trough concentrations of growth hormone in amenorrheic compared to eumenorrheic athletes. *Journal of Clinical Endocrinology and Metabolism, 86(3)*, 1013–1019.

Yildiz, B.O., Suchard, M.A., Wong, M.L., McCann, S.M., and Licinio, J. (2004). Alterations in the dynamics of circulating ghrelin, adiponectin, and leptin in human obesity. *Proceedings of the National Academy of Sciences, 101(28)*, 10434–10439.

Young, E.A. and Veldhuis, J.D. (2006). Disordered adrenocorticotropin secretion in women with major depression. *Journal of Clinical Endocrinology and Metabolism, 91(5)*, 1924–1928.

Zarkovi, M., Ciri, J., Penezi, Z., Trbojevi, B., and Drezgi, M. (2000). Effect of weight loss on the pulsatile insulin secretion. *Journal of Clinical Endocrinology and Metabolism, 85(10)*, 3673–3677.

Zarkovi, M., Ciri, J., Stojanovi, M., Penezi, Z., Trbojevi, B., Dresgi, M., and Nesovi, M. (1999). Effect of insulin sensitivity on pulsatile insulin secretion. *European Journal of Endocrinology, 141(5)*, 494–501.

Zwart, A.D., Iranmanesh, A., and Veldhuis, J.D. (1997). Disparate serum free testosterone concentrations and degrees of hypothalamo-pituitary-luteinizing hormone suppression are achieved by continuous versus pulsatile intravenous androgen replacement in men: A clinical experimental model of ketoconazole-induced reversible hypoandrogenemia with controlled testosterone add-back. *Journal of Clinical Endocrinology and Metabolism, 82(7)*, 2062–2069.

READING LIST: PSYCHOLOGY/NEUROSCIENCE

Abásolo, D., Hornero, R., Espino, P., Escudero, J., and Gómez, C. (2007a). Electroencephalogram background activity characterization with approximate entropy and auto mutual information in Alzheimer's disease patients. *Conference Proceedings: Annual International Conference of the IEEE Engineering in Medicine and Biology Society*, Lyon, 2007, pp. 6192–6195.

Abásolo, D., Hornero, R., Espino, P., Poza, J., Sánchez, C.I., and de la Rosa, R. (2005). Analysis of regularity in the EEG background activity of Alzheimer's disease patients with approximate entropy. *Clinical Neurophysiology, 116(8)*, 1826–1834.

Abásolo, D., James, C.J., and Hornero, R. (2007b). Non-linear analysis of intracranial electroencephalogram recordings with approximate entropy and Lempel-Ziv complexity for epileptic seizure detection. *Conference Proceedings: Annual International Conference of the IEEE Engineering in Medicine and Biology Society*, Lyon, 2007, pp. 1953–1956.

Acharya, U.R., Faust, O., Kannathal, N., Chua, T., and Laxminarayan, S. (2005). Non-linear analysis of EEG signals at various sleep stages. *Computer Methods and Programs in Biomedicine, 80(1)*, 37–45.

Alesci, S., Martinez, P.E., Kelkar, S., Ilias, I., Ronsaville, D.S., Listwak, S.J., Ayala, A.R. et al. (2005). Major depression is associated with significant diurnal elevations in plasma interleukin-6 levels, a shift of its circadian rhythm, and loss of physiological complexity in its secretion: Clinical implications. *Journal of Clinical Endocrinology and Metabolism, 90(5)*, 2522–2530.

Bär, K.J., Boettger, M.K., Koschke, M., Boettger, S., Grotelüschen, M., Voss, A., and Yeragani, V.K. (2007a). Increased QT interval variability index in acute alcohol withdrawal. *Drug and Alcohol Dependence, 89(2–3)*, 259–266.

Bär, K.J., Boettger, M.K., Koschke, M., Schulz, S., Chokka, P., Yeragani, V.K., and Voss, A. (2007b). Non-linear complexity measures of heart rate variability in acute schizophrenia. *Clinical Neurophysiology, 118(9)*, 2009–2015.

Bär, K.J., Koschke, M., Boettger, M.K., Berger, S., Kabisch, A., Sauer, H., Voss, A., and Yeragani, V.K. (2007c). Acute psychosis leads to increased QT variability in patients suffering from schizophrenia. *Schizophrenia Research, 95(1–3)*, 115–123.

Beaumont, A. and Marmarou, A. (2002). Approximate entropy: A regularity statistic for assessment of intracranial pressure. *Acta Neurochirurgica Supplement, 81*, 193–195.

Bhattacharya, J. (2000). Complexity analysis of spontaneous EEG. *Acta Neurobiologiae Experimentalis, 60(4)*, 495–501.

Bruhn, J., Bouillon, T.W., Hoeft, A., and Shafer, S.L. (2002). Artifact robustness, inter- and intraindividual baseline stability, and rational EEG parameter selection. *Anesthesiology, 96(1)*, 54–59.

Bruhn, J., Bouillon, T.W., Radulescu, L., Hoeft, A., Bertaccini, E., and Shafer, S.L. (2003). Correlation of approximate entropy, bispectral index, and spectral edge frequency 95 (SEF95) with clinical signs of "anesthetic depth" during coadministration of propofol and remifentanil. *Anesthesiology, 98(3)*, 621–627.

Bruhn, J., Bouillon, T.W., and Shafer, S.L. (2001a). Onset of propofol-induced burst suppression may be correctly detected as deepening of anaesthesia by approximate entropy but not by bispectral index. *British Journal of Anaesthesia, 87(3)*, 505–507.

Bruhn, J., Lehmann, L.E., Röpcke, H., Bouillon, T.W., and Hoeft, A. (2001b). Shannon entropy applied to the measurement of the electroencephalographic effects of desflurane. *Anesthesiology, 95(1)*, 30–35.

Bruhn, J., Röpcke, H., and Hoeft, A. (2000a). Approximate entropy as an electroencephalographic measure of anesthetic drug effect during desflurane anesthesia. *Anesthesiology, 92(3)*, 715–726.

Bruhn, J., Röpcke, H., Rehberg, B., Bouillon, T., and Hoeft, A. (2000b). Electroencephalogram approximate entropy correctly classifies the occurrence of burst suppression pattern as increasing anesthetic drug effect. *Anesthesiology, 93(4),* 981–985.

Burioka, N., Cornélissen, G., Maegaki, Y., Halberg, F., Kaplan, D.T., Miyata, M., Fukuoka, Y., Endo, M., Suyama, H., Tomita, Y., and Shimizu, E. (2005a). Approximate entropy of the electroencephalogram in healthy awake subjects and absence epilepsy patients. *Clinical EEG and Neuroscience, 36(3),* 188–193.

Burioka, N., Miyata, M., Cornélissen, G., Halberg, F., Takeshima, T., Kaplan, D.T., Suyama, H. et al. (2005b). Approximate entropy in the electroencephalogram during wake and sleep. *Clinical EEG and Neuroscience, 36(1),* 21–24.

Caldirola, D., Bellodi, L., Cammino, S., and Perna, G. (2004a). Smoking and respiratory irregularity in panic disorder. *Biological Psychiatry, 56(6),* 393–398.

Caldirola, D., Bellodi, L., Caumo, A., Migliarese, G., and Perna, G. (2004b). Approximate entropy of respiratory patterns in panic disorder. *American Journal of Psychiatry, 161(1),* 79–87.

Carroll, B.J., Cassidy, F., Naftolowitz, D., Tatham, N.E., Wilson, W.H., Iranmanesh, A., Liu, P.Y., and Veldhuis, J.D. (2007). Pathophysiology of hypercortisolism in depression. *Acta Psychiatrica Scandinavica Supplementum, 433,* 90–103.

Cavanaugh, J.T., Guskiewicz, K.M., Giuliani, C., Marshall, S., Mercer, V., and Stergiou, N. (2005a). Detecting altered postural control after cerebral concussion in athletes with normal postural stability. *British Journal of Sports Medicine, 39(11),* 805–811.

Cavanaugh, J.T., Guskiewicz, K.M., Giuliani, C., Marshall, S., Mercer, V., and Stergiou, N. (2006). Recovery of postural control after cerebral concussion: New insights using approximate entropy. *Journal of Athletic Training, 41(3),* 305–313.

Cavanaugh, J.T., Guskiewicz, K.M., and Stergiou, N. (2005b). A nonlinear dynamic approach for evaluating postural control: New directions for the management of sport-related cerebral concussion. *Sports Medicine, 35(11),* 935–950.

Cavanaugh, J.T., Mercer, V.S., and Stergiou, N. (2007). Approximate entropy detects the effect of a secondary cognitive task on postural control in healthy young adults: A methodological report. *Journal of Neuroengineering and Rehabilitation, 4,* 42.

Darbin, O., Soares, J., and Wichmann, T. (2006). Nonlinear analysis of discharge patterns in monkey basal ganglia. *Brain Research, 1118(1),* 84–93.

Darzy, K.H., Pezzoli, S.S., Thorner, M.O., and Shalet, S.M. (2005). The dynamics of growth hormone (GH) secretion in adult cancer survivors with severe GH deficiency acquired after brain irradiation in childhood for nonpituitary brain tumors: Evidence for preserved pulsatility and diurnal variation with increased secretory disorderliness. *Journal of Clinical Endocrinology and Metabolism, 90(5),* 2794–2803.

Escudero, J., Hornero, R., Abásolo, D., Fernández, A., and Poza, J. (2007). Magnetoencephalogram blind source separation and component selection procedure to improve the diagnosis of Alzheimer's disease patients. *Conference Proceedings: Annual International Conference of the IEEE Engineering in Medicine and Biology Society,* Lyon, *2007,* pp. 5437–5440.

Esmaeili, V., Shamsollahi, M.B., Arefian, N.M., and Assareh, A. (2007). Classifying depth of anesthesia using EEG features, a comparison. *Conference Proceedings: Annual International Conference of the IEEE Engineering in Medicine and Biology Society,* Lyon, *2007,* pp. 4106–4109.

Fang, S., Chan, H., and Chen, W. (2005). Combination of linear and nonlinear methods on electroencephalogram state recognition. *Conference Proceedings: Annual International Conference of the IEEE Engineering in Medicine and Biology Society,* Shanghai, Vol. *5,* pp. 4604–4605.

Fang, S.C., Chan, H.L., and Chen, W.H. (2004). Approximate entropy analysis of electroencephalogram in vasovagal syncope on tilt table test. *Conference Proceedings: Annual International Conference of the IEEE Engineering in Medicine and Biology Society,* San Francisco, CA, Vol. *1,* pp. 590–592.

Ferenets, R., Lipping, T., Anier, A., Jäntti, V., Melto, S., and Hovilehto, S. (2006a). Comparison of entropy and complexity measures for the assessment of depth of sedation. *IEEE Transactions on Biomedical Engineering, 53(6),* 1067–1077.

Ferenets, R., Lipping, T., Suominen, P., Turunen, J., Puumala, P., Jäntti, V., Himanen, S.L., and Huotari, A.M. (2006b). Comparison of the properties of EEG spindles in sleep and propofol anesthesia. *Conference Proceedings: Annual International Conference of the IEEE Engineering in Medicine and Biology Society,* New York, NY, Vol. *1,* pp. 6356–6359.

Ferenets, R., Vanluchene, A., Lipping, T., Heyse, B., and Struys, M.M. (2007). Behavior of entropy/complexity measures of the electroencephalogram during propofol-induced sedation: Dose-dependent effects of remifentanil. *Anesthesiology, 106(4),* 696–706.

Ge, M., Guo, H., Dong, G., Sun, M., Jia, W., Shen, X., and Yan, W. (2004). A theoretical study for the chaos and complexity of the synchronous oscillations in electrically coupled abnormal neurons. *Conference Proceedings: Annual International Conference of the IEEE Engineering in Medicine and Biology Society,* San Francisco, CA, Vol. *1,* pp. 550–553.

Glenn, T., Whybrow, P.C., Rasgon, N., Grof, P., Alda, M., Baethge, C., and Bauer, M. (2006). Approximate entropy of self-reported mood prior to episodes in bipolar disorder. *Bipolar Disorders, 8(5 Pt 1),* 424–429.

Gurney, K.N. (2001). Information processing in dendrites II. Information theoretic complexity. *Neural Networks, 14(8),* 1005–1022.

He, W.X., Yan, X.G., Chen, X.P., and Liu, H. (2005). Nonlinear feature extraction of sleeping EEG signals. *Conference Proceedings: Annual International Conference of the IEEE Engineering in Medicine and Biology Society,* Shanghai, *5,* 4614–4617.

Hornero, R., Abásolo, D., Jimeno, N., Sánchez, C.I., Poza, J., and Aboy, M. (2006a). Variability, regularity, and complexity of time series generated by schizophrenic patients and control subjects. *IEEE Transactions on Biomedical Engineering, 53(2),* 210–218.

Hornero, R., Aboy, M., Abásolo, D., McNames, J., and Goldstein, B. (2005). Interpretation of approximate entropy: Analysis of intracranial pressure approximate entropy during acute intracranial hypertension. *IEEE Transactions on Biomedical Engineering, 52(10),* 1671–1680.

Hornero, R., Aboy, M., Abasolo, D., McNames, J., Wakeland, W., and Goldstein, B. (2006b). Complex analysis of intracranial hypertension using approximate entropy. *Critical Care Medicine, 34(1),* 87–95.

Huang, L., Wang, Y., Liu, J., and Wang, J. (2004). Approximate entropy of EEG as a measure of cerebral ischemic injury. *Conference Proceedings: Annual International Conference of the IEEE Engineering in Medicine and Biology Society,* Vol. *6,* San Francisco, CA, pp. 4537–4539.

Hudetz, A.G. (2002). Effect of volatile anesthetics on interhemispheric EEG cross-approximate entropy in the rat. *Brain Research, 954(1),* 123–131.

Hudetz, A.G., Wood, J.D., and Kampine, J.P. (2003). Cholinergic reversal of isoflurane anesthesia in rats as measured by cross-approximate entropy of the electroencephalogram. *Anesthesiology, 99(5),* 1125–1131.

Ihmsen, H., Schywalsky, M., Plettke, R., Priller, M., Walz, F., and Schwilden, H. (2008). Concentration-effect relations, prediction probabilities (Pk), and signal-to-noise ratios of different electroencephalographic parameters during administration of desflurane, isoflurane, and sevoflurane in rats. *Anesthesiology, 108(2),* 276–285.

Jausovec, N. and Jausovec, K. (2000). Correlations between ERP parameters and intelligence: A reconsideration. *Biological Psychology, 55*(2), 137–154.

Jeleazcov, C., Egner, S., Bremer, F., and Schwilden, H. (2004). Automated EEG preprocessing during anaesthesia: New aspects using artificial neural networks. *Biomedizinische Technik/Biomedical Engineering, 49*(5), 125–131.

Jeleazcov, C., Schmidt, J., Schmitz, B., Becke, K., and Albrecht, S. (2007). EEG variables as measures of arousal during propofol anaesthesia for general surgery in children: Rational selection and age dependence. *British Journal of Anaesthesia, 99*(6), 845–854.

Jordan, D., Schneider, G., Hock, A., Hensel, T., Stockmanns, G., and Kochs, E.F. (2006). EEG parameters and their combination as indicators of depth of anaesthesia. *Biomedizinische Technik/Biomedical Engineering, 51*(2), 89–94.

Kojima, M., Hayano, J., Fukuta, H., Sakata, S., Mukai, S., Ohte, N., Seno, H., Toriyama, T., Kawahara, H., Furukawa, T.A., and Tokudome, S. (2008). Loss of fractal heart rate dynamics in depressive hemodialysis patients. *Psychosomatic Medicine, 70*(2), 177–185.

Koskinen, M., Seppänen, T., Tong, S., Mustola, S., and Thakor, N.V. (2006). Monotonicity of approximate entropy during transition from awareness to unresponsiveness due to propofol anesthetic induction. *IEEE Transactions on Biomedical Engineering, 53*(4), 669–675.

Kumar, A., Anand, S., Chari, P., Yaddanapudi, L.N., and Srivastava, A. (2007). A set of EEG parameters to predict clinically anaesthetized state in humans for halothane anaesthesia. *Journal of Medical Engineering & Technology, 31*(1), 46–53.

Lee, M.S., Rim, Y.H., Jeong, D.M., Kim, M.K., Joo, M.C., and Shin, S.H. (2005). Nonlinear analysis of heart rate variability during Qi therapy (external Qigong). *American Journal of Chinese Medicine, 33*(4), 579–588.

Levy, W.J., Pantin, E., Mehta, S., and McGarvey, M. (2003). Hypothermia and the approximate entropy of the electroencephalogram. *Anesthesiology, 98*(1), 53–57.

Lin, M., Chan, H., and Fang, S. (2005). Linear and nonlinear EEG indexes in relation to the severity of coma. *Conference Proceedings: Annual International Conference of the IEEE Engineering in Medicine and Biology Society*, Shanghai, Vol. 5, pp. 4580–4583.

Lipping, T., Ferenets, R., Mortier, E.P., and Struys, M.M. (2007). A new method for evaluating the performance of depth-of-hypnosis indices—The D-value. *Conference Proceedings: Annual International Conference of the IEEE Engineering in Medicine and Biology Society*, Lyon, *2007*, pp. 6488–6491.

Mantini, D., Franciotti, R., Romani, G.L., and Pizzella, V. (2008). Improving MEG source localizations: An automated method for complete artifact removal based on independent component analysis. *NeuroImage, 40*(1), 160–173.

McComb, J.J., Qian, X.P., Veldhuis, J.D., J. McGlone, J., and Norman, R.L. (2006). Neuroendocrine responses to psychological stress in eumenorrheic and oligomenorrheic women. *Stress, 9*(1), 41–51.

Naguib, M., Schmid, P.G. 3rd, and Baker, M.T. (2003). The electroencephalographic effects of IV anesthetic doses of melatonin: Comparative studies with thiopental and propofol. *Anesthesia and Analgesia, 97*(1), 238–243, table of contents.

Naritoku, D.K., Casebeer, D.J., and Darbin, O. (2003). Effects of seizure repetition on postictal and interictal neurocardiac regulation in the rat. *Epilepsia, 44*(7), 912–916.

Natarajan, K., Acharya, U.R., Alias, F., Tiboleng, T., and Puthusserypady, S.K. (2004). Nonlinear analysis of EEG signals at different mental states. *Biomedical Engineering Online, 3*(1), 7.

Newlin, D.B., Wong, C.J., Stapleton, J.M., and London, E.D. (2000). Intravenous cocaine decreases cardiac vagal tone, vagal index (derived in lorenz space), and heart period complexity (approximate entropy) in cocaine abusers. *Neuropsychopharmacology, 23*(5), 560–568.

Noh, G.J., Kim, K.M., Jeong, Y.B., Jeong, S.W., Yoon, H.S., Jeong, S.M., Kang, S.H., Linares, O., and Kern, S.E. (2006). Electroencephalographic approximate entropy changes in healthy volunteers during remifentanil infusion. *Anesthesiology, 104*(5), 921–932.

Otto, K.A. (2008). EEG power spectrum analysis for monitoring depth of anaesthesia during experimental surgery. *Laboratory Animals, 42(1)*, 45–61.

Palaniappan, R. (2008). Two-stage biometric authentication method using thought activity brain waves. *International Journal of Neural Systems, 18(1)*, 59–66.

Papadelis, C., Chen, Z., Kourtidou-Papadeli, C., Bamidis, P.D., Chouvarda, I., Bekiaris, E., and Maglaveras, N. (2007a). Monitoring sleepiness with on-board electrophysiological recordings for preventing sleep-deprived traffic accidents. *Clinical Neurophysiology, 118(9)*, 1906–1922.

Papadelis, C., Kourtidou-Papadeli, C., Bamidis, P.D., Maglaveras, N., and Pappas, K. (2007b). The effect of hypobaric hypoxia on multichannel EEG signal complexity. *Clinical Neurophysiology, 118(1)*, 31–52.

Perentos, N., Croft, R.J., McKenzie, R.J., Cvetkovic, D., and Cosic, I. (2007). Comparison of the effects of continuous and pulsed mobile phone like RF exposure on the human EEG. *Australasian Physical and Engineering Sciences in Medicine, 30(4)*, 274–280.

Pincus, S.M. (2006). Approximate entropy as a measure of irregularity for psychiatric serial metrics. *Bipolar Disorders, 8(5 Pt 1)*, 430–440.

Pincus, S.M., Schmidt, P.J., Palladino-Negro, P., and Rubinow, D.R. (2008). Differentiation of women with premenstrual dysphoric disorder, recurrent brief depression, and healthy controls by daily mood rating dynamics. *Journal of Psychiatric Research, 42(5)*, 337–347.

Posener, J.A., Charles DeBattista, Veldhuis, J.D., Province, M.A., Williams, G.H., and Schatzberg, A.F. (2004). Process irregularity of cortisol and adrenocorticotropin secretion in men with major depressive disorder. *Psychoneuroendocrinology, 29(9)*, 1129–1137.

Pravitha, R., Sreenivasan, R., and Nampoori, V.P. (2005). Complexity analysis of dense array EEG signal reveals sex difference. *International Journal of Neuroscience, 115(4)*, 445–460.

Sarà, M., Sebastiano, F., Sacco, S., Pistoia, F., Onorati, P., Albertini, G., and Carolei, A. (2008). Heart rate non linear dynamics in patients with persistent vegetative state: A preliminary report. *Brain Injury, 22(1)*, 33–37.

Schneider, G., Hollweck, R., Ningler, M., Stockmanns, G., and Kochs, E.F. (2005). Detection of consciousness by electroencephalogram and auditory evoked potentials. *Anesthesiology, 103(5)*, 934–943.

Sleigh, J.W. and Donovan, J. (1999). Comparison of bispectral index, 95% spectral edge frequency and approximate entropy of the EEG, with changes in heart rate variability during induction of general anaesthesia. *British Journal of Anaesthesia, 82(5)*, 666–671.

Sree Hari Rao, V., Raghvendra Rao, C., and Yeragani, V.K. (2006). A novel technique to evaluate fluctuations of mood: Implications for evaluating course and treatment effects in bipolar/affective disorders. *Bipolar Disorders, 8(5 Pt 1)*, 453–466.

Srinivasan, V., Eswaran, C., and Sriraam, N. (2007). Approximate entropy-based epileptic EEG detection using artificial neural networks. *IEEE Transactions on Information Technology in Biomedicine, 11(3)*, 288–295.

Vigo, D.E., Nicola Siri, L., Ladrón De Guevara, M.S., Martínez-Martínez, J.A., Fahrer, R.D., Cardinali, D.P., Masoli, O., and Guinjoan, S.M. (2004). Relation of depression to heart rate nonlinear dynamics in patients > or =60 years of age with recent unstable angina pectoris or acute myocardial infarction. *American Journal of Cardiology, 93(6)*, 756–760.

Voss, L.J., Ludbrook, G., Grant, C., Sleigh, J.W., and Barnard, J.P. (2006). Cerebral cortical effects of desflurane in sheep: Comparison with isoflurane, sevoflurane and enflurane. *Acta Anaesthesiologica Scandinavica, 50(3)*, 313–319.

Voss, L.J., Ludbrook, G., Grant, C., Upton, R., and Sleigh, J.W. (2007). A comparison of pharmacokinetic/pharmacodynamic versus mass-balance measurement of brain concentrations of intravenous anesthetics in sheep. *Anesthesia and Analgesia, 104(6)*, 1440–1446, table of contents.

Wang, L., Xu, G., Wang, J., Yang, S., and Yan, W. (2007). Feature extraction of mental task in BCI based on the method of approximate entropy. *Conference Proceedings: Annual International Conference of the IEEE Engineering in Medicine and Biology Society,* Lyon, *2007,* pp. 1941–1944.

Yang, H.J., Hu, S.J., Han, S., Liu, G.P., Xie, Y., and Xu, J.X. (2002). Relation between responsiveness to neurotransmitters and complexity of epileptiform activity in rat hippocampal CA1 neurons. *Epilepsia, 43(11),* 1330–1336.

Yeragani, V.K., Pohl, R., Mallavarapu, M., and Balon, R. (2003). Approximate entropy of symptoms of mood: An effective technique to quantify regularity of mood. *Bipolar Disorders, 5(4),* 279–286.

Yeragani, V.K., Radhakrishna, R.K., Tancer, M., and Uhde, T. (2002). Nonlinear measures of respiration: Respiratory irregularity and increased chaos of respiration in patients with panic disorder. *Neuropsychobiology, 46(3),* 111–120.

Yeragani, V.K., Rao, R., Tancer, M., and Uhde, T. (2004). Paroxetine decreases respiratory irregularity of linear and nonlinear measures of respiration in patients with panic disorder. A preliminary report. *Neuropsychobiology, 49(2),* 53–57.

Young, E.A. and Veldhuis, J.D. (2006). Disordered adrenocorticotropin secretion in women with major depression. *Journal of Clinical Endocrinology and Metabolism, 91(5),* 1924–1928.

Zhang, T. and Turner, D. (2001). A visuomotor reaction time task increases the irregularity and complexity of inspiratory airflow pattern in man. *Neuroscience Letters, 297(1),* 41–44.

Zhang, X.S., Roy, R.J., and Jensen, E.W. (2001). EEG complexity as a measure of depth of anesthesia for patients. *IEEE Transactions on Biomedical Engineering, 48(12),* 1424–1433.

Zhao, L., Liang, Z., Hu, G., and Wu, W. (2005). Nonlinear analysis in treatment of intractable epilepsy with EEG biofeedback. *Conference Proceedings: Annual International Conference of the IEEE Engineering in Medicine and Biology Society,* San Francisco, CA, Vol. *5,* pp. 4568–4571.

Zheng, J.H., Chen, J., and Arendt-Nielsen, L. (2004). Complexity of tissue injury-induced nociceptive discharge of dorsal horn wide dynamic range neurons in the rat, correlation with the effect of systemic morphine. *Brain Research, 1001(1–2),* 143–149.

Zhou, W., Zhong, L., and Zhao, H. (2005). Feature attraction and classification of mental EEG using approximate entropy. *Conference Proceedings: Annual International Conference of the IEEE Engineering in Medicine and Biology Society,* San Francisco, CA, Vol. *6,* pp. 5975–5978.

READING LIST: BIOMECHANICS/GAIT/POSTURE

Buzzi, U.H. and Ulrich, B.D. (2004). Dynamic stability of gait cycles as a function of speed and system constraints. *Motor Control, 8(3),* 241–254.

Cavanaugh, J.T., Guskiewicz, K.M., Giuliani, C., Marshall, S., Mercer, V., and Stergiou, N. (2005a). Detecting altered postural control after cerebral concussion in athletes with normal postural stability. *British Journal of Sports Medicine, 39(11),* 805–811.

Cavanaugh, J.T., Guskiewicz, K.M., Giuliani, C., Marshall, S., Mercer, V., and Stergiou, N. (2006). Recovery of postural control after cerebral concussion: New insights using approximate entropy. *Journal of Athletic Training, 41(3),* 305–313.

Cavanaugh, J.T., Guskiewicz, K.M., and Stergiou, N. (2005b). A nonlinear dynamic approach for evaluating postural control: New directions for the management of sport-related cerebral concussion. *Sports Medicine, 35(11),* 935–950.

Cavanaugh, J.T., Mercer, V.S., and Stergiou, N. (2007). Approximate entropy detects the effect of a secondary cognitive task on postural control in healthy young adults: A methodological report. *Journal of Neuroengineering and Rehabilitation, 4,* 42.

Challis, J.H. (2006). Aging, regularity and variability in maximum isometric moments. *Journal of Biomechanics, 39(8)*, 1543–1546.

Chen, W.T., Wang, Z.Z., and Ren, X.M. (2006). Characterization of surface EMG signals using improved approximate entropy. *Journal of Zhejiang University Science B, 7(10)*, 844–848.

Donker, S.F., Ledebt, A., Roerdink, M., Savelsbergh, G.J., Beek, P.J. (2008). Children with cerebral palsy exhibit greater and more regular postural sway than typically developing children. *Experimental Brain Research. 184(3)*, 363–370.

Georgoulis, A.D., Moraiti, C., Ristanis, S., and Stergiou, N. (2006). A novel approach to measure variability in the anterior cruciate ligament deficient knee during walking: The use of the approximate entropy in orthopaedics. *Journal of Clinical Monitoring and Computing, 20(1)*, 11–18.

Harbourne, R.T. and Stergiou, N. (2003). Nonlinear analysis of the development of sitting postural control. *Developmental Psychobiology, 42(4)*, 368–377.

Hong, S.L., Bodfish, J.W., and Newell, K.M. (2006). Power-law scaling for macroscopic entropy and microscopic complexity: Evidence from human movement and posture. *Chaos, 16(1)*, 013135.

Hong, S.L., Manor, B., and Li, L. (2007). Stance and sensory feedback influence on postural dynamics. *Neuroscience Letters, 423(2)*, 104–108.

Karmakar, C.K., Khandoker, A.H., Begg, R.K., Palaniswami, M., and Taylor, S. (2007). Understanding ageing effects by approximate entropy analysis of gait variability. *Conference Proceedings: Annual International Conference of the IEEE Engineering in Medicine and Biology Society, Lyon, 2007*, pp. 1965–1968.

Khandoker, A.H., Palaniswami, M., and Begg, R.K. (2008). A comparative study on approximate entropy measure and poincaré plot indexes of minimum foot clearance variability in the elderly during walking. *Journal of Neuroengineering and Rehabilitation, 5*, 4.

Kovacs, N., Balas, I., Illes, Z., Kellenyi, L., Doczi, T.P., Czopf, J., Poto, L., and Nagy, F. (2006). Uniform qualitative electrophysiological changes in postoperative rest tremor. *Movement Disorders, 21(3)*, 318–324.

Mackenzie, S.J., Getchell, N., Deutsch, K., Wilms-Floet, A., Clark, J.E., and Whitall, J. (2008). Multi-limb coordination and rhythmic variability under varying sensory availability conditions in children with DCD. *Human Movement Science, 27(2)*, 256–269.

Meng, Y., Liu, Y., and Liu, B. (2005). Test nonlinear determinacy of electromyogram. *Conference Proceedings: Annual International Conference of the IEEE Engineering in Medicine and Biology Society, San Francisco, CA, Vol. 5(1)*, pp. 4592–4595.

Morrison, S. and Keogh, J. (2001). Changes in the dynamics of tremor during goal-directed pointing. *Human Movement Science, 20(4–5)*, 675–693.

Sabatini, A.M. (2000). Analysis of postural sway using entropy measures of signal complexity. *Medical and Biological Engineering and Computing, 38(6)*, 617–624.

Schiffman, J.M., Luchies, C.W., Piscitelle, L., Hasselquist, L., and Gregorczyk, K.N. (2006). Discrete bandwidth visual feedback increases structure of output as compared to continuous visual feedback in isometric force control tasks. *Clinical Biomechanics, 21(10)*, 1042–1050.

Slifkin, A.B. and Newell, K.M. (1999). Noise, information transmission, and force variability. *Journal of Experimental Psychology: Human Perception and Performance, 25(3)*, 837–851.

Slifkin, A.B. and Newell, K.M. (2000). Variability and noise in continuous force production. *Journal of Motor Behavior, 32(2)*, 141–150.

Sosnoff, J.J., Valantine, A.D., and Newell, K.M. (2006). Independence between the amount and structure of variability at low force levels. *Neuroscience Letters, 392(3)*, 165–169.

Vaillancourt, D.E. and Newell, K.M. (2000). The dynamics of resting and postural tremor in Parkinson's disease. *Clinical Neurophysiology, 111(11)*, 2046–2056.

Vaillancourt, D.E., Slifkin, A.B., and Newell, K.M. (2001). Regularity of force tremor in Parkinson's disease. *Clinical Neurophysiology, 112(9)*, 1594–1603.

Vaillancourt, D.E., Slifkin, A.B., and Newell, K.M. (2002). Inter-digit individuation and force variability in the precision grip of young, elderly, and Parkinson's disease participants. *Motor Control, 6(2)*, 113–128.

READING LIST: OTHER TOPICS

Aboy, M., Cuesta-Frau, D., Austin, D., and Mico-Tormos, P. (2007). Characterization of sample entropy in the context of biomedical signal analysis. *Conference Proceedings: Annual International Conference of the IEEE Engineering in Medicine and Biology Society,* Lyon, *2007*, pp. 5943–5946.

Abundo, M., Accardi, L., Rosato, N., and Stella, L. (2002). Analysing protein energy data by a stochastic model for cooperative interactions: Comparison and characterization of cooperativity. *Journal of Mathematical Biology, 44(4)*, 341–359.

Aghazadeh, B.S., Khadivi, H., and Nikkhah-Bahrami, M. (2007). Nonlinear analysis and classification of vocal disorders. *Conference Proceedings: Annual International Conference of the IEEE Engineering in Medicine and Biology Society,* Lyon, *2007*, pp. 6200–6203.

Bandt, C. and Pompe, B. (2002). Permutation entropy: A natural complexity measure for time series. *Physical Review Letters. 88(17)*, 174102.

Cuesta, D., Varela, M., Miró, P., Galdós, P., Abásolo, D., Hornero, R., and Aboy, M. (2007). Predicting survival in critical patients by use of body temperature regularity measurement based on approximate entropy. *Medical and Biological Engineering and Computing, 45(7)*, 671–678.

Ferrario, M., Signorini, M.G., Magenes, G. (2009). Complexity analysis of the fetal heart rate variability: Early identification of severe intrauterine growth-restricted fetuses. *Medical & Biological Engineering & Computing. 47(9)*, 911–919.

Jiang, X., Wei, R., Zhao, Y., and Zhang, T. (2008). Using Chou's pseudo amino acid composition based on approximate entropy and an ensemble of AdaBoost classifiers to predict protein subnuclear location. *Amino Acids, 34(4)*, 669–675.

Johnson, M.L., Lampl, M., and Straume, M. (2000). Distinguishing models of growth with approximate entropy. *Methods in Enzymology, 321,* 196–207.

Johnson, M.L. and Straume, M. (2000). Approximate entropy as indication of goodness-of-fit. *Methods in Enzymology, 321,* 207–216.

Johnson, M.L., Straume, M., and Lampl, M. (2001). The use of regularity as estimated by approximate entropy to distinguish saltatory growth. *Annals of Human Biology, 28(5)*, 491–504.

Karamanos, K., Dakopoulos, D., Aloupis, K., Peratzakis, A., Athanasopoulou, L., Nikolopoulos, S., Kapiris, P., and Eftaxias, K. (2006). Preseismic electromagnetic signals in terms of complexity. *Physical Review E, 74(1 Pt 2)*, 016104.

Moore, C., Manickam, K., Willard, T., Jones, S., Slevin, N., and Shalet, S. (2004). Spectral pattern complexity analysis and the quantification of voice normality in healthy and radiotherapy patient groups. *Medical Engineering & Physics, 26(4)*, 291–301.

National Center for Biotechnology Information, U.S. National Library of Medicine. (2015). http://www.ncbi.nlm.nih.gov/pubmed) (Accessed on October 27, 2015.)

Physionet.org. (2011). http://www.physionet.org/. (Accessed on October 27, 2015).

Pincus, S. and Kalman, R.E. (1997). Not all (possibly) "random" sequences are created equal. *Proceedings of the National Academy of Sciences, 94(8)*, 3513–3518.

Pincus, S. and Kalman, R.E. (2004). Irregularity, volatility, risk, and financial market time series. *Proceedings of the National Academy of Sciences, 101(38)*, 13709–13714.

Pincus, S. and Singer, B.H. (1996). Randomness and degrees of irregularity. *Proceedings of the National Academy of Sciences, 93(5)*, 2083–2088.

Riedl, M., Muller, A., Wessel, N. (2013). Practical considerations of permutation entropy. *European Physical Journal-Special Topics. 222(2)*, 249–262.

Pincus, S. and Singer, B.H. (1998). A recipe for randomness. *Proceedings of the National Academy of Sciences, 95(18)*, 10367–10372.

Pincus, S.M. (1992). Approximating Markov chains. *Proceedings of the National Academy of Sciences, 89(10)*, 4432–4436.

Semenov, A.V., Franz, E., van Overbeek, L., Termorshuizen, A.J., and van Bruggen, A.H. (2008). Estimating the stability of *Escherichia coli* O157:H7 survival in manure-amended soils with different management histories. *Environmental Microbiology, 10(6)*, 1450–1459.

Singer, B.H. and Pincus, S. (1998). Irregular arrays and randomization. *Proceedings of the National Academy of Sciences, 95(4)*, 1363–1368.

Souza, G.M., Ribeiro, R.V., Santos, M.G., Ribeiro, H.L., and Oliveira, R.F. (2004). Approximate entropy as a measure of complexity in sap flow temporal dynamics of two tropical tree species under water deficit. *Anais da Academia Brasileira de Ciencias, 76(3)*, 625–630.

Van der Kloot, W., Andricioaei, I., and Balezina, O.P. (1999). Examining the timing of miniature endplate potential releases at the frog and mouse neuromuscular junctions for deviations from Poisson expectations. *Pflügers Archiv, European Journal of Physiology, 438(5)*, 578–586.

Vandierendonck, A. (2000). Analyzing human random time generation behavior: A methodology and a computer program. *Behavior Research Methods, Instruments, and Computers, 32(4)*, 555–565.

Varela, M., Calvo, M., Chana, M., Gomez-Mestre, I., Asensio, R., and Galdos, P. (2005). Clinical implications of temperature curve complexity in critically ill patients. *Critical Care Medicine, 33(12)*, 2764–2771.

Varela, M., Churruca, J., Gonzalez, A., Martin, A., Ode, J., and Galdos, P. (2006). Temperature curve complexity predicts survival in critically ill patients. *American Journal of Respiratory and Critical Care Medicine, 174(3)*, 290–298.

Varela, M., Jimenez, L., and Fariña, R. (2003). Complexity analysis of the temperature curve: New information from body temperature. *European Journal of Applied Physiology, 89(3–4)*, 230–237.

Weinstein, M., Gorrindo, T., Riley, A., Mormino, J., Niedfeldt, J., Singer, B., Rodríguez, G., Simon, J., and Pincus, S. (2003). Timing of menopause and patterns of menstrual bleeding. *American Journal of Epidemiology, 158(8)*, 782–791.

Zhang, T.L., Ding, Y.S., and Chou, K.C. (2008). Prediction protein structural classes with pseudo-amino acid composition: Approximate entropy and hydrophobicity pattern. *Journal of Theoretical Biology, 250(1)*, 186–193.

7 Fractals

Denise McGrath

CONTENTS

Introduction 261
Fractals 262
What Do Broccoli and Coastlines Have to Do with Human Movement? 265
Revision of Logarithms and Power Laws 266
Distributions 270
What Is the Significance of a Power-Law Distribution? 272
Fractal Methods 274
　Fractional Brownian Motion and Fractional Gaussian Noise 274
　Fractal Analysis in Human Movement 277
　　Gait 277
　　Ambulatory Activity 280
　　Upper Limb Movement 280
　　Postural Control 281
　Procedure for Detrended Fluctuation Analysis 282
Practical Considerations 283
　Study Design 285
　Data Collection 285
　Data Analysis 287
　Reporting 289
Future of Fractal Analysis in Human Movement 289
　Current State of the Art 289
　Paradigm Shift in Health Care 289
　Fractal Scaling as a Measure of Physiologic Reserve 291
　Technology 292
Exercises 292
References 295

God used beautiful mathematics in creating the world.

Paul Dirac (1902–1984)

INTRODUCTION

A Polish-born, French–American mathematician by the name of Benoit Mandelbrot (1924–2010) was requested, as an IBM employee in 1961, to work on the problem of transmitting computer data over telephone lines, where bursts of white noise continuously interrupted the clean flow of the signal [1]. The seemingly random bursts of noise contained within the signal were a source of frustration for the company. Mandelbrot, who had always approached mathematics from a visual perspective, examined the temporal patterns generated by the bursts of noise, and made a significant discovery. He found that the patterning of periods of noise to periods of clean information transmission was similar, whether he plotted the time series across months, days, or even seconds. The seemingly erratic appearance of noise within the signal actually demonstrated a very clear order that did not vary when examined across different time scales.

This chapter will describe how and why we analyze human movement data, recorded over a period of time, that is, minutes, hours or days, to see whether we can identify patterns within the fluctuations of the data that are repeated over time. The approach that we describe is called "fractal analysis." If we record a healthy adult walking, uninterrupted, over a period of minutes, we will observe a very well-controlled walking gait. However, closer examination of the data will show that the individual's stride time, stride length, and step width will all change ever so slightly for every step that is taken. Fluctuations in continuous movement data like this have often been treated as unwanted "outliers" or "errors" or "noise." Traditionally, summary statistics such as the mean and standard deviation have been used to describe these data sets, which convey a useful picture of a person's movement, but do not provide us with the complete picture. In the analysis approach described in this chapter, we are expressly interested in the nature of the moment-to-moment fluctuations that occur when steady-state, continuous movement is being performed. We believe that understanding the nature of these fluctuations can lead us to important insights into the state of a person's health. In the words of Mandelbrot (1963), "it is very desirable that both 'trend' and 'noise' be aspects of the same deeper 'truth,' which may not be explainable today, but which can be adequately described." Harvesting the richness contained within human movement data, rather than looking only at averages of time series, should bring us closer to the "deeper truth" to which Mandelbrot referred.

FRACTALS

In order to understand fractal analysis techniques, it is useful to first learn about geometric fractals. A fractal can be thought of as an object that when magnified, reveals smaller features that appear to resemble the whole object. Take the example of a coastline. If you look at a coastline on a map from a particular scale, you will see an irregular, jagged line that separates the land from the sea (Figure 7.1) [2]. If you magnify a portion of this image, you will see a similarly irregular, jagged line as smaller bays and inlets are revealed through the magnification process. If you repeat this process again, you will again see an irregular, jagged line that represents outcrops of rock and even smaller inlets. This example highlights two important properties of a fractal: self-similarity and scale-free. In other words, no matter what scale you examine the object from, its structure on a large scale looks similar to its structure on a small scale.

Another interesting example of fractal geometry in nature is the Romanesco broccoli. This beautifully shaped vegetable is composed of smaller florets that resemble

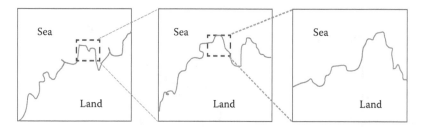

FIGURE 7.1 A representation of a coastline that, when magnified, reveals finer and finer features (bays, inlets) that look similar to the bigger features (harbors, peninsulas), all represented by an irregular, jagged line, that is, a self-similar, scale-free fractal.

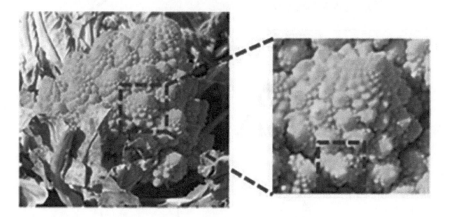

FIGURE 7.2 Romanesco Broccoli, an example of a naturally occurring fractal shape that exhibits self-similarity at smaller scales.

the entire object, and these florets are, in turn, composed of smaller florets again (Figure 7.2). The self-similarity is observable on four levels of magnification, which means that across these ranges, the shape is scale-free (i.e., it does not matter at what scale you look at it, it always looks similar) and this scale-free property is due to its inherent self-similarity. Other naturally occurring fractal objects include trees and branching networks such as the winding paths of rivers and their tributaries, blood vessels in the body, or the branching from the trachea to the bronchi, bronchioles, and alveoli in the lungs. Of course not everything is fractal. If you take a part out of your computer, the part does not represent a smaller version of your computer. Similarly, if you magnify a piece of a circle or a square, the magnified portion does not reveal smaller circular or square features, it just reveals a portion of the shape's perimeter (Figure 7.3).

As well as naturally occurring fractal objects, exact geometric fractals can also be constructed using simple formula that are repeated over and over again. Well-known mathematical, or geometric fractals include the Sierpinski triangle (Figure 7.4). The basic rule for the construction of this triangle is as follows: connect the midpoints of each side of the equilateral triangle to form four separate triangles, and differentially color the triangle in the center (the downward pointing triangle). When this rule is

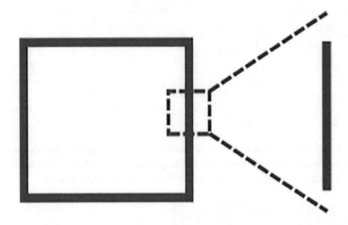

FIGURE 7.3   Magnification of a square does not reveal self-similarity at smaller scales.

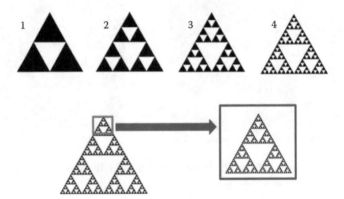

FIGURE 7.4   The process of constructing the Sierpinski Triangle. Note that magnifying a portion of the final triangle leaves the original shape unchanged. The Sierpinski triangle shows how fractal geometry provides a framework in which a simple process, involving a basic operation repeated many-times, can give rise to a rather complex result.

iterated, that is, repeated, as illustrated in steps 1–4 of Figure 7.4, an interesting shape begins to emerge. If the process is continued (e.g., using a computer program), a rather intricate object appears. Also illustrated in Figure 7.4 is the fact that magnifying a portion of the Sierpinski triangle produces an exact copy of the original shape. This magnification process can conceptually go on to infinity in a geometric fractal. However, fractals found in nature are not so exact. They naturally include elements of randomness and the fractal scaling exists over a finite range of scales, as is the case with the Romanesco Broccoli.

Fractal geometry is a curious type of geometry that is different from the classic shapes of Euclidean geometry. Euclidean geometry has certainly proved to be very useful when straight or curved lines are in question, such as triangles or circles. However, natural, irregular shaped objects that we find in nature such as mountains cannot be measured precisely using Euclidean geometry. They could perhaps be approximated by triangular representations, but they have rough surfaces with pits and mounds that are ignored if approximated by a triangle. Fractal geometry, made famous by Mandelbrot, provides us with a way to very precisely measure the natural world in which we live. The word fractal comes from the Latin word *fractus* meaning broken. It is a general description for a large class of irregular objects. It is a geometry of roughness, a geometry of the entwined. It enables us to see patterns not at one scale or another, but across every scale, and reveals a strange kind of symmetry therein.

WHAT DO BROCCOLI AND COASTLINES HAVE TO DO WITH HUMAN MOVEMENT?

If you are reading this chapter, the chances are that you have previously analyzed human movement in some way. You have probably used sophisticated equipment like force plates, optical motion capture, inertial sensors, load cells, or electrogoniometers to capture various aspects of human movement. Using this equipment, you probably have produced some sort of signal that represents the movement you have observed. In many cases, human movement scientists are interested in observing a movement over time, for example, examining a person's postural control, walking/running gait or ambulatory behavior over a period of minutes, hours, or even days. If, for example, we are interested in investigating stride times, we might calculate a person's stride times over time, and then plot the series of stride times on a graph, that is, stride times on the y-axis and number of strides on the x-axis. We know that healthy human movement is variable, so we would not expect each stride time to be the exact same. We would expect to see variations of the order of milliseconds across individual strides. When plotting the data points for each stride time, the variation inherent in a person's movement would start to create a particular shape in the graph—a seemingly irregular, jagged line, not unlike the coastline we described before. With enough stride-time observations, as in Figure 7.5 where the gait of

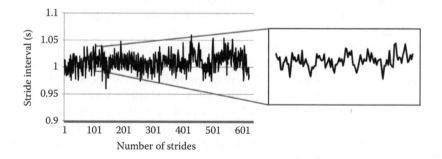

FIGURE 7.5 A healthy gait signal can exhibit fractal scaling of stride intervals when the pattern of the stride interval signal is repeated over time and at different time scales, that is, one can discern a repeated pattern with a relatively large amplitude, but if a smaller segment of the signal is magnified, a similar repeated pattern could be observed at this smaller scale. These different scales may represent different neuromuscular control processes that are coordinated through this fractal structure.

a healthy young person is depicted, we can see that there seems to be a repeating structure to this kind of time series. Furthermore, when we magnify a portion of the graph, a similar, jagged and repeating structure is apparent at this smaller scale. Therefore, from what we already know about fractals, we can say that the pattern of stride-time observations over a relatively large time scale (10 min in the case of Figure 7.5) exhibits fractal scaling (i.e., the curve looks the same at different scales) and is thus self-similar.

However, this is somewhat of a simplification. We can see in Figure 7.5 that the magnified curve's structure is not an exact copy of the original curve, unlike what we saw in the Sierpinksi triangle. Rather, the statistical properties of the magnified curve, for example, the amount of variation present, is proportional to the statistical properties of the whole curve. This is called "statistical self-similarity," and this is what we mean when we refer to self-similarity or "fractal scaling" in a physiological time series, such as human movement. When measuring statistical self-similarity of a time series, the properties of the signal are examined at different scales, that is, the time dimension is rescaled. This reveals a particular property of physiological time series known as self-affinity which means that the statistical properties of the fractal time series scale differently along different dimensions. Before we discuss further the fractality of human movement, we need to explore some mathematical concepts that will enable us to employ methods of fractal analysis with greater clarity.

REVISION OF LOGARITHMS AND POWER LAWS

Consider the equation in the following, and solve for x:

$$10^x = 50 \tag{7.1}$$

Assuming that we do not know about logarithms, we first have to guess what x could be. If x was 1, we would get $10^1 = 10$, if x were 2, we would get $10^2 = 100$. Therefore, x must be a value between 1 and 2, in order to satisfy Equation 7.1. If we plot the function $y = 10^x$ (Figure 7.6), we can estimate from the graph that, indeed, x lies somewhere between 1.6 and 1.8.

We can see from this graph that x is related to y in some way [3]. If $y = 10^x$, then we can say that the exponent x is the logarithm of y, that is, $x = \log(y)$. Substituting this into Equation 7.1, we get $10^{\log(y)} = y$, which illustrates how the logarithm is the inverse of the exponential function. This mathematical rule can be said as follows: the logarithm of a number to a given base equals the power (exponent) to which the base must be raised in order to produce the number. In our example, we can now say that the logarithm of 50 to base 10 will give us our answer, which we can easily compute using a calculator, that is, $\log_{10} 50 = 1.699$, or putting it the other way, $10^{1.699} = 50$. This confirms that the value for x is between 1.6 and 1.8, as suggested by Figure 7.6. Mathematically, this relationship is given as follows:

$$b^x = y \quad x = \log_b y \tag{7.2}$$

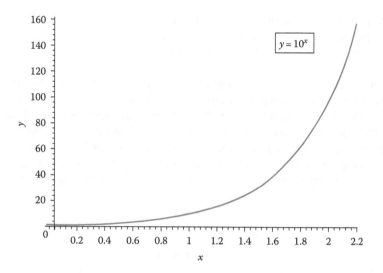

FIGURE 7.6   Plotting the function $y = 10^x$, we can locate 50 on the y-axis and estimate that x lies somewhere between 1.6 and 1.8.

Some key properties of logarithms that can be derived from Equation 7.2 are as follows:

$$\log(AB) = \log A + \log B$$

$$\log\left(\frac{A}{B}\right) = \log(A) - \log(B)$$

$$\log A^n = n \log A$$

Consider the equation $y = Ax^\alpha$. This is a power curve, as the variable x is raised to the power of α. If $A = 1$ and $\alpha = 2$, then $y = x^2$. This means that for

$$x = 1, y = 1$$

$$x = 2, y = 4$$

$$x = 3, y = 9$$

$$x = 4, y = 16$$

...etc.

The plot of $y\,x = 2$ would thus look like this Figure 7.7.
The plot of $y\,x = -2$ would look like this Figure 7.8.
The plot of $y\,x = -9$ would look like this Figure 7.9.

It is not that easy to tell what the power law (or exponent) is by simply looking at the graphs in Figures 7.7 through 7.9. However, we can use logarithms to reformulate the power curves as straight lines that will enable us to extract both α and A values to solve the equation $y = Ax^\alpha$, using the equation of a line ($y = b + ax$). We can draw new graphs called log–log plots, which ensures that the points in the graph are evenly spaced, compared to how they look on the power curves. From the properties of logarithms derived from Equation 7.2, we can rewrite the power-curve equation as follows:

$$y = Ax^n$$

$$\log y = \log Ax^n$$

$$\log y = \log A + \log x^n y$$

$$\log y = \log A + n \log x \tag{7.3}$$

Note that Equation 7.3 has the same format as the equation of a line ($y = b + ax$), where log y is y, log A is b, n is a, and log x is x. Therefore, when we plot our log–log plot, we can easily identify the slope of the line (Figure 7.10). This information

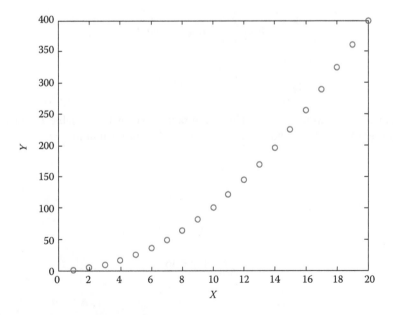

FIGURE 7.7 Power law with a positive exponent of 2.

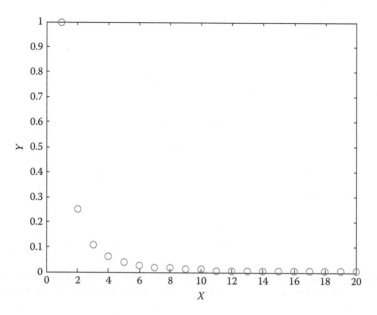

FIGURE 7.8   Power law with a negative exponent of 2.

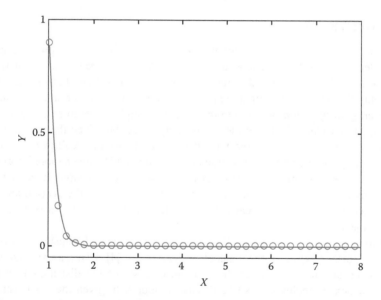

FIGURE 7.9   Power law with a negative exponent of 9.

is critical in understanding how we can measure the fractal properties of a human movement time series. Investigating whether data appear as a straight line on a log–log scale can be instructive in detecting possible power laws. In the next section, we will explore what kind of data need to be plotted on a log–log plot, and what power laws mean for human movement.

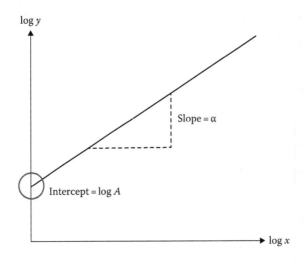

FIGURE 7.10 The slope of a log–log plot provides us with the scaling exponent α that describes the power law governing the data (provided that the data are accurately represented by a power law).

DISTRIBUTIONS

If I were to ask you to describe the triangles that make up the Sierpinski Triangle, illustrated in Figure 7.4, what would you say? You might say that the Sierpinksi triangle is made up of many different triangles of many different sizes, the biggest one being the outer triangle that creates a boundary for the other smaller triangles. However, *quantification* of the Sierpinski triangle might prove to be more difficult. One might consider calculating the mean triangle size, but given the very large differences in size between the largest and smallest triangles, this really would not be a very meaningful description of this fractal object. It would be much more informative to describe the Sierpinksi triangle in terms of how many very large, large, medium, small, tiny triangles comprise the whole shape. In other words, the distribution of the various triangle sizes that appear within the shape provides a clearer picture of the fractal object.

Similarly, we can look at the Romanesco broccoli and, for instance, a box of apples to further explicate the concept of distribution [4]. Using an average value, such as the arithmetic mean or the median, to describe the distribution of apple sizes in a box of apples seems like a sensible approach, given the small variation that exists in sizes of apples. The vast majority of apple sizes will fall close to the mean apple size, with a small number falling a little further from the mean. This is a typical Gaussian distribution, or "normal" distribution, which most people have encountered in the course of their studies. This distribution comes as a result of the apples having a "characteristic" or typical size. On the other hand, the various florets on the Romanesco broccoli exhibit a large range in size. The largest size is the whole vegetable itself, and then, smaller and smaller florets appear as you zoom closer and closer. There is, therefore, no characteristic size of florets because the smallest visible floret is vastly different from the largest. Again, the most informative description of this fractal object, like the Sierpinski Triangle, would be to describe the distribution of sizes of florets. The object is best described by how the particular property being measured, for example, size, depends upon the resolution, or scale, at which it is measured. This relationship is characterized by a parameter called the fractal dimension. The fractal dimension, or the relationship between the statistical properties of an object measured at small scales and the statistical properties of the object measured at large scales, is the focus of this chapter; where the "object" in question becomes a time series from movement data.

The following is a simplistic example of how we can use the log–log plots described earlier to understand the statistics of a distribution. If we take the stylized "fractal tree" in Figure 7.11, we can calculate the distribution of different sized branches in the tree. To put it another way, we are asking, how often does each branch size appear in this tree? This is known as the probability density function. From looking at the tree, we can see that big branches appear less frequently than smaller branches. This tree consists of 10 different sized branches. When we plot the number of branches at each branch size, we get Figure 7.12a, that is, a power-law distribution, similar to Figures 7.8 and 7.9. Recasting this plot as a log–log plot, we observe that the data then appear along a straight line. We can observe from the log–log plot that the statistics for the larger branches are similar to the statistics for the

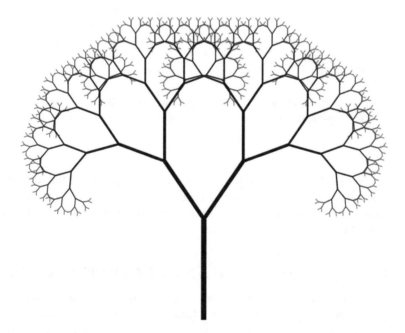

FIGURE 7.11 A computer-generated fractal "tree."

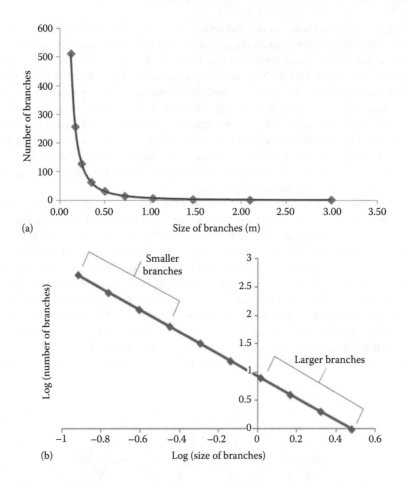

FIGURE 7.12 (a) Distribution of branches in the fractal tree demonstrating a power-law relationship. (b) Log–log plot illustrating similar statistical properties for branches at different scales.

smaller branches, that is, statistically self-similar. The slope of this line will reveal the scaling relation that exists between the size of the branches and how often they appear. The slope of the line is −1.943, and the intercept is 0.927, therefore, the probability that a branch has length $y = 0.927x^{-1.943}$.

WHAT IS THE SIGNIFICANCE OF A POWER-LAW DISTRIBUTION?

A fundamental characteristic of fractal objects is that their measured metric properties, such as length or area, are a function of the scale of measurement. The classic example of this is measuring the length of a coastline. The smaller the measuring tool that you use to measure a coastline, the longer the coastline appears. If you use a meter stick to measure a coastline compared to measuring in kilometers, you will discover finer features to measure with the meter stick. The length of a coastline will, therefore, be greater when the smaller inlets are included using the meter stick, compared to measuring it in kilometers. When we are seeking to quantify human movement variability, we are measuring the fluctuations that occur over time. As in the case of the coastline, we know that the magnitude of fluctuations depends on what timescale we are observing. A large body of research [5–7] has shown that the magnitude of fluctuations in gait parameters at small time scales is correlated with the magnitude of fluctuations at larger time scales, in a power-law fashion.

A power-law distribution is said to decay slowly (Figure 7.12), that is, there is a "long-tail" that extends to the right of the graph. Power-law distributions are suitable models for fractal processes because, like fractals, they do not have a meaningful average or typical size or scale. They are sometimes called scaling distributions, because they describe phenomena that scale, that is, appear statistically the same as one observes a phenomenon at different ranges. A typical pattern in a fractal time series, for example, a positive trend between successive values, appears nested with similar positive trends being expressed at larger scales. Statistically similar fluctuations can be observed across a range of time scales from seconds to minutes to hours to days, depending on what data are being collected. The current trend, therefore, is said to possess the "memory" of the preceding values of the series [8]. This phenomenon is termed long-term memory, long-range dependence, long-range correlations, fractal process, or $1/f$ noise. These different terms can often cause confusion for the uninitiated reader. "$1/f$ noise" means that in the power spectrum of a time series, each frequency has energy proportional to its period of oscillation. Energy is, therefore, distributed across the entire spectrum and not concentrated at a certain portion (i.e., there is no "average"). Many phenomena are believed to be distributed according to a power law, including biological rhythms, such as heart rate [9], respiration [10], and walking strides [11]. These biological signals examined over time reveal the presence of power laws, or long-range correlations in healthy systems, and a loss of this structure in aging and across a range of illnesses [10–23]. This means that in healthy human movement time series such as gait or tapping sequences, the time intervals between events are not equal, nor are they independent. Rather, there is a relationship between these fluctuating intervals that holds beyond consecutive intervals, extending far forward and backward in time. The structure of these multiscale interactions are, therefore, ordered, because they are related in a power-law fashion yet flexible because the pattern fluctuates across different time scales. This relates to the concept in nonlinear dynamics known as "complexity" [24]. The complexity of a system is closely linked to its organization, or coordination. Complexity requires a certain level of coordination between the multiple components that compose the system. Interactions between the components are thought to be more important than the components themselves, and the whole is greater than the sum of its parts.

To recap, long-range correlations that characterize fractal scaling refer to the statistical relationship that exists between fluctuations measured at tiny time scales all the way up to fluctuations measured at very large time scales. The exact cause and function of these long-range correlations, commonly observed in highly functioning biological processes, and less frequently in systems that have been compromised by degeneration or disease, is currently not clear. It is widely suggested that fractal scaling confers enhanced connectivity between biological processes [25], while a breakdown in fractal scaling arises from a gradual deterioration in the number of "functioning elements of a given system and/or a decrease in the interactions between these components" [14,26]. From this perspective, there is no particular component that causes fractal scaling to occur. Instead, it is an emergent property that stems from the interactions across the many spatiotemporal scales of organization instantiated within an organism [27], giving rise to a "nimble" but coordinated biological system. This complexity is thought to be biologically adaptive because it is flexible, allowing organisms to cope with stress and unpredictable environments [11,14,26,28–31]. Complexity is, therefore, conceived as an essential property, which could be lost with aging and disease, yielding maladaptation and lack of flexibility, and regained with rehabilitation and learning [32]. Nonetheless, while the conceptual power of this analysis is widely accepted, detailed knowledge of the neurophysiologically relevant mechanisms that explain the presence of fractal fluctuations is still lacking [33]. Understanding fractal properties in human movement time series has important implications and could lead to fundamentally new theoretical and applied models of motor control in health and disease.

FRACTAL METHODS

FRACTIONAL BROWNIAN MOTION AND FRACTIONAL GAUSSIAN NOISE

The definition of complexity as an optimal region between order and disorder was mapped to time series modeling by Mandelbrot and van Ness in 1968 [34]. Their model was based on two well-known stochastic processes: white noise and Brownian motion, that is, series with uncorrelated data and increments, respectively. The model they proposed consisted of fractional Brownian motions (fBm) based on Brownian motion, and fractional Gaussian noise (fGn) based on white noise. The main difference between fBm and ordinary Brownian motion is that in fBm, successive increments are correlated. A positive correlation indicates that an increasing trend in the past is likely to be followed by an increasing trend in the future. In terms of movement parameters this would mean that, for example, an increasing trend in stride length will be followed by an increasing trend in stride length. The series is said to be persistent. Conversely, a negative correlation indicates that an increasing trend in the past is likely to be followed by a decreasing trend. The series is then said to be antipersistent. fGn relates to another type of fractal process and is defined as the series of successive increments in an fBm. fGn and fBm are, therefore, interrelated: when an fGn is cumulatively summed, the resultant series constitutes an fBm. However, these two processes possess fundamentally different properties: fBm is nonstationary, while fGn is a stationary process. A stationary process, or stationarity, exhibits a constant mean value and constant variance over time (see Chapter 2). Stationarity is an important concept to be

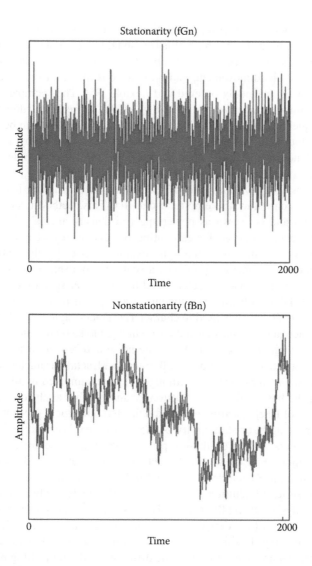

FIGURE 7.13   Illustration of stationarity (fGn) and nonstationarity (fBn). Differencing the increments of a nonstationary fBn time series will result in a stationary fGn time series.

aware of in any biological series, including human movement, because time series of this sort are frequently not stationary. How you go about calculating the fractal scaling of a time series can depend on what type of process, fGn or fBm, your data represents. Figure 7.13 illustrates fGn and fBn. The fGn exhibits a flat, random signal with no real discernible pattern. The fBn on the other hand exhibits a clear nonstationary process, where the mean is clearly drifting up and down.

Interestingly, healthy physiological time series, including human movement, generally fall somewhere between the fGn or fBm dichotomy, in a region known as "pink" noise, which is another representation of $1/f$ fluctuations, long-range correlations or fractal scaling. Therefore, in this fractional noise framework, white noise is considered to represent incoherent movement, brown noise is considered to represent overly constrained movement, and pink noise is thought to represent complex movement, that is, optimally ordered and flexible [35]. The "complex" portion of this continuum is characterized by a scaling law, in the frequency domain, relating power to frequency: $S(f) \propto f^{-\beta}$. This scaling law (or power law) can be revealed by the log–log plot of the power spectrum, which is characterized by a linear shape of slope $-\beta$. The linear relation must span a range of at least two decades of frequency to be considered as a possible power-law distribution (i.e., 2 log units, or 100 frequencies [36,37]). The value of the scaling exponent then indicates where on the "noise" continuum the empirical data lie. This method relates to the frequency domain and is known as power spectral density analysis; however, other methods have been proposed for estimating the exponent that governs the scaling of fluctuations in the time domain, for example, detrended fluctuation analysis (described later). This method produces a scaling exponent, α, which is linearly related to the power exponent β determined by the power spectral density method (i.e., $\alpha = (\beta + 1)/2$). Both these exponents α and β can be used to calculate the Hurst coefficient, H, which is used to characterize fractal signals. Pink noise, or the range of $1/f$ fluctuations in biological data are thought to be represented by an α-value approaching 1, while the exponent for white noise and brown noise is found near 0.5 and 1.5, respectively. Therefore, H, β, α, are all fractal parameters that express the same statistical characteristics, although they are computed in different ways.

Choosing the best method(s) to accurately and reliably analyze empirical time series in terms of fractal scaling is not trivial. Methodological precautions regarding the nature, length, or stationarity of the series have been advised, with many informative papers written on these topics [32,38–48]. These considerations will be expanded upon under the section "Practical Considerations." Many other methods exist, which have been developed and refined to identify long-range correlations in time series in addition to power spectral density analysis and detrended fluctuation analysis (DFA) [49], such as Hurst's rescaled range analysis (R/S) [50], dispersional analysis [51], detrending moving average algorithm [52], to name a few. The preliminary classification of empirical time series as fGn or fBm is a crucial step in fractal analysis. However, the difficulty in distinguishing between fGn and fBm around the $1/f$ boundary is problematic particularly in human movement data, as empirical time series produced by the motor system often fall into this range. It can, therefore, be difficult to decide which fractal analysis method to use, one that is based on fGn type signals, or one that is based upon fBn type signals. Delignieres and colleagues investigated a range of fractal analysis methods and concluded that for behavioral or psychological data, methods that are insensitive to the fGn/fBm dichotomy are recommended, and favored DFA for this purpose [39]. Indeed, DFA has become the predominant method of fractal analysis in the human movement literature and was recently reported as being the "method of choice" in determining fractal scaling of a time series [46]. However, other studies have questioned the supposed advantage of using DFA for short time series that are common in human movement [43,48].

FRACTAL ANALYSIS IN HUMAN MOVEMENT

Gait

Many studies have investigated the fractal scaling of human gait and have found that long-range correlations do exist in healthy gait. Stride interval has been the most researched parameter, where an α-value of 1 is theoretically anticipated, as it corresponds to pink noise, or $1/f$ fluctuations in the time series, indicating an idealized level of complexity that leads to both stable and flexible movement patterns. Table 7.1 summarizes selected research on long-range correlations in stride intervals. This is not an exhaustive list. Rather, the studies have been chosen to highlight some pertinent points relating to the investigation of fractal dynamics in human gait. The studies described in the table focus on walking gait, but fractal analysis has also been applied to running gait in terms of speed variability in a race, and the effect of running speed on long-range correlations [53,54]. DFA is the method that has been used in all of these studies to quantify fractal scaling, which highlights the current popularity of this approach.

On examining Table 7.1, you should note a number of things:

- $1/f$ fluctuations are not observed at the level of exactly $\alpha = 1$. Rather, $1/f$ fluctuations encompass a range for α between 0.7 and 1.2. These values mean that there are persistent correlations in the stride interval time series, that is, an increase in stride time is followed by an increase in stride time.
- There is significant variation between studies in the size of α for the walking stride interval of young healthy adults. There are, therefore, factors other than age, and the health of the neuromuscular control system can influence fractal scaling of normal walking.
- Gait trials need to be long enough to ensure valid application of fractal analysis. This is feasible for young healthy adults, but less so for older or infirm individuals.
- In order to capture sufficient data that is representative of the steady state dynamics of the neuromuscular system, experiments often need to be carried out on a treadmill. Using a treadmill alters fractal scaling in walking compared to over-ground walking [55]. If a treadmill is not used, it can often be challenging to find a suitable facility that enables over-ground steady-state walking.
- Speed of movement greatly influences fractal scaling.
- Elderly adults and certain neurological diseases appear to exhibit a scaling exponent that moves away from the pink noise region and closer to uncorrelated (white) noise ($\alpha = 0.5$), suggesting more random movement patterns compared to young healthy adults.
- Walking in time to an isochronous metronome changes the fractal dynamics of walking. Some studies have shown a trend towards uncorrelated movement patterns when walking with a traditional metronome, that is, the exponent α is moving towards 0.5, while other studies have shown antipersistent correlations, that is $0 < \alpha < 0.5$.
- Fractal scaling can be engendered by fractal stimuli, which opens up new possibilities in gait rehabilitation.

TABLE 7.1

List of Selected Studies That Have Investigated Fractal Fluctuations in Walking Gait

Authors	Nature of Investigation	Protocol	Fractal Exponents of Stride Times, Mean (SD)
Marmelat et al. [105]	Can synchronization with a human partner modify the fractal exponent of stride intervals of the "follower" toward that of the "leader"?	16 healthy participants aged 26.5 ± 2.8 years walked on a large treadmill at a speed of 4.5 km/h for 11 min.	Intrasession reliability of participants walking alone on treadmill: • Session 1: α = 0.81(0.10) • Session 2: α = 0.83(0.11)
Rhea et al. [106]	Are fractal gait patterns retained for up to 15 min after entraining gait to a visual fractal stimulus?	12 healthy participants aged 23.56 ± 4.5 years walked on a treadmill at a self-selected walking speed (mean = 1.08 m/s) for three 15 min consecutive phases.	First 15 min baseline phase: α = 0.72 Second 15 min synchronization phase with fractal visual metronome with an α exponent of 0.98: α = 0.86
Marmelat et al. [107]	Does a persistent, long-range correlated auditory metronome preserve the fractal dynamics of stride intervals in healthy subjects?	12 healthy participants aged 28 ± 6 years walked on a treadmill at a self-selected walking speed for 6 min.	Control, no auditory metronome condition: α = 0.73(0.12) Isochronous metronome: α = 0.25(0.15)
Hunt et al. [7]	Do fractal gait dynamics depend on the fractal structure of music that participants listen to while walking?	10 healthy participants aged 28.16 ± 5.3 years walked over ground for ~6 min on an empty indoor running track at a self-selected speed.	Control, no music condition: α = 0.98(0.14) Metronomic music condition: α = 0.74(0.16)
Kaipust et al. [108]	Does listening to different auditory stimuli, that is, with isochronous, random and chaotic temporal structures affect gait variability in younger and older adults?	27 healthy young participants (25.7 ± 3.0 years) and 27 healthy elderly (71.4 ± 4.4 years) walked on a treadmill for 5 min at a self-selected speed.	Control, no auditory stimulus condition: Elderly α = 0.85(0.22) Young α = 0.6(0.20) Metronome: Elderly α = 0.72(0.32) Young α = 0.54(0.20)

(Continued)

TABLE 7.1 (*Continued*)
List of Selected Studies That Have Investigated Fractal Fluctuations in Walking Gait

Authors	Nature of Investigation	Protocol	Fractal Exponents of Stride Times, Mean (SD)
Terrier and Deriaz [55]	Does the constraint of a treadmill induce a less persistent pattern in stride interval, similar to the constraint induced by a metronome?	20 healthy participants (35 ± 7 years) walked on a treadmill for 10 min at 4.5 km/h, and walked for 10 min along an 800 m indoor circuit consisting of hospital corridors that included turns and other hospital workers.	Over ground walking: $\alpha = 0.81(0.09)$ Treadmill walking: $\alpha = 0.72(0.13)$
Jordan et al. [109]	What is the influence of walking speed on the amount and structure of stride-to-stride fluctuations of the gait cycle?	11 healthy participants aged 24.9 ± 2.4 years walked on a treadmill for 5 × 12 min trials at each of the following percentages of preferred walking speed: 80%, 90%, 100%, 110% and 120%.	α exponents ranged from ~0.72 to 0.79 across speeds, lowest α-value observed near preferred walking speed.
Hausdorff et al. [19]	Is the locomotor system's ability to produce stride-interval long-range correlations diminished in elderly subjects and in subjects with Huntington's disease?	10 elderly aged >70 years, 20 healthy young aged 24.6 ± 1.9 years walked over ground at a self-selected pace for 6 min around a 160 m, roughly circular path. 17 patients with Huntington's disease walked up and down a 77 m hallway at a self-selected speed for 5 min	Elderly: $\alpha = 0.68(0.14)$ Control: $\alpha = 0.87(0.15)$ Huntington's disease: $\alpha = 0.60(0.24)$

All studies report the exponent α value derived from detrended fluctuation analysis, illustrating that this method is currently the most prevalent in gait studies.

Ambulatory Activity

Recent research [16,17,56] strongly suggests that nonlinear analysis of the patterns of locomotor activity—also referred to as ambulatory activity—can assist in developing a deeper understanding of adaptive behaviors that characterize health, and the deterioration of these behaviors in degeneration or disease. Critically, the analysis of these patterns provides additional and unique information that is not available from measures of "*average*" activity duration or intensity counts. When referring to "patterns of locomotor activity," we are referring to, for example, the durations or amplitudes of rest/activity bouts over days/weeks. There are compelling findings—in both animal and human studies—indicating that the complexity of locomotor patterns provide a rich source of information that could be very relevant to the diagnosis and management of a variety of diseases. Our previous research has shown that highly active older adults exhibit more complex patterns of locomotor activity than less active older adults, despite the absence of differences between these groups in the variability of step counts [17]. Furthermore, the natural locomotor activity patterns of older adults, particularly those with functional limitations, have been associated with a loss of complexity compared to a healthy, young group [16]. Hu and colleagues have recently shown that older adults and dementia patients have disrupted fractal activity patterns [57] and the degree of disruption is positively related to the burden of amyloid plaques—a marker of Alzheimer's disease severity [56]. Using DFA, they have previously shown that activity fluctuations of healthy young individuals possess robust fractal correlations characterized by a power-law function, with the scaling exponent $\alpha \sim 0.9$ [57], that breaks down in older adults. They have also found that fractal scaling of activity fluctuations is unrelated to extrinsic scheduled events and, importantly, is unrelated to the *average* level of activity as assessed within and between subjects [58]. A loss of complexity in the patterns of locomotor activity has also been found in bipolar disorder [59], schizophrenia and depression [60–62], chronic pain [63,65], cognitive impairment [65], and chronic fatigue syndrome [66]. A study of primates suggests a loss of complexity in locomotor behavior that is associated with illness and aging reduces the efficiency with which an animal is able to cope with heterogeneity in its natural environment [67]. Japanese quail became less periodic and more complex in their locomotor behavior when they were stimulated to explore without commensurate changes in the percentage of total time-spent walking or in the average duration of the walking events [68]. Additionally, fractal scaling has been observed in the locomotor activity of young, healthy small mammals, a feature that is less evident in aged animals [69]. Despite the growing evidence for the existence of long-range correlations in a variety of biological signals, studies of locomotor activity in humans are relatively underrepresented. This, however, could be an interesting area of research going forward, as recent progress in wearable technologies enables the capture of long-term ambulatory data.

Upper Limb Movement

Investigations of fractal scaling in upper limb movement have focused predominantly on self-paced finger tapping, tapping in time to a metronome or bimanual hand coordination. These studies have reported fractal fluctuations that reliably reflect the functional relationships of the processes underlying task performance [70–72]. Interestingly, pen grip forces in drawing and handwriting have also been shown to exhibit fractal fluctuations [73]. The purpose of fractal fluctuations has been investigated in wielding behavior of the upper limbs, that is, holding an object in the hand and waving it around. Stephen and colleagues have shown that fractal fluctuations of exploratory behavior (i.e., trying to estimate the length of an unseen object held in the hand by wielding) can modulate information detection. They showed that exploratory movements were fractal in nature and that a fractal-scaling exponent calculated using DFA predicts individual differences in haptic judgments [74,75]. The authors interpret these intriguing findings within the framework of a flexible perceptual system that processes sensory information at different timescales. The fractal fluctuations instantiated at different time scales map to the use of information at differing perceptual time scales such as instantaneous detection in the very short term combined with long-term information about calibration and attunement.

Postural Control

The idea of fractal fluctuations being a functional model to explore the environment has also been proposed in investigations of postural sway. Postural sway has been identified as being representative of a fBm process, which, as explained previously, is a special type of nonstationary process with long-range correlations [76]. Accordingly, Duarte and Zatsiorsky have shown that quiet standing exhibits fractal fluctuations over a range of time scales from 10 s to 10 min in healthy young adults in both mediolateral and anterior/posterior directions. The α exponents in this experiment ranged from 0.68 to 1.47 [77]. Data reported in a later study by Duarte and Sternad show slightly higher α exponents, particularly for anterior–posterior sway in young adults, and demonstrate differences between elderly and young adults in extended standing trials up to 600 s [78]. Many studies that have investigated center-of-pressure excursions in postural sway using monofractal methods (consistent with the fGn–fBm framework) have identified not one, but two (or more) scaling regions on the log–log plot. This phenomenon of different scaling regions evident on a log–log plot is known as a "cross-over," where fluctuations cross over between persistent and antipersistent COP fluctuations, that is, the slope of the scaling region is not uniform. For an ideal fGn–fBm process, one would expect to see a single scaling region. While the reasons behind this cross-over have been debated [79,80], recent research suggests that a monofractal model may not be the best model to capture the fractal dynamics of postural control. A recent study using adaptive fractal analysis in fact observed three scaling regions in quiet standing data, which calls into question the best methods and models that should be applied to understanding the dynamics of postural control [80]. The authors of that study suggest that an on/off intermittency model might be more appropriate than the fGn–fBm framework. An expanded description of the fluctuations observed in postural control is provided by Palatinus et al., who showed that the fractal fluctuations indicate cascade-like nonlinear interactions across different scales. They use the term multifractality to capture the cascade dynamics that reflect a movement system in the act of coordinating low-dimensional, relatively stable patterns with the high-dimensional, relatively fleeting field of perturbations and stimulations [81]. It may be the case, therefore, that postural control dynamics should be additionally assessed with a multifractal method, as well as a mono-fractal method, where nonlinear interactions across many scales are suspected. Crucially, this study demonstrated that fractality is a key property of postural control fluctuations that are harnessed to detect perceptual information in the environment.

PROCEDURE FOR DETRENDED FLUCTUATION ANALYSIS

The DFA procedure is a method that is commonly used to measure fractal scaling in physiological time series. It is a monofractal method that is based on the idea that fractal data have a characteristic statistical form that can be described by a power law. The method is outlined in detail as follows to assist the reader in understanding the associated MATLAB® code accompanying this chapter.

The original time series $y(i)$ is integrated from its mean, $\bar{y}$, for every time point i, such that

$$y(k) = \sum_{i=1}^{k} [y(i) - \bar{y}] \quad \text{for } k = 1, \ldots, N$$

where N is the length of the time series (Figure 7.14).

This integrated time series, $y(k)$, is then divided up into nonoverlapping box sizes of length n (Figure 7.15).

The next stage of the technique requires you to

1. "Detrend" the signal in each box
2. Calculate the magnitude of fluctuation in each box
3. Calculate the average fluctuation across all of the boxes of length n

To detrend the signal in each box, a least-squares line, $y_n(k)$ is fitted to the segment of the signal that appears in each box. This line is representative of the trend in each box. A root-mean-square (RMS) computation is then used to calculate the magnitude of fluctuation, $F(n)$, of $y(k)$, around the least square trend line within each box. This is done for every box of length n. Each RMS value per box is then averaged to quantify the average fluctuation measured in boxes of length n.

Steps 1–3 are repeated across a range of different box sizes $n_1 \ldots n_m$, to get a range of associated fluctuation values $F(n_1) \ldots F(n_m)$.

The functions $\log F(n_i)$ versus $\log n_i$ for $i = 1, \ldots, m$ are plotted on a graph. If there is a clear linear relationship between them, the slope of the line provides an estimate of the scaling exponent, α. A linear relationship on a log-log plot confirms that $\log F(n)$ is related to n to by a power law: $F(n) \propto n^{\alpha}$

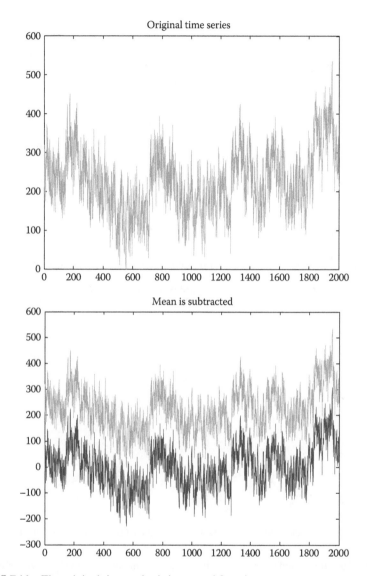

FIGURE 7.14 The original time series is integrated from its mean.

PRACTICAL CONSIDERATIONS

Fractal analysis methods in the field of human movement have demonstrated a remarkable growth in popularity in the past three decades. These novel approaches to movement analysis have revealed intriguing properties of the motor control system and have given rise to new ways of thinking about variability, adaptability, health, and motor learning. The current theoretical framework suggests that $1/f$ fluctuations represent an optimal "middle-ground" between order and disorder

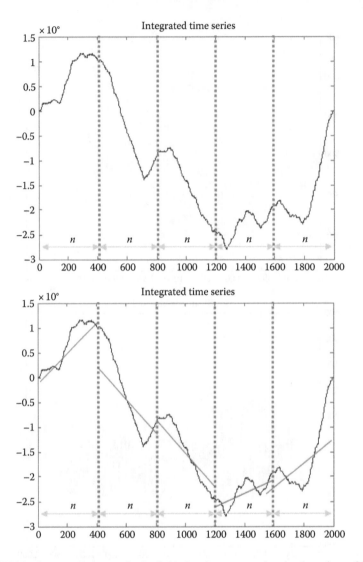

FIGURE 7.15 Integrated time series is divided up into nonoverlapping box sizes of length n (upper). The signal is each box is then "detrended" (lower).

where a rich repertoire of movement potential exists [82,83]. It is tempting, therefore, to simply apply fractal methods and interpret the results in terms of deviation from the optimal $1/f$ noise. Indeed, this is the prevalent approach in the current human movement literature. Increasingly though, prominent authors in this field, and in other fields, where these techniques are also employed, are cautioning against this rather simplistic application of the techniques. Marmelat and colleagues [40,41] remind us that a number of methodological points continue to be debated, and there is still much work left to be performed on the theoretical side of this field to avoid erroneous interpretation of these findings. This assertion is echoed in others' fields, in works such as Clauset et al. [42] where a widespread lack of robust empirical evidence to support the presence of power-law behavior in a variety of disciplines (e.g., physics, biology, engineering, computer science, economics) was revealed. It is against this backdrop of cautious optimism that we encourage you to embrace these new approaches to human movement analysis, but in doing so, we advise both prudent and innovative thinking in the design and execution of your experiments. Figure 7.16 describes a research journey that focuses on fractal analysis, specifically on the implementation of DFA, as this is currently the most popular method appearing in the human movement literature. The goal of this roadmap is to help you plan and execute theoretically and methodologically sound research in this area.

STUDY DESIGN

Given the emerging nature of this approach in human movement analysis, it is not surprising that much of the previous research has been based on observation studies that have sought to provide evidence for the presence of long-range correlations in movement data. However, it is noted that the field is progressing rapidly, and we must aspire to deeper theoretical discourse that can be tested in targeted, mechanistic experiments. Examples of some research questions that go beyond descriptive accounts of scaling exponents in various cohorts are as follows: Does fractal organization enable motor learning? Does motor learning lead to more robust fractal scaling? If $1/f$ fluctuations are restored, does this affect a person's adaptive behavior? Does the degree of fractality in movement patterns predict responders to rehabilitation interventions? Is fractal scaling a potential biomarker for use in clinical trials? And are power-law distributions the best available model to describe continuous, steady-state human movement? As suggested in Figure 7.16, you are encouraged to think through your hypotheses carefully in a bottom-up approach [84], rather than including fractal scaling as a cursory outcome variable, simply because you can.

DATA COLLECTION

An important thing to note when reading about fractal analysis in human movement is that, generally speaking, fractal analysis is not carried out on true "time series." Instead, successive events are computed, for example, intertap intervals/interstride intervals, giving rise to a temporally ordered sequence of measures. In these examples, we would therefore be conducting fractal analysis on event series, rather than time series, which captures the cycle-to-cycle fluctuations that are the essence of movement variability [40]. Thus, one whole cycle of movement represents one data point. All fractal analysis techniques require relatively large data sets, given the fundamentals of the techniques, that is, quantifying fluctuations across a range of scales. Some studies have recommended a minimum of 500–600 data points for valid use of fractal analysis techniques in short physiological data sets [38,47]. In terms of gait, this represents 500–600 strides, so approximately 10–12 min of walking. This is

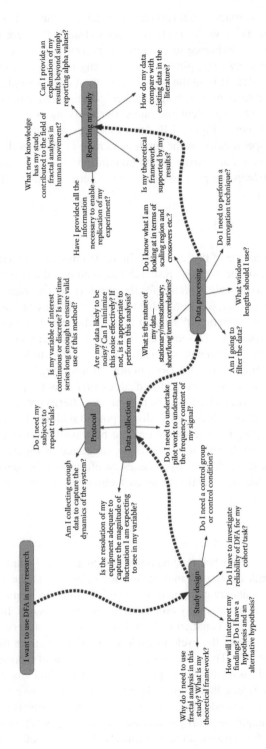

FIGURE 7.16 A research journey with fractal analysis.

often not possible if the subject of our investigation is aging or affected by a disease, as individuals with pathological gait would not be able to manage trials of such length. Pierrynowski et al. have suggested that data from four 3 min, three 6 min or two 8 min walk duration trials provide reliable α estimates from short series of treadmill walks [85].

It is easy to conceive how an event series can be constructed when investigating cyclical events. However, data such as center of pressure excursions in a given environment, for example, on a force plate during standing balance, pose a challenge. In this case, the center of pressure time series can be converted to a series of successive increments, and this would be based on the sampling rate. When undertaking this approach, the appropriate sampling frequency has to be selected. Additionally, the fractal analysis should be performed on the data at different sampling frequencies (i.e., down sampling the data) in the postprocessing phase to ensure that the observed fractal scaling is not merely an artifact of sampling frequency (e.g., Stephen et al. [74]).

Applying filters to noisy signals has been shown to affect the long-range correlation properties of a signal [45,86]. Therefore, special care needs to be taken in minimizing experimental noise so that the use of filters is not required. This is feasible in some types of human movement experimentation, but perhaps not in others. It is important to know the limitations of your equipment, for example, more error introduced at the limits of field of view in optical motion capture, and to minimize these effects on the data. Additionally, you need to know what order of fluctuations you expect to see in your data—for example, milliseconds/microseconds—and ensure that the resolution of the recording equipment is adequate in this regard.

DATA ANALYSIS

There is no such thing as a "cookbook" type approach for applying fractal methods to human movement data, or indeed any data. The main challenge with these methods is that specific preconditions exist that have to be satisfied before these methods are applied to the data. Determining if these specific conditions exist is not always straightforward. For example, it is necessary to decipher which class of signal best represents your data, that is, fGn or fBn, stationary or nonstationary. Some fractal methods are only suitable for one type of signal or another, for example, dispersional analysis is thought to be valid for signals that represent fGn or differenced fBm, whereas DFA is thought to be useful for both classes of signals.

Methodological issues have challenged the existence of true long-range correlations in movement time series. If a researcher goes in search of a power law in his or her data by applying fractal analysis when the data are not actually governed by a power law, these methods will always give a result, but the result might very well be misleading. This is somewhat analogous to applying parametric statistical tests to nonparametric data. The tests will yield a result, but the result may not be valid. It is therefore advised that researchers include a number of safeguards in their data analysis to ensure that they have correctly identified long-range temporal correlations, as opposed to short-range correlations, which can also be found in biological data. Multiple measures of the fractal dimension are recommended in order to corroborate evidence of long-range correlations. Additionally, it has been recommended that a relevant null hypothesis for testing for the presence of long-range correlations should consider the possible short-range nature of serial correlations [40,87]. An inferential test for the presence of long-range dependence in time series, based on ARFIMA (autoregressive fractionally integrated moving average) modeling has been proposed to test this hypothesis. While this method constitutes a valuable, complementary solution for addressing some of the challenges of fractal estimation, it is not without its problems either [88]. Finally, a surrogation method is recommended when using any of the fractal methods. This is where the original, experimental time series is shuffled multiple times so that the presumed temporal correlations are destroyed, and then the fractal methods are applied to the surrogate time series. Hypothesis testing reveals whether or not the shuffled time series are different from the original time series, suggesting that the empirical time series indeed possesses a different fractal structure to a randomly shuffled time series.

Since natural fractals exhibit self-affinity across only a finite range of scales, the power-law scaling relation may break down at either the highest or lowest frequencies, or both. It is therefore important to understand how the size of the windows are represented on the log–log plot and to understand what represents the natural dynamics of the system, and what might be an artifact of window size. For very small window sizes, the slope of the log–log plot of fluctuations versus window size is sampling the dynamics of the system on short time scales and is likely to be contaminated by experimental noise. For very large window sizes, the slope of the log–log plot of fluctuations versus window size is altered because the window size is of the order of the length of the data time series. An experimentally acquired log–log plot of fluctuations versus window size may therefore not be linear at very high and/ or very low window size values (Figure 7.17). It is very important to visualize the

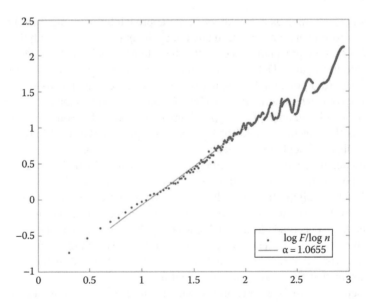

FIGURE 7.17 Example of a log–log plot exhibiting a nonlinear slope at high and low window sizes.

data and to understand the effect of parameter selection. Damouras et al. proposed the use of box sizes from 16 to $N/9$ for gait analysis, where N is the number of stride intervals [47]. As stated previously, the linear scaling region in a log–log plot should hold over a range of at least two decades of frequency (i.e., 2 log units, or 100 frequencies [36,37]).

Reporting

Now that you have finished the study, you will hopefully want to share your findings with the wider community so that the field can continue to progress. Be clear about what new information your experiment has added to the field and whether or not your findings support the existing theoretical framework.

FUTURE OF FRACTAL ANALYSIS IN HUMAN MOVEMENT

The term "fractal" was first coined by Mandelbrot in the 1960s. In 1985, Goldberger et al. introduced the notion of fractal patterns in biological rhythms with their paper on cardiac electrical stability [89]. Ten years later, in 1995, the first paper on fractal dynamics in human gait appeared in the scientific literature [90]. Now, 21 years on in 2016, where do we stand?

Current State of the Art

A review of the current literature in the area of fractal analysis in human movement reveals that the majority of studies to date are observational, reporting the existence of fractal patterns in gait, postural control, and upper limb movements in a variety of populations or conditions. Another significant portion of the research in this field focuses on the examination and/or development of methods for more appropriate quantification and interpretation of fractal scaling in movement data. A small but emerging body of research seeks to translate fractal theory to the rehabilitation setting, specifically, using fractal auditory rhythms as a model to rehabilitate pathological gait. Finally, taking a broader view of fractal analysis that goes beyond the field of human movement to include psychology, one finds important theoretical discourse on the origins of fractal fluctuations in human biology. The scope of the existing literature on this topic thus suggests that this area is still very much in its infancy. A clear causal link between fractal patterns in human movement and the health status of an individual has not yet been definitively established. The field of fractal dynamics applied to human movement is open for expansion and to the challenge of empirical testing. For scientists who are interested in developing this field, exemplary levels of rigor in the design, implementation, and interpretation of experimental data is a must.

Paradigm Shift in Health Care

Oftentimes, the long-term goal of human movement research is to create new knowledge that translates to meaningful clinical impact. We are currently living through a very interesting time in which a paradigm shift in the way health research is undertaken and the way health care is delivered is imminent. We do not yet have a full-fledged alternate paradigm to move to, but there are strong indications that the concepts of "complexity" and nonlinear science, including fractal dynamics, are poised to play a significant role both in terms of a conceptual paradigm shift and also from an applied perspective. In the following, we highlight some of the challenges that are facing the status quo.

An important and widely debated question is: When are experimental data deemed to possess clinical utility? The cornerstone of evidence-based medicine is the randomized controlled trial (RTC), where a well-characterized group of patients with a particular condition are randomly assigned to an intervention or control group. Given the homogeneity and control that is required in this experimental design, the concern as to whether RTCs can produce results that are applicable to everyday practice is being carefully considered. Recently, a more "pragmatic" approach has been advocated, where maximal heterogeneity in all aspects of the trial is encouraged, that is, patients, treatments, clinical settings, and so forth. However, this heterogeneity is then "averaged" through traditional inferential statistics, and the effectiveness of an intervention in a real world setting is evaluated for the "average" person, with statistics such as "minimally important clinical change," or "minimal detectable difference" computed on large scales.

While the pragmatic approach may be preferable to the traditional RCT, it still does not capture the complexity of real life in the way to which it purports. This model is not sufficient to deal with the current prevalence of "chronicity." Chronicity has been defined as a value-laden term implying incurability, difficulty in living, dependency and cost [91]. The traditional, reductionist model of health, with disease symptoms as its focus, appears to be floundering in its efforts to adopt new mindsets that require a broader understanding of a person's complex health journey. The reality of chronic disease is that each disease entity, or indeed multiple disease entities, manifests in a unique individual who experiences it in her unique personal way, in her unique social context [91]. Despite an increasingly sophisticated understanding of differences among patients, the application of "average" disease data to explain or predict a particular individual's health outcome continues to be standard practice. This is not person-centered and does not make economic or mathematical sense. An understanding of fractal dynamics and the nature of power laws applied to human health should elucidate the fact that uncertainty is inherent in these systems and that predictive power is very much limited at a population level.

The standard idea of disease is highly dichotomic—either you have the disease or not—and this tendency to dichotomize applies to almost every medical sign or symptom. Even obviously continuous variables are dichotomized using an often arbitrarily drawn threshold, for example, blood pressure being hypertensive/normotensive [92]. It is hard to break the habit of thinking of things in terms of how big/small they are, how high/low they are, but what we have learned from fractal geometry is that, for many elements of nature, looking for a characteristic scale becomes a distraction. Take, for example, the quantification of postural sway as an indicator of physical function. Hundreds of experiments have been conducted that attempt to answer the question of how much sway is too much sway and yet we still do not have a definitive answer that is clinically useful. Indeed, recent work shows that a singular clinical measurement of balance, taken at one point in time, is not reflective of the global functioning of the system [93]. The fractal scaling patterns that are observed in healthy biological systems suggest that health/disease can never be fully explained on the basis of specific local events.

FRACTAL SCALING AS A MEASURE OF PHYSIOLOGIC RESERVE

The concept of disease is deeply rooted in medical practice. Both doctors and patients race to find the appropriate label for the deficit a person is experiencing, and once this has been agreed upon (often erroneously), a particular course of action, usually pharmacological, is pursued. A health and wellness approach that is based upon fractal dynamics would be less concerned with the label, and all it brings with it, and more concerned with the bigger picture. The enormous challenge of demographic aging that we now face provides us with a good example of how this could be implemented. Mobility is a highly relevant health outcome in many chronic diseases. Causes of gait and balance disturbances in the elderly are multifactorial. For example, abnormal gait can be due to single diseases or multiple diseases developing simultaneously across all sensorimotor levels, atrophy or disease of brain structures involved in central mechanisms [94], degeneration of neurotransmitter systems [95,96], reduced muscle mass and/or muscle quality [97], psychosocial factors [98], medication use [99,100], or reduced "physiological reserve" as is thought to be the case in the clinical syndrome of frailty. Compensatory postures, slower gait speeds, and cautious gait are all trademarks of abnormal gait in the elderly.

The capacity to maintain balance when walking through unpredictably changing environments is critical to independent living for elderly populations. Reduced adaptive capacity in the locomotor system has been linked to falls due to the difficulty that older adults experience in recovering quickly from a loss of dynamic balance [101,102]. Newell and colleagues demonstrated that any behavioral performance results from the coordination of the degrees of freedom available to the individual with respect to constraints imposed from the neuromuscular system, the task, and the environment [103]. In the fractal dynamics framework of health, it is possible that the nature of the specific physiological limitation present in the system is less important than the solution adopted by the older individual in the coordination of the available degrees of freedom. It is very plausible that measures of fractal dynamics could ultimately lead to a quantification of physiologic reserve and resilience, both of which are strongly associated with successful aging [104]. Mandelbrot's advice to the engineers at IBM on the problem of eradicating the bothersome noise in the telephone lines was that instead of trying to increase signal strength to drown out the noise, engineers should accept the inevitability of noise and use a strategy of redundancy to catch and correct the errors. Analogous to this, our health care system needs to become proactive in galvanizing wellness by providing prehabilitation strategies that are based on the notion of complexity, that is, ensuring that a person is able to flexibly cope across the broad spectrum of biopsychosocial domains. Treating disorders may depend on broadening a system's spectral reserve, that is, its ability to range over many frequencies without falling into a "locked" behavior or state.

TECHNOLOGY

The preceding discussion highlights the limitations of the traditional, reductionist models of health research and healthcare delivery. In the emerging field of personalized, "patient-centered" medicine, one of the biggest catalysts in merging the science of fractals with human movement and healthcare is going to be the proliferation of sensing technologies. Fractal analysis of human movement, whether it may be gait parameters (micro) or ambulatory movement (macro), is going to be transformed by the global trend of people choosing to record and upload their own movement/health data through a wide range of wearable devices. Companies, such as Apple and Google, are producing accessible suites of sensors that can be used by both healthy individuals and patient groups to enable them to monitor and learn about their health. This trend is going to give rise to completely new types of time series. Individual trajectories, that are inherently self-referential, will easily be constructed for each person, unlocking the potential of fractal analysis as a means of understanding our own individual behaviors, what influences them, and how we can influence these patterns.

EXERCISES

1. Describe two important properties of a fractal.
2. What is the difference between a geometric fractal and a natural fractal?
3. How is the concept of fractal dimension applied in human movement?
4. What is meant by a stationary process?
5. Figure 7.18 shows two graphs a and b. Match the titles "Stationary fGn" and "Nonstationary fBn" with the correct signal. Explain your choice.
6. What is the difference between "time series" and "event series" with respect to human movement data and give an example of both.
7. Using a log–log plot and the equation of a straight line, find the scaling exponent of the power law that is represented by the following data set:
8. When using detrended fluctuation analysis to calculate the fractal dimension of a movement time series, $\alpha > 0.5$ indicates the presence of persistent long-range correlations in the time series, while $\alpha < 0.5$ indicates antipersistence in the time series. Explain what this mean in terms of walking behavior in the analysis of stride-time intervals.
9. The log–log plots illustrated in Figure 7.19 depict three different types of noise, white noise, pink noise, and brown noise, with $\alpha = 0.5$, $\alpha = 1$ and $\alpha = 1.5$, respectively. Match the type of noise to the correct plot. Remember that α refers to the slope of the log–log plot.

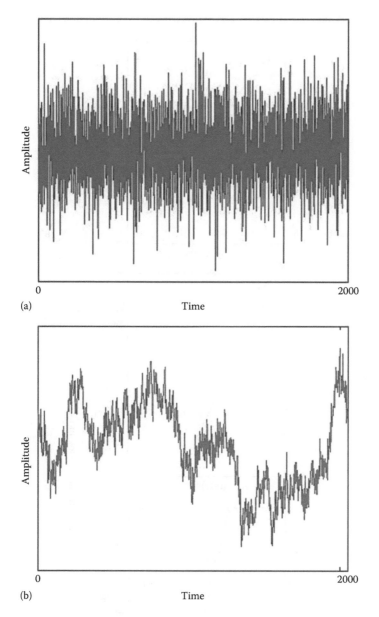

FIGURE 7.18 Activity: Match stationary fGn and nonstationary fBn with the correct signal shown in graphs (a) and (b).

10. You have been presented the results of a case–control study where the fractal dimension of a center of pressure event series has been investigated. You have been told that one group has a clinically relevant balance deficit and one group does not, which group would you attribute the following results to:
    Group 1: $\alpha = 0.98(0.12)$
    Group 2: $\alpha = 0.65(0.23)$

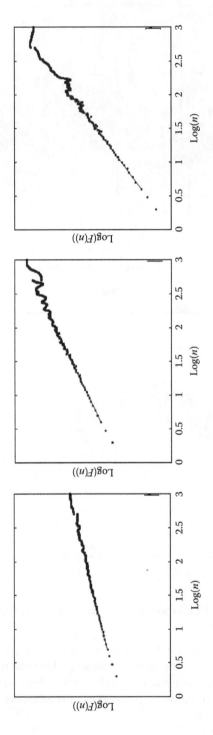

FIGURE 7.19 Activity: Match the type of noise to the log–log plots.

REFERENCES

1. IBM Corporation. Fractal geometry. http://www-03.ibm.com/ibm/history/ibm100/us/en/icons/fractal/.
2. Liebovitch, L.S. (1998). *Fractals and Chaos: Simplified for the Life Sciences*, New York: Oxford University Press.
3. David P. Feldman. (2012). *Chaos and Fractals: An Elementary Introduction*, Oxford, UK: Oxford University Press.
4. Hardstone, R., S.S. Poil, G. Schiavone, R. Jansen, V.V. Nikulin, H.D. Mansvelder, and K. Linkenkaer-Hansen. (2012). Detrended fluctuation analysis: A scale-free view on neuronal oscillations. *Frontiers in Physiology*, 30(3):450.
5. Delignieres, D. and K. Torre. (2009). Fractal dynamics of human gait: A reassessment of the 1996 data of Hausdorff et al. *Journal of Applied Physiology*, 106(4):1272–1279.
6. Hausdorff, J.M. (2005). Gait variability: Methods, modeling and meaning. *Journal of Neuroengineering and Rehabilitation*, 20(2):19.
7. Hunt, N., D. McGrath, and N. Stergiou. (2014). The influence of auditory-motor coupling on fractal dynamics in human gait. *Scientific Reports*, 1(4):5879.
8. Diniz, A., M.L. Wijnants, K. Torre, J. Barreiros, N. Crato, A.M. Bosman, F. Hasselman, R.F. Cox, G.C. Van Orden, and D. Delignières. (2010). Contemporary theories of 1/f noise in motor control. *Human Movement Science*, 30(5):889–905.
9. Costa, M., A.L. Goldberger, and C.K. Peng, (2002). Multiscale entropy analysis of complex physiologic time series. *Physical Review Letters*, 89(6):068102.
10. Peng, C.K., J.E. Mietus, Y. Liu, C. Lee, J.M. Hausdorff, H.E. Stanley, A.L. Goldberger, and L.A. Lipsitz. (2002). Quantifying fractal dynamics of human respiration: Age and gender effects. *Annals of Biomedical Engineering*, 30(5):683–692.
11. Buzzi, U.H., N. Stergiou, M.J. Kurz, P.A. Hageman, and J. Heidel. (2003). Nonlinear dynamics indicates aging affects variability during gait. *Clinical Biomechanics*, 18(5):435–443.
12. Bystritsky, A., A.A. Nierenberg, J.D. Feusner, and M. Rabinovich. (2012). Computational non-linear dynamical psychiatry: A new methodological paradigm for diagnosis and course of illness. *Journal of Psychiatric Research*, 46(4):428–435.
13. Yang, A.C., C.C. Huang, H.L. Yeh, M.E. Liu, C.J. Hong, P.C. Tu, J.F. Chen et al. (2013). Complexity of spontaneous BOLD activity in default mode network is correlated with cognitive function in normal male elderly: A multiscale entropy analysis. *Neurobiology of Aging*, 34(2):428–438.
14. Goldberger, A.L., L.A. Amaral, J.M. Hausdorff, P.Ch. Ivanov, C.K. Peng, and H.E. Stanley. (2002). Fractal dynamics in physiology: Alterations with disease and aging. *Proceedings of the National Academy of Sciences of the United States of America*, 99(Suppl. 1):2466–2472.
15. Goldberger, A.L. (1996). Non-linear dynamics for clinicians: Chaos theory, fractals, and complexity at the bedside. *Lancet*, 347(9011):1312–1314.
16. Cavanaugh, J.T., K.L. Coleman, J.M. Gaines, L. Laing, and M.C. Morey. (2007). Using step activity monitoring to characterize ambulatory activity in community-dwelling older adults. *Journal of the American Geriatrics Society*, 55(1):120–124.
17. Cavanaugh, J.T., N. Kochi, and N. Stergiou. (2010). Nonlinear analysis of ambulatory activity patterns in community-dwelling older adults. *The Journals of Gerontology Series A: Biological Sciences and Medical Sciences*, 65(2):197–203.
18. Hausdorff, J.M., M.E. Cudkowicz, R. Firtion, J.Y. Wei, and A.L. Goldberger. (1998). Gait variability and basal ganglia disorders: Stride-to-stride variations of gait cycle timing in Parkinson's disease and Huntington's disease. *Movement Disorders*, 13(3):428–437.

19. Hausdorff, J.M., S.L. Mitchell, R. Firtion, C.K. Peng, M.E. Cudkowicz, J.Y. Wei, and A.L. Goldberger. (1997). Altered fractal dynamics of gait: Reduced stride-interval correlations with aging and Huntington's disease. *Journal of Applied Physiology*, 82(1):262–269.

20. Decker, L., C. Moraiti, N. Stergiou, and A.D. Georgoulis. (2011). New insights into anterior cruciate ligament deficiency and reconstruction through the assessment of knee kinematic variability in terms of nonlinear dynamics. *Knee Surgery, Sports Traumatology, Arthroscopy*, 19(10):1620–1633.

21. Deffeyes, J.E., N. Kochi, R.T. Harbourne, A. Kyvelidou, W.A. Stuberg, and N. Stergiou. (2009). Nonlinear detrended fluctuation analysis of sitting center-of-pressure data as an early measure of motor development pathology in infants. *Nonlinear Dynamics, Psychology and Life Sciences*, 13(4):351–368.

22. Myers, S.A., I.I. Pipinos, J.M. Johanning, and N. Stergiou. (2011). Gait variability of patients with intermittent claudication is similar before and after the onset of claudication pain. *Clinical Biomechanics*, 26(7):729–734.

23. Smith, B.A., N. Stergiou, and B.D. Ulrich. (2011). Patterns of gait variability across the lifespan in persons with and without Down syndrome. *Journal of Neurologic Physical Therapy*, 35(4):170–177.

24. Goldberger, A.L., D.R. Rigney, and B.J. West. (1990). Chaos and fractals in human physiology. *Scientific American*, 262(2):42–49.

25. Vaillancourt, D.E. and K.M. Newell. (2003). Aging and the time and frequency structure of force output variability. *Journal of Applied Physiology*, 94(3):903–912.

26. Goldberger, A.L. (2001). Heartbeats, hormones, and health: Is variability the spice of life? *American Journal of Respiratory Critical Care Medicine*, 163(6):1289–1290.

27. Van Orden, G.C., J.G. Holden, and M.T. Turvey. (2005). Human cognition and 1/f scaling. *Journal of Experimental Psychology: General*, 134(1):117–123.

28. Goldberger, A.L., C.K. Peng, and L.A. Lipsitz. (2002). What is physiologic complexity and how does it change with aging and disease? *Neurobiology of Aging*, 23(1):23–26.

29. Lipsitz, L. and A. Goldberger. (1992). Loss of 'complexity' and aging. Potential applications of fractals and chaos theory to senescence. *Journal of the American Medical Association*, 267(13):1806–1809.

30. Lipsitz, L.A. (2002). Dynamics of stability: The physiologic basis of functional health and frailty. *The Journals of Gerontology Series A: Biological Sciences and Medical Sciences*, 57(3):115–125.

31. Manor, B., M.D. Costa, K. Hu, E. Newton, O. Starobinets, H.G. Kang, C.K. Peng, V. Novak, and L.A. Lipsitz. (2010). Physiological complexity and system adaptability: Evidence from postural control dynamics of older adults. *Journal of Applied Physiology*, 109(6):1786–1791.

32. Delignieres, D. and V. Marmelat. (2012). Fractal fluctuations and complexity: Current debates and future challenges. *Critical Reviews in Biomedical Engineering*, 40(6):485–500.

33. Pittman-Polletta, B.R., F.A. Scheer, M.P. Butler, S.A. Shea, and K. Hu. (2013). The role of the circadian system in fractal neurophysiological control. *Biological Reviews*, 88(4):873–894.

34. Mandelbrot, B.B. and J.W. van Ness. (1968). Fractional Brownian motions, fractional noises and applications. *SIAM Review*, 10(4):422–437.

35. Stergiou, N., R.T. Harbourne, and J.T. Cavanaugh. (2006). Optimal movement variability: A new theoretical perspective for neurologic physical therapy. *Journal of Neurological Physical Therapy*, 30(3):120–129.

36. Eke, A., P. Hermán, J.B. Bassingthwaighte, G.M. Raymond, D.B. Percival, M. Cannon, I. Balla, and C. Ikrényi. (2000). Physiological time series: Distinguishing fractal noises from motions. *Pflugers Arch: European Journal of Physiology*, 439(4):403–415.

37. Eke, A., P. Herman, L. Kocsis, and L.R. Kozak. (2002). Fractal characterization of complexity in temporal physiological signals. *Physiological Measurement*, 23(1):R1–R38.

38. Delignieres, D., S. Ramdani, L. Lemoine, K. Torre, M. Fortes, and G. Ninot. (2006). Fractal analyses for 'short' time series: A re-assessment of classical methods. *Journal of Mathematical Psychology*, 50(6):525–544.

39. Delignières, D., K. Torre, and L. Lemoine. (2005). Methodological issues in the application of monofractal analyses in psychological and behavioral research. *Nonlinear Dynamics, Psychology, and Life Sciences*, 9(4):435–461.

40. Marmelat, V. and D. Delignières. (2011). Complexity, coordination, and health: Avoiding pitfalls and erroneous interpretations in fractal analyses. *Medicina (Kaunas)*, 47(7):393–398.

41. Marmelat, V., K. Torre, and D. Delignieres. (2012). Relative roughness: An index for testing the suitability of the monofractal model. *Frontiers in Physiology*, 3:208.

42. Clauset, A., C.R. Shalizi, and M.E.J. Newman. (2009). Power-law distributions in empirical data. *SIAM Review*, 51(4):661–703.

43. Bryce, R.M. and K.B. Sprague. (2012). Revisiting detrended fluctuation analysis. *Scientific Reports*, 2:315.

44. Chen, Z., P.Ch. Ivanov, K. Hu, and H.E. Stanley. (2002). Effect of nonstationarities on detrended fluctuation analysis. *Physical Review E*, 65(4):041107.

45. Chen, Z., K. Hu, P. Carpena, P. Bernaola-Galvan, H.E. Stanley, and P.Ch. Ivanov. (2005). Effect of nonlinear filters on detrended fluctuation analysis. *Physical Review E: Statistical Nonlinear and Soft Matter Physics*, 71(1 Pt 1):011104.

46. Shao, Y.-H., G.F. Gu, Z.Q. Jiang, W.X. Zhou, and D. Sornette. (2012). Comparing the performance of FA, DFA and DMA using different synthetic long-range correlated time series. *Scientific Reports*, 2:835.

47. Damouras, S., M.D. Chang, E. Sejdić, and T. Chau. (2010). An empirical examination of detrended fluctuation analysis for gait data. *Gait Posture*, 31(3):336–340.

48. Schaefer, A., J.S. Brach, S. Perera, and E. Sejdić. (2014). A comparative analysis of spectral exponent estimation techniques for $1/f\hat{I}^2$ processes with applications to the analysis of stride interval time series. *Journal of Neuroscience Methods*, 222:118–130.

49. Peng, C.K., J. Mietus, J.M. Hausdorff, S. Havlin, H.E. Stanley, and A.L. Goldberger. (1993). Long-range anticorrelations and non-Gaussian behavior of the heartbeat. *Physical Review Letters*, 70(9):1343–1346.

50. Hurst, H.E., R.P. Black, and Y.M. Simaika. (1965). *Long-Term Storage: An Experimental Study*. London, U.K.: Constable Publisher.

51. Bassingthwaighte, J.B. (1988). Physiological heterogeneity: Fractals link determinism and randomness in structures and functions. *News in Physiological Sciences*, 3(1):5–10.

52. Arianos, S. and A. Carbone. (2007). Detrending moving average algorithm: A closed-form approximation of the scaling law. *Physica A: Statistical Mechanics and Its Applications*, 382(1):9–15.

53. Hoos, O., T. Boeselt, M. Steiner, K. Hottenrott, and R. Beneke. (2014). Long-range correlations and complex regulation of pacing in long-distance road racing. *International Journal of Sports Physiology and Performance*, 9(3):544–553.

54. Jordan, K., J.H. Challis, and K.M. Newell. (2007). Speed influences on the scaling behavior of gait cycle fluctuations during treadmill running. *Human Movement Science*, 26(1):87–102.

55. Terrier, P. and O. Deriaz. (2011). Kinematic variability, fractal dynamics and local dynamic stability of treadmill walking. *Journal of NeuroEngineering and Rehabilitation*, 8:12.

56. Hu, K., D.G. Harper, S.A. Shea, E.G. Stopa, and F.A. Scheer. (2013). Noninvasive fractal biomarker of clock neurotransmitter disturbance in humans with dementia. *Scientific Reports*, 3:2229.

57. Hu, K., E.J. Van Someren, S.A. Shea, and F.A. Scheer. (2009). Reduction of scale invariance of activity fluctuations with aging and Alzheimer's disease: Involvement of the circadian pacemaker. *Proceedings of the National Academy of Sciences*, 106(8):2490–2494.

58. Hu, K., P.Ch. Ivanov, Z. Chen, M.F. Hilton, H.E. Stanley, and S.A. Shea. (2004). Nonrandom fluctuations and multi-scale dynamics regulation of human activity. *Physica A*, 337(1–2):307–318.

59. Indic, P., P. Salvatore, C. Maggini, S. Ghidini, G. Ferraro, R.J. Baldessarini, and G. Murray (2011). Scaling behavior of human locomotor activity amplitude: Association with bipolar disorder. *PLoS One*, 6(5):e20650.

60. Hauge, E.R., J.Ø. Berle, K.J. Oedegaard, F. Holsten, and O.B. Fasmer. (2011). Nonlinear analysis of motor activity shows differences between schizophrenia and depression: A study using Fourier analysis and sample entropy. *PLoS One*, 6(1):e16291.

61. Nakamura, T., K. Kiyono, K. Yoshiuchi, R. Nakahara, Z.R. Struzik, and Y. Yamamoto. (2007). Universal scaling law in human behavioral organization. *Physical Review Letters*, 99(13):138103.

62. Aybek, S., A. Ionescu, A. Berney, O. Chocron, K. Aminian, and F.J. Vingerhoets. (2012). Fractal temporal organisation of motricity is altered in major depression. *Psychiatry Research*, 200(2–3):288–293.

63. Paraschiv-Ionescu, A., E. Buchser, B. Rutschmann, and K. Aminian. (2008). Nonlinear analysis of human physical activity patterns in health and disease. *Physical Review E*, 77(2):021913.

64. Paraschiv-Ionescu, A., E. Buchser, and K. Aminian. (2013). Unraveling dynamics of human physical activity patterns in chronic pain conditions. *Scientific Reports*, 3:2019.

65. Kearns, W.D., V.O. Nams, and J.L. Fozard. (2010). Tortuosity in movement paths is related to cognitive impairment: Wireless fractal estimation in assisted living facility residents. *Methods of Information in Medicine*, 49(6):592–598.

66. Ohashi, K., G. Bleijenberg, S. van der Werf, J. Prins, L.A. Amaral, B.H. Natelson, and Y. Yamamoto. (2004). Decreased fractal correlation in diurnal physical activity in chronic fatigue syndrome. *Methods of Information in Medicine*, 43(1):26–29.

67. MacIntosh, A.J., C. L. Alados, and M.A. Huffman. (2011). Fractal analysis of behaviour in a wild primate: Behavioural complexity in health and disease. *Journal of the Royal Society Interface*, 8(63):1497–1509.

68. Kembro, J.M., M.A. Perillo, P.A. Pury, D.G. Satterlee, and R.H Marín. (2009). Fractal analysis of the ambulation pattern of Japanese quail. *British Poultry Science*, 50(2):161–170.

69. Anteneodo, C. and D.R. Chialvo. (2009). Unraveling the fluctuations of animal motor activity. *Chaos*, 19(3): 033123–033127.

70. Coey, C., J. Hassebrock, H. Kloos, and M.J. Richardson. (2015). The complexities of keeping the beat: Dynamical structure in the nested behaviors of finger tapping. *Attention, Perception, & Psychophysics*, 77(4):1423–1439.

71. Delignieres, D., K. Torre, and L. Lemoine. (2008). Fractal models for event-based and dynamical timers. *Acta Psychologica*, 127(2):382–397.

72. Marmelat, V. and D. Delignieres. (2012). Strong anticipation: Complexity matching in interpersonal coordination. *Experimental Brain Research*, 222(1–2):137–148.

73. Fernandes, D.N. and T. Chau. (2008). Fractal dimensions of pacing and grip force in drawing and handwriting production. *Journal of Biomechanics*, 41(1):40–46.

74. Stephen, D.G., R. Arzamarski, and C.F. Michaels. (2010). The role of fractality in perceptual learning: Exploration in dynamic touch. *Journal of Experimental Psychology: Human Perception and Performance*, 36(5):1161–1173.

75. Stephen, D.G. and A. Hajnal. (2011). Transfer of calibration between hand and foot: Functional equivalence and fractal fluctuations. *Attention, Perception, & Psychophysics*, 73(5):1302–1328.

76. Collins, J.J. and C.J. De Luca. (1994). Random walking during quiet standing. *Physical Review Letters*, 73(5):764–767.
77. Duarte, M. and V.M. Zatsiorsky. (2001). Long-range correlations in human standing. *Physics Letters A*, 283:124–128.
78. Duarte, M. and D. Sternad. (2008). Complexity of human postural control in young and older adults during prolonged standing. *Experimental Brain Research*, 191(3):265–276.
79. Delignieres, D., K. Torre, and P.L. Bernard. (2011). Transition from persistent to anti-persistent correlations in postural sway indicates velocity-based control. *PLoS Computational Biology*, 7(2):e1001089.
80. Kuznetsov, N., S. Bonnette, J. Gao, and M.A. Riley. (2012). Adaptive fractal analysis reveals limits to fractal scaling in center of pressure trajectories. *Annals of Biomedical Engineering*, 41(8):1646–1660.
81. Palatinus, Z., J. Dixon, and D. Kelty-Stephen. (2013). Fractal fluctuations in quiet standing predict the use of mechanical information for haptic perception. *Annals of Biomedical Engineering*, 41(8):1625–1634.
82. Harbourne, R.T. and N. Stergiou. (2009). Movement variability and the use of nonlinear tools: Principles to guide physical therapist practice. *Physical Therapy*, 89(3):267–282.
83. Stergiou, N. and L.M. Decker. (2011). Human movement variability, nonlinear dynamics, and pathology: Is there a connection? *Human Movement Science*, 30(5):869–888.
84. Platt, J.R. (1964). Strong inference: Certain systematic methods of scientific thinking may produce much more rapid progress than others. *Science*, 146(3642):347–353.
85. Pierrynowski, M.R., A. Gross, M. Miles, V. Galea, L. McLaughlin, and C. McPhee. (2005). Reliability of the long-range power-law correlations obtained from the bilateral stride intervals in asymptomatic volunteers whilst treadmill walking. *Gait Posture*, 22(1):46–50.
86. Valencia, M., J. Artieda, M. Alegre, and D. Maza. (2008). Influence of filters in the detrended fluctuation analysis of digital electroencephalographic data. *Journal of Neuroscience Methods*, 170(2):310–316.
87. Wagenmakers, E.J., S. Farrell, and R. Ratcliff. (2004). Estimation and interpretation of 1/f noise in human cognition. *Psychonomic Bulletin and Review*, 11(4):579–615.
88. Torre, K., D. Delignières, and L. Lemoine. (2007). Detection of long-range dependence and estimation of fractal exponents through ARFIMA modelling. *British Journal of Mathematical and Statistical Psychology*, 60:85–106.
89. Goldberger, A.L., V. Bhargava, B.J. West, and A.J. Mandell. (1985). On a mechanism of cardiac electrical stability. The fractal hypothesis. *Biophysical Journal*, 48(3):525–528.
90. Hausdorff, J.M., C.K. Peng, Z. Ladin, J.Y. Wei, and A.L. Goldberger. (1995). Is walking a random walk? Evidence for long-range correlations in stride interval of human gait. *Journal of Applied Physiology*, 78(1):349–358.
91. Martin, C. and J. Sturmberg. (2009). Complex adaptive chronic care. *Journal of Evaluation in Clinical Practice*, 15(3):571–577.
92. Vargas, B. and M. Varela. (2013). Facing a shift in paradigm at the bedside? *International Journal of Clinical Medicine*, 4(1):35–40.
93. McGrath, D., B.R. Greene, K. Sheehan, L. Walsh, R.A. Kenny, and B. Caulfield. (2015). Stability of daily home-based measures of postural control over an 8-week period in highly functioning older adults. *European Journal of Applied Physiology*, 115(2):437–449.
94. Seidler, R.D., J.A. Bernard, T.B. Burutolu, B.W. Fling, M.T. Gordon, J.T. Gwin, Y. Kwak, and D.B. Lipps. (2010). Motor control and aging: Links to age-related brain structural, functional, and biochemical effects. *Neuroscience Biobehavioral Reviews*, 34(5):721–733.
95. Cham, R., S. Perera, S.A. Studenski, and N.I. Bohnen. (2007). Striatal dopamine denervation and sensory integration for balance in middle-aged and older adults. *Gait Posture*, 26(4):516–525.

96. Cham, R., S.A. Studenski, S. Perera, and N.I. Bohnen. (2008). Striatal dopaminergic denervation and gait in healthy adults. *Experimental Brain Research*, 185(3):391–398.
97. Shin, S., R.J. Valentine, E.M. Evans, and J.J. Sosnoff. (2012). Lower extremity muscle quality and gait variability in older adults. *Age and Ageing*, 41(5):595–599.
98. Baik, J.S. and A.E. Lang. (2007). Gait abnormalities in psychogenic movement disorders. *Movement Disorders*, 22(3):395–399.
99. Boudreau, R.M., J.T. Hanlon, Y.F. Roumani, S.A. Studenski, C.M. Ruby, R.M. Wright, S.N. Hilmer, R.I. Shorr, D.C. Bauer, E.M. Simonsick, and A.B. Newman. (2009). Central nervous system medication use and incident mobility limitation in community elders: The health, aging, and body composition study. *Pharmacoepidemiology and Drug Safety*, 18(10):916–922.
100. Hilmer, S.N. and Health ABC Study. (2009). Drug burden index score and functional decline in older people. *The American Journal of Medicine*, 122(12):1142–1149.
101. Wojcik, L.A., D.G. Thelen, A.B. Schultz, J.A. Ashton-Miller, and N.B. Alexander. (1999). Age and gender differences in single-step recovery from a forward fall. *The Journals of Gerontology Series A: Biological Sciences and Medical Sciences*, 54(1):M44–M50.
102. Madigan, M.L. and E.M. Lloyd. (2005). Age and stepping limb performance differences during a single-step recovery from a forward fall. *The Journals of Gerontology Series A: Biological Sciences and Medical Sciences*, 60(4):481–485.
102. Vaillancourt, D.E., J.J. Sosnoff, and K.M. Newell. (2004). Age-related changes in complexity depend on task dynamics. *Journal of Applied Physiology*, 97(1):454–455.
104. Jeste, D.V., G.N. Savla, W.K. Thompson, I.V. Vahia, D.K. Glorioso, A.S. Martin, B.W. Palmer, D. Rock, S. Golshan, H.C. Kraemer, and C.A. Depp. (2013). Older age is associated with more successful aging: Role of resilience and depression. *The American Journal of Psychiatry*, 170(2):188–196.
105. Marmelat, V., D. Delignières, K. Torre, P.J. Beek, and A. Daffertshofer. (2014). "Human paced" walking: Followers adopt stride time dynamics of leaders. *Neuroscience Letters*, 564:67–71.
106. Rhea, C.K., A.W. Kiefer, M.W. Wittstein, K.B. Leonard, R.P. MacPherson, W.G. Wright, and F.J. Haran. (2014). Fractal gait patterns are retained after entrainment to a fractal stimulus. *PLoS One*, 9(9):e106755.
107. Marmelat, V., K. Torre, P.J Beek, and A. Daffertshofer. (2014). Persistent fluctuations in stride intervals under fractal auditory stimulation. *PLoS One*, 9(3):e91949.
108. Kaipust, J.P., D. McGrath, M. Mukherjee, and N. Stergiou. (2013). Gait variability is altered in older adults when listening to auditory stimuli with differing temporal structures. *Annals of Biomedical Engineering*, 41(8):1595–1603.
109. Jordan, K., J.H. Challis, and K.M. Newell. (2007). Walking speed influences on gait cycle variability. *Gait Posture*, 26(1):128–134.

8 Autocorrelation Function, Mutual Information, and Correlation Dimension

Nathaniel H. Hunt

CONTENTS

Autocorrelation Function 301
Mutual Information 316
Correlation Dimension 331
Practical Applications 339
Exercises 340
References 340

> Some of nature's most exquisite handiwork is on a miniature scale, as anyone knows who has applied a magnifying glass to a snowflake.
>
> **Rachel Carson (1907–1964)**

In this chapter, we will discuss in greater detail the autocorrelation function and the mutual information we mentioned in Chapter 3 on the reconstruction of the state space. We will also cover a new measure called the correlation dimension, which quantifies the dimensionality of an attractor.

AUTOCORRELATION FUNCTION

Before defining the autocorrelation function, let us go over the concepts of covariance and correlation that are necessary to understand the autocorrelation function. So what is covariance? Covariance is the measure of how much two variables vary. Suppose we have two variables (e.g., height and weight), and each variable has N observations. Let $x_1, x_2, x_3, \ldots, x_N$ be observations on variable x, while $y_1, y_2, y_3, \ldots, y_N$ be observations on variable y. We have pairs of N observations (Figure 8.1). Now, we can calculate the mean of the two variables x, y and call them $\bar{x}$ and $\bar{y}$ (Figure 8.2).

We subtract the mean from each data point of both x and y and multiply the differences to get the products. If the values of both x and y are above its mean respectively or below its mean, then the product of the differences will be positive because they vary together in the same direction from their means. However, if one of them has a value that is above its mean, while the other has a value that is below

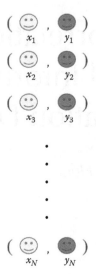

FIGURE 8.1   *N* pairs of observations on two variables, *x* and *y*.

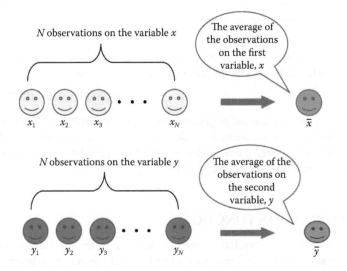

FIGURE 8.2   Means are calculated from both variables, *x* and *y*.

its mean, then the product will be negative because *x* and *y* vary in opposite directions from their means. We calculate this product of differences between each pair of data points x_i and y_i and take the average, which is called covariance (Figure 8.3 and Equation 8.1).

$$\text{Cov}(x_i, y_i) = \frac{\sum (x_i - \bar{x})(y_i - \bar{y})}{N-1} = \frac{\sum x_i y_i - \dfrac{\sum x_i \sum y_i}{N}}{N-1} \tag{8.1}$$

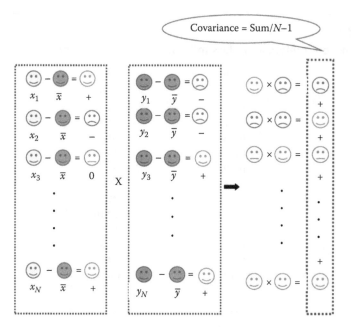

FIGURE 8.3   Covariance of variable x and y is calculated.

Thus, covariance measures how the relationship between x and y changes on the average; specifically, it measures a linear association between the two variables. If the covariance is zero, there is no linear relationship between the two variables, positive values of the products of the differences between x and y being canceled by negative values of the products of the differences.

However, the limitation of covariance is its dependency on the unit of data. If the data sets have different scales, then it is difficult to make comparisons. For example, Tables 8.1 and 8.2 show the height and weight of 12 people. In Table 8.1, the heights of 12 people are expressed in centimeters (X_1) and the weights are expressed in kilograms (Y_1). In Table 8.2, the heights of the same 12 people are expressed in inches (X_2) and the weights are expressed in pounds (Y_2). The covariance of X_1 and Y_1, $\text{Cov}(X_1$ and $Y_1)$ and the covariance of X_2 and Y_2, $\text{Cov}(X_2$ and $Y_2)$ are calculated as follows:

$$\text{Cov}(X_1, Y_1) = \frac{\sum (X_1 - \bar{X}_1)(Y_1 - \bar{Y}_1)}{N-1} = \frac{\sum X_1 Y_1 - (\Sigma X_1 \Sigma Y_1 / N)}{N-1}$$

$$= \frac{114{,}135.99 - (1{,}993.90(684.94)/12)}{11} = 29.83$$

$$\text{Cov}(X_2, Y_2) = \frac{\sum (X_2 - \bar{X}_2)(Y_2 - \bar{Y}_2)}{N-1} = \frac{\sum X_2 Y_2 - (\Sigma X_2 \Sigma Y_2 / N)}{N-1}$$

$$= \frac{99{,}064 - (785(1{,}510)/12)}{11} = 25.89$$

TABLE 8.1
Height in Centimeters and Mass in Kilograms of 12 Subjects

Subject	X_1 (cm)	Y_1 (kg)	$(X_1)(Y_1)$
1	175.26	48.99	8,585.78
2	154.94	58.97	9,136.50
3	172.72	61.24	10,576.68
4	167.64	61.24	10,265.60
5	167.64	54.43	9,124.98
6	160.02	52.16	8,347.28
7	182.88	68.04	12,443.16
8	157.48	47.63	7,500.46
9	157.48	52.16	8,214.79
10	170.18	65.77	11,193.08
11	167.64	59.88	10,037.48
12	160.02	54.43	8,710.21
Sum	1993.90	684.94	114,136.00

TABLE 8.2
Height in Inches and Mass in Pounds of the 12 Subjects from Table 8.1

Subject	X_2 (in)	Y_2 (lb)	$(X_2)(Y_2)$
1	69.00	108.00	7,452.00
2	61.00	130.00	7,930.00
3	68.00	135.00	9,180.00
4	66.00	135.00	8,910.00
5	66.00	120.00	7,920.00
6	63.00	115.00	7,245.00
7	72.00	150.00	10,800.00
8	62.00	105.00	6,510.00
9	62.00	115.00	7,130.00
10	67.00	145.00	9,715.00
11	66.00	132.00	8,712.00
12	63.00	120.00	7,560.00
Sum	785	1510	99,664

Even though the relationship between X_1 and Y_1 and relationship between X_2 and Y_2 are the same, the values of covariance are different due to the differences in scales. This indicates that little information is obtained from covariance regarding the relationship between variables.

Instead of covariance, correlation which does not depend on the unit of data can be used to overcome this limitation. Correlation r is simply dividing the covariance of the two variables by the product of their standard deviations. It ranges between -1 and 1 with $r = 1$ indicating a positive linear relationship, $r = 0$ no linear relationship and $r = -1$ a negative linear relationship. For the example given earlier, the correlation of X_1 and Y_1, $\text{Corr}(X_1$ and $Y_1)$ is calculated by dividing $\text{Cov}(X_1$ and $Y_1)$ by products of standard deviations of X_1 and Y_1, and $\text{Corr}(X_2$ and $Y_2)$ is calculated by dividing $\text{Cov}(X_2$ and $Y_2)$ by products of standard deviations of X_2 and Y_2:

$$\text{Corr}(X_1, Y_1) = \frac{\text{Cov}(X_1, Y_1)}{SD(X_1, Y_1)} = \frac{29.83}{(8.42)(6.46)} = 0.55$$

$$\text{Corr}(X_2, Y_2) = \frac{\text{Cov}(X_2, Y_2)}{SD(X_2, Y_2)} = \frac{25.89}{(3.32)(14.24)} = 0.55$$

As this result indicates, correlation could rightly assess the relationship between X_1 and Y_1 and between X_2 and Y_2 by returning the same value, and in this case, it is concluded that the height and weight have a positive linear relationship.

Now we know what covariance and correlation are. But how can we apply these concepts to a time series with one variable? A scalar time series such as we discuss here has no pairs of observations. For this purpose, we can use the autocovariance instead of the covariance and the autocorrelation function instead of the correlation. Our focus is on the autocorrelation function which is the correlation of time series with itself. The autocorrelation has an advantage over autocovariance because autocorrelation is also independent of scales.

Suppose a time series consists of $x_1, x_2, x_3, \dots, x_N$ with the mean $\bar{x}$. First, we create pairs from this time series as $(x_1, x_2), (x_2, x_3), (x_3, x_4), \dots, (x_{N-1}, x_N)$ and calculate covariance (autocovariance) and correlation (autocorrelation) in the same way as we did with observations on the two variables (Figure 8.4). However, this is not the only way to create pairs from the same time series. For example, we can create pairs as $(x_1, x_5), (x_2, x_6), (x_3, x_7), \dots, (x_{N-4}, x_N)$ and calculate autocorrelations (Figure 8.5). The difference of the index in each pair is called lag k; in the first example (Figure 8.4) we have $k = 1$, and in the second example, $k = 4$ (Figure 8.5). The lag k autocorrelation function is defined as follows:

$$r(k) = \frac{\sum_{i=1}^{N-k} (x_i - \bar{x})(x_{i+k} - \bar{x})}{\sum_{i=1}^{N} (x_i - \bar{x})^2} \tag{8.2}$$

Autocorrelation is the correlation between data points x_i and x_{i+k}. The same variable at different times instead of two variables is used to calculate autocorrelation, and the autocorrelation function is only defined at integer values of k. When $k = 0$, the numerator and denominator have the same value. Therefore, autocorrelation always has the value of 1 when $k = 0$. Autocorrelation also ranges between 1 and -1 just as correlation between two variables.

Now let us examine an autocorrelation plot by using a simple example. Let the original time series be a sequence, $x_i = 1, 2, 3, 1, 2, 3, 1, 2, 3, 1, 2, 3, i = 1, 2, \dots, 12$.

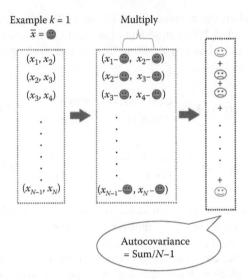

FIGURE 8.4 Autocovariance of a single variable x with lag $k = 1$ is calculated.

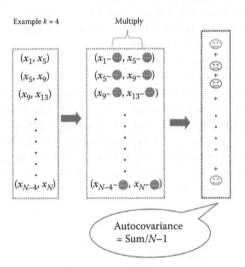

FIGURE 8.5 Autocovariance of a single variable x with lag $k = 4$ is calculated.

This time series is periodic (Figure 8.6) and has data length $N = 12$ and the mean $= 2$. We calculate the denominator of Equation 8.1 as follows:

$$\sum_{i=1}^{12} (x_i - \bar{x})^2 = (x_1 - \bar{x})^2 + (x_2 - \bar{x})^2 + \cdots + (x_{12} - \bar{x})^2$$

$$= (1 - 2)^2 + (2 - 2)^2 + \cdots + (3 - 2)^2 = 8$$

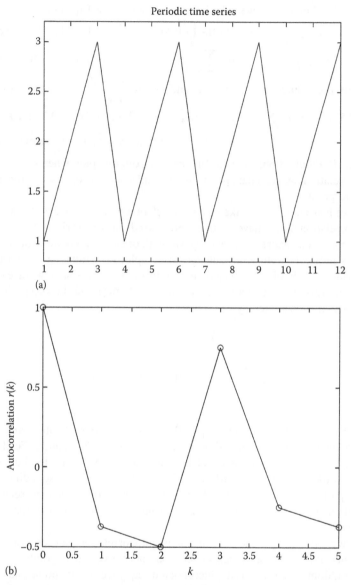

FIGURE 8.6   (a) A plot of a periodic sequence. (b) An autocorrelation plot of the periodic sequence. When $k = 4$, there is a strong positive correlation among data points.

Now, let us find autocorrelations for $k = 0, 2,..., 5$. Since $r(0) = 1$ always holds, we calculate $r(k)$ for $k = 1, 2,..., 5$. First, we calculate $x_i - \overline{x}$ for $i = 1, 2,..., 12$, and we obtain a sequence of values $-1, 0, 1, -1, 0, 1, -1, 0, 1, -1, 0, 1$. For $k = 1$, the numerator of Equation 8.1 is $\sum_{i=1}^{12-1} (x_i - \overline{x})(x_{i+1} - \overline{x}) = 0 + 0 - 1 + 0 + 0 - 1 + 0 + 0 - 1 + 0 + 0 = -3.$

Then, we divide $\sum_{i=1}^{12-1} (x_i - \overline{x})(x_{i+1} - \overline{x}) = -3$ by $\sum_{i=1}^{12} (x_i - \overline{x})^2 = 8$ and we obtain

$r(1) = -0.375$. For $k = 2$, we calculate the numerator of Equation 8.1 and obtain,

$\sum_{i=1}^{12-2} (x_i - \bar{x})(x_{i+2} - \bar{x}) = -1+0+0-1+0+0-1+0+0-1 = -4$. Then, we divide

$\sum_{i=1}^{12-2} (x_i - \bar{x})(x_{i+2} - \bar{x}) = -4$ by $\sum_{i=1}^{12} (x_i - \bar{x})^2 = 8$ and obtain $r(2) = -0.5$. We

repeat this procedure for $k = 3, 4, 5$ and obtain $\sum_{i=1}^{12-3} (x_i - \bar{x})(x_{i+3} - \bar{x}) = 6$ and

$r(3) = 0.75$ for $k = 3$, $\sum_{i=1}^{12-4} (x_i - \bar{x})(x_{i+4} - \bar{x}) = -2$ and $r(4) = -0.25$ for $k = 4$, and

$\sum_{i=1}^{12-5} (x_i - \bar{x})(x_{i+5} - \bar{x}) = -3$ and $r(5) = -0.375$ for $k = 5$. Then, we make a plot of

$r(k)$ versus k (Figure 8.6b). As you can observe from this plot, when $k = 3$, there is a strong correlation between data points as it should since this time series repeats itself every third point.

We have learned how to make an autocorrelation plot; next, we will examine how an autocorrelation plot behaves with different kinds of time series. The autocorrelation function is a measure of the average strength of each data point with data point k time steps away. Therefore, an autocorrelation plot of a time series that contains some periodicity should have peaks at certain intervals, displaying waves passing through zero repeatedly and not decaying to zero. Figure 8.7a shows a periodic time series y, which is generated by

$$y = \sin\left(\frac{x}{5}\right) + 2\sin\left(\frac{x}{3}\right) + 0.5\sin\left(\frac{3x}{4}\right) \tag{8.3}$$

where $x = 1, 2,..., 10,000$ at time step of 0.05. Figure 8.7b is an autocorrelation plot of $r(k)$ versus k for this periodic time series, where $k = 1, 2,..., 5000$. Furthermore, Figure 8.8a shows the time series of the joint angle for the ankle obtained from a subject walking on a treadmill, and Figure 8.8b is the corresponding autocorrelations plot for this time series. Wave-like patterns of the autocorrelations are identified in Figures 8.7b and 8.8b, indicating that repeating patterns exist in a time series.

Next, we will examine the behavior of an autocorrelation plot for a random time series. Since autocorrelations measure correlations between data points, and by definition, a random time series is an uncorrelated sequence of data points, autocorrelations for the random time series should be near zero for all k's. In other words, if one or more autocorrelations have values significantly greater than zero except $k = 0$, then we can assume that the time series is not random. For example, there are two time series, data 1 and data 2 (Figure 8.9a and b). Data 1 is a random time series (white noise), while data 2 is an autoregressive model generated by the following equation:

$$y_n = 0.9y_{n-1} + \varepsilon \tag{8.4}$$

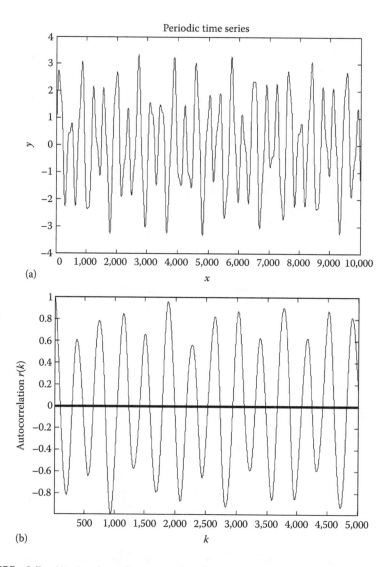

FIGURE 8.7 (a) A plot of a periodic time series generated by Equation 8.3. (b) An autocorrelation plot of the periodic time series, which also contains repeating patterns.

where ε is Gaussian white noise. The plots of data 1 and data 2 look both noisy, and it is hard to tell if both time series are generated by a random process or not. However, autocorrelations plots for these time series clearly show the difference. The autocorrelations for data 1 (Figure 8.10a) are all close to zero for all $k = 1, 2,..., 100$, while not many autocorrelations for data 2 (Figure 8.10b) are close to zero, indicating data 2 is not a random time series. Furthermore, for a random time series, 95% of the k values should have autocorrelations $r(k)$ within two standard deviations of a time series ($-2/\sqrt{N}$ and $2/\sqrt{N}$, where N is the data length; Box

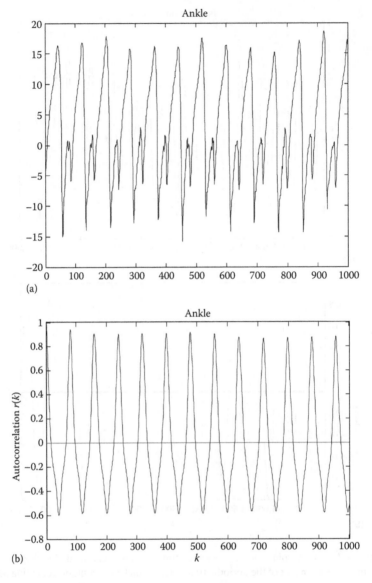

FIGURE 8.8 (a) A plot of a time series of joint angles for ankle obtained from a subject walking on a treadmill. (b) An autocorrelation plot of the time series of joint ankles for ankle.

et al. 1994). Therefore, for a random time series with $N = 2000$ and k from 0 to 100, less than five autocorrelations should be above 0.0447 and below −0.0447. In this example, only at $k = 47$ and $k = 54$, autocorrelation values exceed 0.0447 for data 1 (Figure 8.10a).

So far, we have examined autocorrelation plots of periodic and random time series, but can we always identify them by using an autocorrelations plot? When an

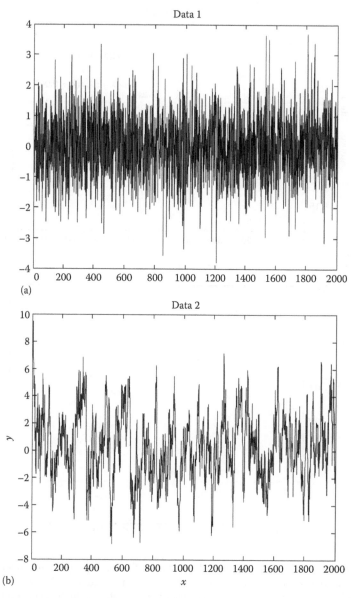

FIGURE 8.9   (a) A plot of a random time series (data 1). (b) A plot of an autoregressive model (data 2) generated by Equation 8.4.

autocorrelations plot exhibits wavelike patterns, should we always expect the time series to be periodic? Or if we have autocorrelations close to zero for all k values, then can we conclude that the time series is random for sure? In fact, there are exceptions to what we have seen regarding periodicity and randomness in time series identified by autocorrelations.

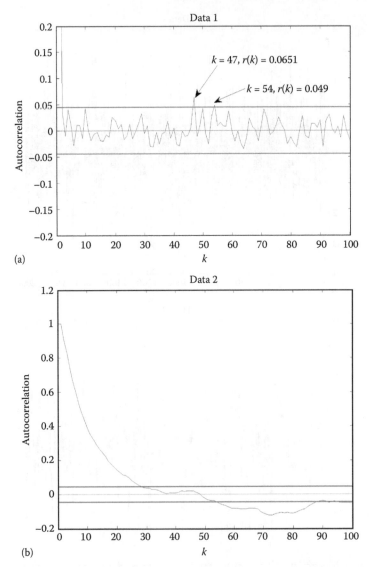

(a)

(b)

FIGURE 8.10   (a) An autocorrelation plot of data 1 (Figure 8.9a). The light gray horizontal lines indicate 0.0447 and −0.0447 respectively. Less than five autocorrelations are outside of these two lines, indicating data points are linearly uncorrelated. (b) An autocorrelation plot of data 2 (Figure 8.9b). Many of autocorrelations fall outside the light gray horizontal lines, indicating some correlations among data points.

Let us examine autocorrelation plots of some chaotic time series. Here, we have theoretical time series of the Rossler and the logistic map. The logistic map is one of the simplest mathematical models often used to study many aspects of chaotic systems and generated by

$$y_{n+1} = 4y_n(1 - y_n) \tag{8.5}$$

The Rossler system is more complicated than a one-dimensional map but simpler than another often-used chaotic attractor, the Lorenz attractor. It is expressed in a simpler set of differential equations than Lorenz's:

$$\frac{dx}{dt} = -y - z$$

$$\frac{dy}{dt} = x + 0.2y \tag{8.6}$$

$$\frac{dz}{dt} = 0.4 + 2(x - 5.7)$$

Figure 8.11a is a plot of Rossler time series. The autocorrelation plot exhibits wave-like patterns as we have observed in the periodic data (Figure 8.11b) even though this Rossler time series is a chaotic system with many repeating patterns. Figure 8.12a is a plot of the logistic map. The autocorrelation plot for this time series is very similar to those for the random time series (Figure 8.12b). In fact, less than 5% of autocorrelations for the logistic map fall outside of the 95% confidence interval. From these results, we can conclude that the autocorrelation function is not sufficient to distinguish the nature of variability that exists in a time series. It cannot distinguish chaotic time series from periodic time series or from random time series. Importantly, the autocorrelation function measures linear dependencies among data points but not nonlinear dependencies.

The autocorrelation function is a linear measure and is used to build a linear autoregressive integrated moving average (ARIMA) model (Makridakis et al. 1983), which will not be discussed here since it is out of the scope of this book. One possible role of an autocorrelation function in nonlinear time series analysis is finding the time lag for the reconstruction of the state space. We will discuss this topic next.

Both the autocorrelation function and the average mutual information are used to find an appropriate time lag for the reconstruction of the state space (see Chapter 3). The value of k at which the first autocorrelation crosses 0 or at which it drops to $1/e$ in an autocorrelations plot can be used as a time lag (Sprott 2003). For example, Figure 8.13b shows an autocorrelations plot of a theoretical time series of the Lorenz system (Figure 8.13a) that represents convective motion of fluid and is expressed in three differential equations:

$$\frac{dx}{dt} = -10(x - y)$$

$$\frac{dy}{dt} = 28x - y - xz \tag{8.7}$$

$$\frac{dz}{dt} = xy - 2x$$

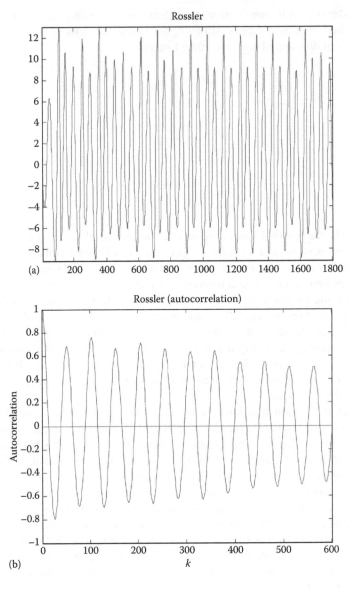

FIGURE 8.11 (a) A plot of Rossler time series. (b) An autocorrelation plot of Rossler time series exhibits wavelike patterns.

In the Figure 8.13b, $r(k)$ is plotted against $k = 0, 1,..., 300$. The autocorrelation is approximately equal to zero at $k = 117$ ($r(117) = 0.0023$), while the autocorrelation falls to approximately $1/e$ at $k = 20$ ($r(20) = 0.3661$) (Figure 8.13b). Since the time lag value should not be too large as discussed in the chapter on the reconstruction of the state space, in this case, $k = 117$ does not seem to be a good value to be used as a time lag. Before using the other value of $k = 20$ as a time lag, the first average mutual information should also be checked since $k = 20$ may still be too large to be used as

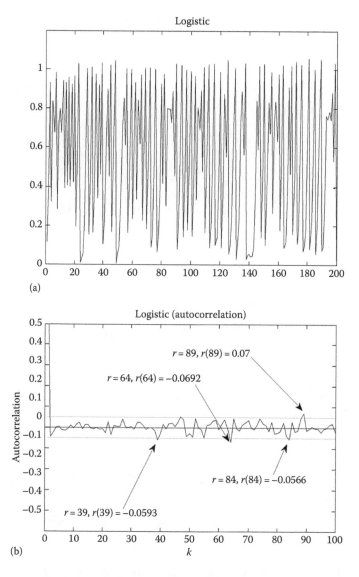

(a)

(b)

FIGURE 8.12 (a) A plot of the time series of the logistic map. (b) An autocorrelation plot of the logistic map. The green lines indicate 0.0447 and −0.0447, respectively, only few auto-correlations fall outside these lines.

a time lag. However, and as we mentioned earlier, the fact that the autocorrelation function measures linear dependencies among data points and not nonlinear depen-dencies should make us skeptical regarding using this approach to find the time lag for the reconstruction of the state space for time series with nonlinear characteristics.

In the next section, we are going to discuss the mutual information (MI), which can be considered as a more general correlation function than the autocorrelation function.

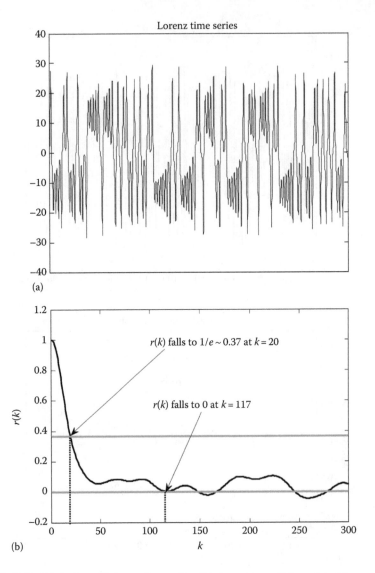

(a)

(b)

FIGURE 8.13 (a) A plot of Lorenz time series. (b) An autocorrelation plot of Lorenz time series. The autocorrelation function falls to $1/e$ at $k = 20$ and falls to 0 at $k = 117$.

MUTUAL INFORMATION

Before describing how you calculate mutual information, let us begin with a toy example to build some intuition. A six-sided cube die has numbers 1–6 on the faces. For a fair die, each face has a 1/6 probability of coming up. So if I roll the die and I tell you that is a 5, how much information am I giving you? The amount of information is simply the number of yes or no questions on average you would have needed to ask me to find out that is a five. You might find out the state of the die by asking three questions:

Is it lower than 4? No
Is it 4? No
Is it 5? Yes

Or maybe you find out the state of the die with only two questions:

Is it lower than 4? No
Is it 5? Yes

If we play this game a 1000 times, the number of yes/no questions you need to ask on average to find the state of the die is between 2 and 3, and is given by Claude Shannon's definition of information:

$$-\log_2(1/6) = 2.58 \text{ bits of information}$$

Every time I roll the die, the amount of information it produces depends on the probability distribution over all states (for a more complete description of the relation between information and probability see Chapter 6).

Let us say the die is also painted in addition to the numbers. The faces containing numbers 1–3 are red and the faces containing numbers 4–6 are blue. When I roll the die, the probability of getting blue is ½ and the probability of getting red is ½. Now, if I roll the die and only tell you the color, then I am giving you $-\log_2(1/2) = 1$ bit of information. By telling you the color, I am also telling you something about what possible numbers could be on the die. Specifically, I am reducing the average number of yes/no questions you need to ask by one from 2.58 to 1.58. This reduction is 1 bit of mutual information (MI) between the colors and the numbers on the faces. If instead you wanted to know the color and I tell you the number you will completely know the color. Thus, I am giving you 1 bit of mutual information, reducing the number of questions you need to ask to determine the color from 1 to 0. So, we can see that mutual information is a symmetric measure that, like covariance and correlation, tells us something about how dependent one process is on another.

Mutual information measures more general dependencies than correlation and covariance, including more importantly for the purposes of this book, nonlinear dependencies among data points (Abarbanel 1996; Fraser 1989; Fraser and Swinney 1986). We can calculate the mutual information of a time series with itself using lag k pairs, just as we did with autocovariance and autocorrelation. It is defined as

$$I(k) = \sum_{t=1}^{n} P(x_t, x_{t+k}) \log_x \frac{P(x_t, x_{t+k})}{P(x_t)P(x_{t+x})} \tag{8.8}$$

where
    $P(x_t)$ is the probability of observing x_t
    $P(x_t, x_{t+k})$ is the probability of observing x_t and x_{t+k}, which is called the joint probability distribution

When $k = 2$, we create pairs from a time series as (x_1, x_3), (x_2, x_4), (x_3, x_5),..., (x_N, x_{N+2}). First, we compute the amount of information and we obtain about x_1 by observing x_3 called I_{13}. Then, we compute the amount of information about x_2 by observing x_4 called I_{24}, and so forth. The amount of mutual information at $k = 2$ is computed by adding all these information I_{13}, I_4,..., and I_{NN+2} together (Figure 8.14). When $k = 3$, we have pairs of (x_1, x_4), (x_2, x_5), (x_3, x_6),.., (x_N, x_{N+3}) and compute the sum of I_{14}, I_{25},..., and I_{NN+3} (Figure 8.15). In this way, we compute $I(k)$ for different k values and make a plot against k just as we did with an autocorrelations plot.

Let us calculate $I(2)$ using a simple example. Let x_i be a binary time series of 0, 1, 0, 0, 1, 0, 1, 1, 0, 0. First, we obtain the probability distributions of x_i. When $x_i = 0$, $P(0) = 6/10$, while $P(1) = 4/10$. Therefore, $P(x_1) = 6/10$, $P(x_2) = 4/10$, $P(x_3) = 6/10$, $P(x_4) = 6/10$, $P(x_5) = 4/10$, $P(x_6) = 6/10$, $P(x_7) = 4/10$, $P(x_8) = 4/10$, $P(x_9) = 6/10$,

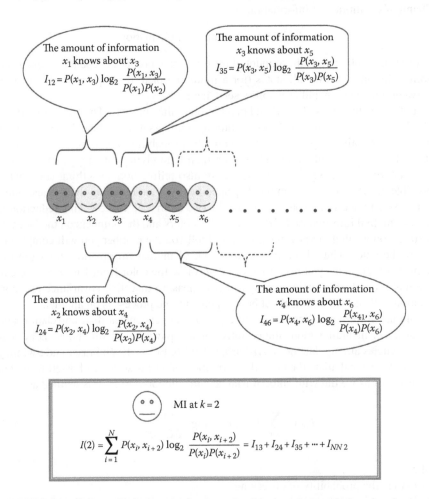

FIGURE 8.14 Create pairs from a time series at $k = 2$ as (x_1, x_3), (x_2, x_4), (x_3, x_5),.., (x_N, x_{N+2}) and compute the amount of mutual information at $k = 2$ by adding $I_{i,i+2}$.

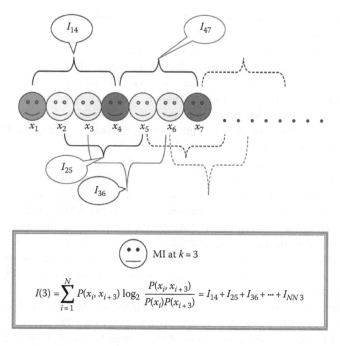

FIGURE 8.15   Create pairs from a time series at $k = 3$ as $(x_1, x_4), (x_2, x_5), (x_3, x_6), \ldots, (x_N, x_{N+3})$ and compute the amount of mutual information at $k = 2$ by adding $I_{i,i+3}$.

$P(x_{10}) = 6/10$. There are four different joint probability distributions obtained from this binary time series: $P(0,0) = 2/9$, $P(0,1) = 3/9$, $P(1,0) = 3/9$, and $P(1,1) = 1/9$. Using Equation 8.8 calculate $I(2)$ as follows:

$$I(2) = \sum_{i=1}^{8} P(x_i, x_{i+2}) \log_2 \frac{P(x_i, x_{i+2})}{P(x_i)P(x_{i+2})}$$

$$= P(x_1, x_3) \log_2 \frac{P(x_1, x_3)}{P(x_1)P(x_3)} + P(x_2, x_4) \log_2 \frac{P(x_2, x_4)}{P(x_2)P(x_4)} \cdots$$

$$+ P(x_8, x_{10}) \log_2 \frac{P(x_8, x_{10})}{P(x_8)P(x_{10})}$$

$$= 2\left(\frac{2}{9}\right) \log_2 \left(\frac{2/9}{(6/10)(6/10)}\right) + 5\left(\frac{3}{9}\right) \log_2 \left(\frac{3/9}{(4/10)(6/10)}\right)$$

$$+ \left(\frac{1}{9}\right) \log_2 \left(\frac{1/9}{(4/10)(4/10)}\right)$$

$$= 0.422$$

In this way, we can find $I(k)$ for $k = 1, 2,...$, and a mutual information (MI) plot can be generated by plotting $I(k)$ against k.

Now, we will examine the behavior of an MI plot with periodic, random and chaotic time series as we did earlier and we will observe whether a plot can be used to identify the variability that exists in a time series like an autocorrelation plot even though it has some limitations. Let us examine some examples.

Figure 8.16 is an MI plot for the same periodic time series as in Figure 8.7a, while Figure 8.17b is for the same periodic time series with noise (Figure 8.17a). Figure 8.18 is an MI plot for the same experimental data of the joint angle for the ankle during walking (Figure 8.8a). Examining these two figures you can see that there is a local maximum that repeats over and over across the plot at regularly spaced intervals. In the autocorrelation plot, this means that each point is highly correlated with the sets of points at regularly spaced intervals, indicating periodicity in the time series. The repetition of local maximums is also observed in the mutual information plot in Figure 8.18. These similarities indicate that visual inspection of a MI plot can also be used to identify whether periodicity exists in a time series. An MI plot for periodic time series also looks periodic, and we can observe peaks at certain intervals (Figure 8.19).

A uniform distribution means that at each point in the time series all values are equally likely. Alternatively, a normal distribution means that the likelihood for each point is greatest at the average and decreases as you move away from the average according to a bell-shaped curve. Both of these random distributions (uniform and normal) imply that there is no serial dependence in the time series since the value that is going to come up next is completely random and not dependent upon the previous point in the time series. Figure 8.20b is a MI plot for a random time series with a uniform distribution (Figure 8.20a), while Figure 8.21b is an MI plot for a random

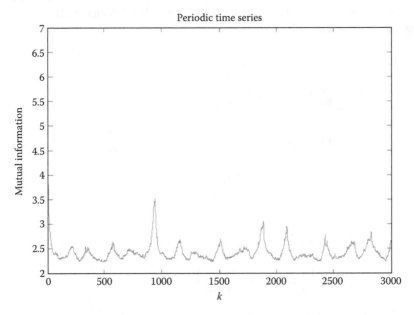

FIGURE 8.16 A plot of the mutual information for the periodic time series in Figure 8.7a.

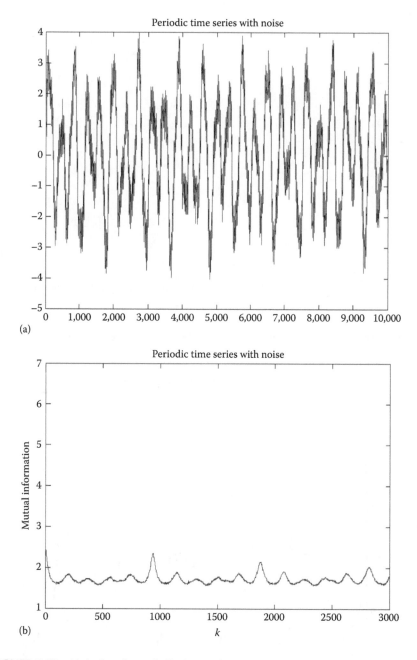

(a)

(b)

FIGURE 8.17   (a) A plot of a periodic time series (Figure 8.7a) with noise. (b) An autocorrelation plot of the periodic time series (Figure 8.17a).

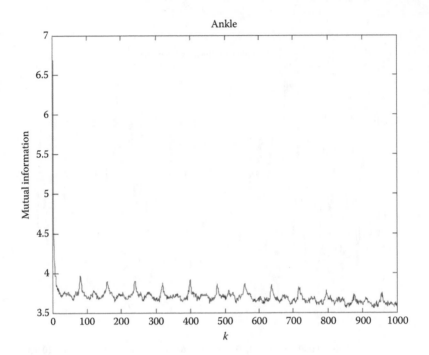

FIGURE 8.18   A plot of the mutual information for the time series of joint angle for ankle (Figure 8.8a).

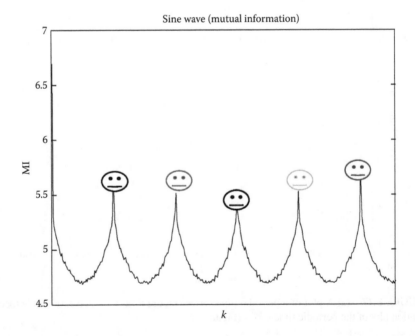

FIGURE 8.19   A plot of the mutual information for periodic time series also looks periodic.

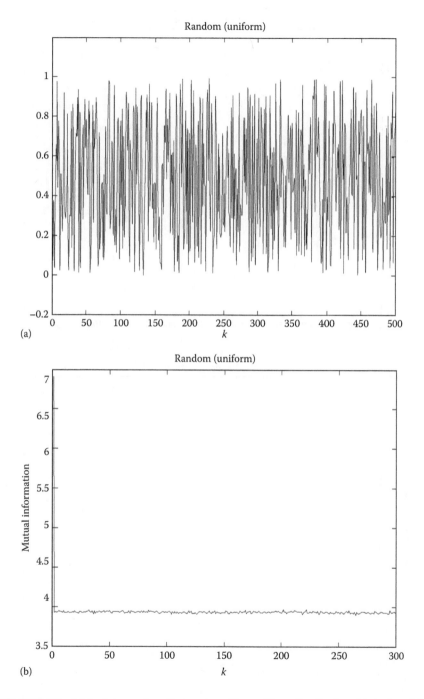

(a)

(b)

FIGURE 8.20   (a) A plot a random time series with a uniform distribution. (b) A plot of the mutual information for random time series with a uniform distribution.

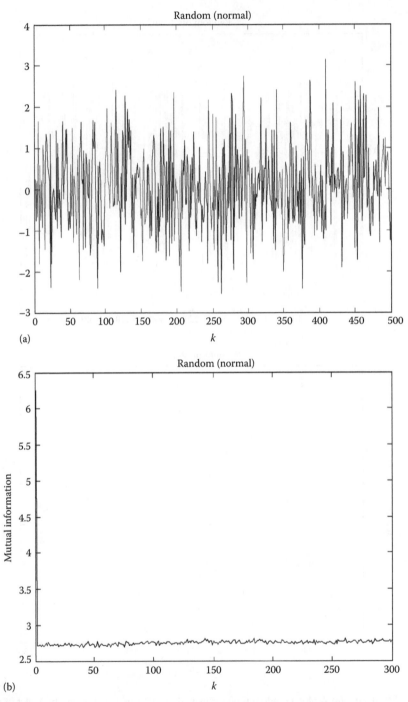

(a)

(b)

FIGURE 8.21   (a) A plot for a random time series with a normal distribution. (b) A mutual information plot for the random time series with a normal distribution.

time series with a normal distribution (Figure 8.21a). In general, it is reasonable to assume that the dependencies among data points will drop as we increase lag values, causing the information obtained from the system to decrease but then after certain k value it is most likely to stay relatively constant. However, since a random time series does not have any dependencies among data points, k values do not affect the amount of information for the system. It drops at $k = 1$ and stays at the same value for the other k's. Figures 8.22a and b show the MI plots for the chaotic time series that we have examined in the previous section, the Rossler and the logistic map, and they are both different from what we have observed in the autocorrelation plots. The MI plot for Rossler time series displays small peaks but not as strong. The MI plot for the logistic map is different from that for a random time series and it has a smooth curve instead of the MI dropping at $k = 1$ and staying there. These results may be an indication that MI plots can be used to differentiate the nature of variability that exists in a time series better than an autocorrelation plot.

Something of notice from the MI plots is the different amounts of MI for the different time series. The MI plots for the periodic time series (Figure 8.16) stay around 2.5–4, while a simple sine wave in Figure 8.23a has MI around 4.5–6 (Figure 8.23b). For the random time series with a uniform distribution, MI stays around 4 (Figure 8.20b), while the random time series with a normal distribution is around 2.5 (Figure 8.21b). For the Rossler time series, the MI values stay around 2.5 (Figure 8.22b) and for the logistic map around 3.5 (Figure 8.22a). Interestingly, there are some differences in the amount of MI for the system, despite the differences in the nature of variability in the data; especially, the random time series has greater MI values than the other one. We will discuss this in detail in the section on entropy, but the MI depends on Shannon's entropy, which takes the highest value when the distribution is uniform. Therefore, the time series of which distribution is closer to uniform has greater MI values. The periodic time series is more uniformly distributed than the simple sine wave (Figure 8.24a and b), and therefore MI values are greater for the periodic time series (Figures 8.7a and 8.23a). The uniformly distributed random time series (Figure 8.25a) has greater MI values than the normally distributed random time series (Figure 8.25b). The logistic map is more uniformly distributed (Figure 8.26a) than the Rossler system (Figure 8.26b), and therefore MI values of the logistic map are greater than the Rossler.

Finally, as it is mentioned earlier, MI can be used to find a time lag for the reconstruction of the state space. The time lag is obtained by finding the first minimum mutual information, which is sometimes mentioned as the first minimum average mutual information. Figure 8.27 is an MI plot for the Lorenz time series (Figure 8.13a). The circle at $k = 11$ in the figure is the first minimum mutual information, which can be used as the time lag for the reconstruction of the state space. When the autocorrelation function was used to find the time lag in the previous section, $k = 20$ and $k = 117$ were found. Let us examine the reconstructed attractors with these different time lag values (Figure 8.28b through d). The reconstructed attractors should look similar to the Lorenz attractor (Figure 8.28a) generated by using differential equations (Equation 8.5). According to these figures, it is clear that time lag = 11 is the best value to be used since the reconstructed attractor best resembles

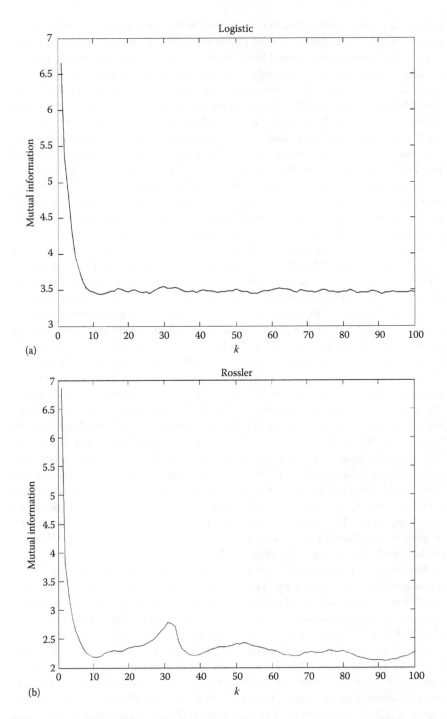

FIGURE 8.22 (a) A mutual information plot for the logistic map. (b) A mutual information plot for the Rossler time series.

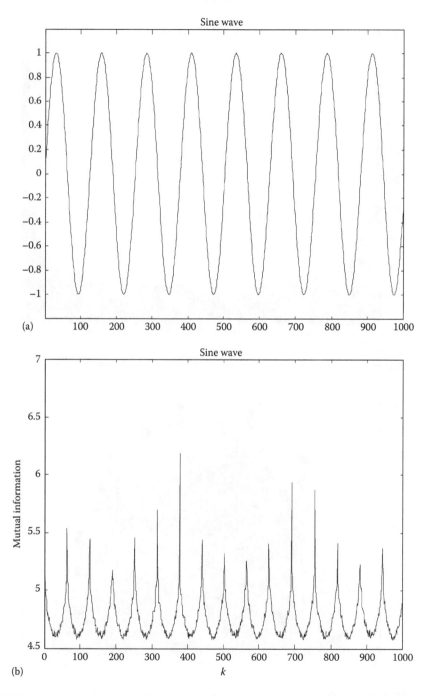

FIGURE 8.23   (a) A plot of a simple sine wave. (b) A mutual information plot for the simple sine wave.

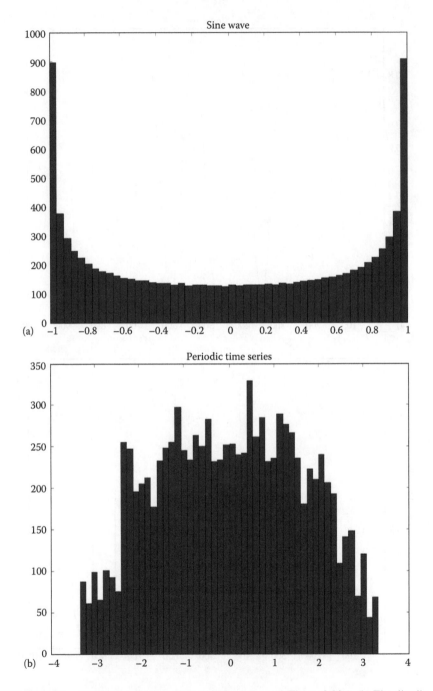

FIGURE 8.24 (a) The distribution of the simple sine wave (Figure 8.23a). (b) The distribution of the periodic time series (Figure 8.7a) is close to normal.

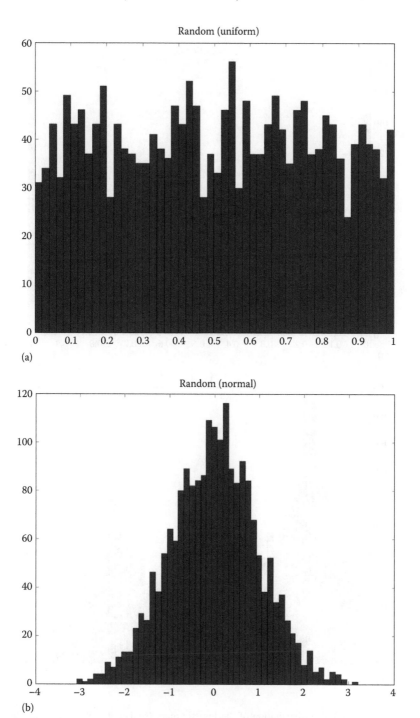

FIGURE 8.25   (a) The uniform distribution of the random time series (Figure 8.20a). (b) The normal distribution of the random time series (Figure 8.21a).

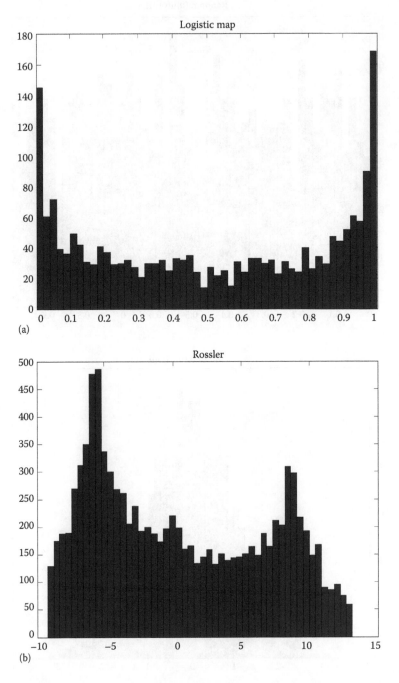

FIGURE 8.26   (a) The distribution of the logistic map. (b) The distribution of the Rossler
time series.

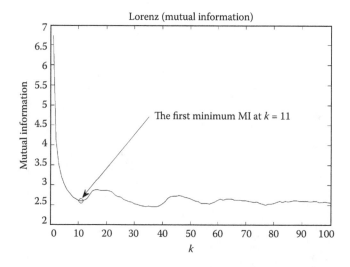

FIGURE 8.27   The first minimum mutual information for the Lorenz time series occurs at $k = 11$, which can be used as a time lag for the reconstruction of the state space.

the Lorenz attractor in Figure 8.28a. With both time lag = 20 and time lag = 117, the attractors are not reconstructed properly and the right structure of the attractor is not preserved. We were suspecting that this may be the case as the autocorrelation function measures linear dependencies among data points and not nonlinear dependencies, while this is not the case with MI. In general, the reconstruction of the state space is an important process for subsequent nonlinear analyses of a time series. Therefore, finding the right parameter values for the reconstruction of the state space is essential.

CORRELATION DIMENSION

Before we go over correlation dimension, let us begin with describing what dimension means and how we might define it. The dimension of some objects is obvious. For example, the dimension of a point is 0, the dimension of a line is 1, the dimension of a square is 2, and the dimension of a cube is 3. But, the dimension of other objects, like fractals may not be obvious. There is a mathematical definition of dimension that can be used for these objects and also for fractal objects. For example, fractal objects are those with a non-integer dimension. Let's start with an example that demonstrates the definition of dimension.

Take a line of length 1 and split that line into three parts, each with length ε. Now let us define $R = 1/\varepsilon$. If we count the total number of parts we have $N = 3$ parts. The Dimension is given by the formula

$$D = \frac{\ln(N)}{\ln(R)} \tag{8.9}$$

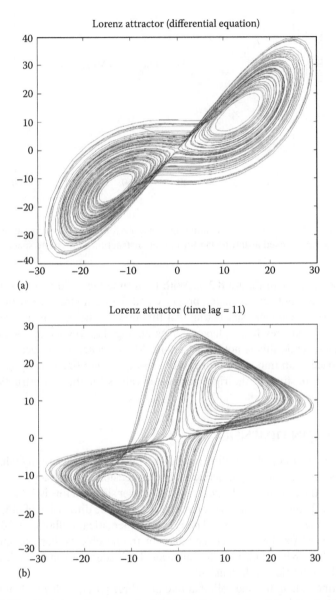

FIGURE 8.28 (a) A two-dimensional plot of the Lorenz attractor generated by the differential equations (Equation 8.6). (b) A two-dimensional plot of the reconstructed Lorenz attractor using the time lag = 11. *(Continued)*

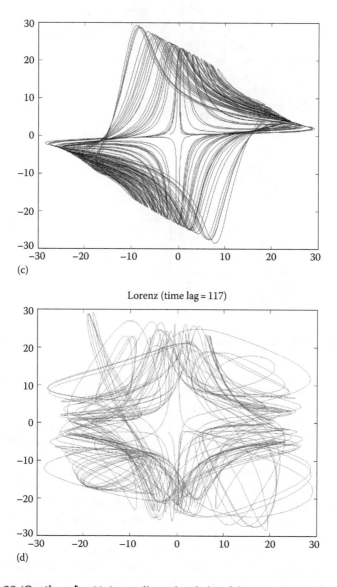

FIGURE 8.28 (*Continued*)   (c) A two-dimensional plot of the reconstructed Lorenz attractor using the time lag = 20. (d) A two-dimensional plot of the reconstructed Lorenz attractor using the time lag = 117.

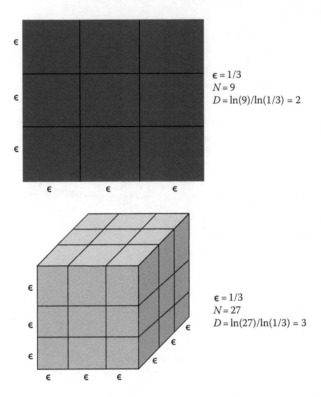

ε = 1/3
N = 9
D = ln(9)/ln(1/3) = 2

ε = 1/3
N = 27
D = ln(27)/ln(1/3) = 3

FIGURE 8.29   Calculating the dimension of a square and a cube gives us integer dimensions.

Therefore, for a line, ln(3)/ln(3) = 1. This definition of the dimension is called the Hausdorff dimension (Mandelbrot 1977). In Figure 8.29, we can see that this definition matches our intuition for a line, a square, and a cube.

Let us calculate the dimension of a fractal object. The Sierpinski triangle is generated by taking a triangle, splitting it into four triangles and taking away the middle triangle (Smith 1988). Then, for each of the remaining triangles you repeat the process, separating them into four triangles and taking away the middle triangle. The Sierpinski triangle is the result of doing this process infinitely many times (Figure 8.30). This is a very strange object. How can we calculate the dimension of such an object? Using our definition of dimension, we can simply ask what is ε and what is N and plug them into our formula. In this case, ε is ½ and N = 3, so D = ln(3)/ln(4) ≈ 1.585 which is a noninteger.

We can use similarity dimension to calculate the dimension of fractal objects that have exact and obvious similarity, like the aforementioned examples. But, we need a more general method that works when the scaling is not immediately apparent, or when the scaling factor is different for different directions. A more general method for calculating the dimension of a fractal object is capacity dimension, sometimes called box-counting dimension (Mandelbrot 1977).

To demonstrate the capacity dimension, we calculate the dimension of the Koch curve (Mandelbrot 1977). The Koch curve is generated by repeating a simple process

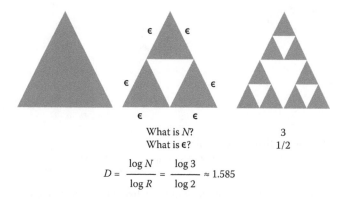

What is N?   3
What is ϵ?   1/2

$$D = \frac{\log N}{\log R} = \frac{\log 3}{\log 2} \approx 1.585$$

FIGURE 8.30 Calculating the dimension of the Sierpinski triangle gives a fractional, or fractal dimension.

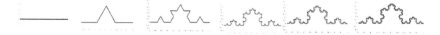

FIGURE 8.31 A first six iterations in an infinite series of iterations that generates the Koch curve.

(Figure 8.31). We take a line, split that line into three equal segments, remove the middle segment, and replace it with two segments that jut out from the line, forming two sides of an equilateral triangle. Then, you take the new object and repeat that process over and over, which generates the Koch curve.

To calculate the capacity dimension of the Koch curve, we place the object on a grid of squares with side length L_1 (Figures 8.32 and 8.33). Then count the number of squares, N, that contain any part of the Koch curve. In this case, we use L_1 of length 1, and find that $N = 22$.

Then place the Koch curve on a grid of smaller squares with side length L_2 and count the number of squares that contain any part of the object. In this case, $L_2 = \frac{1}{2}$

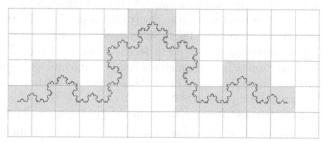

L_1 = the length of a side of tile = 1

N_1 = the minimum number of tiles to cover the object = 22

FIGURE 8.32 We can calculate the capacity dimension of an object by covering it with tiles of different side lengths and counting the number of tiles the object intersects.

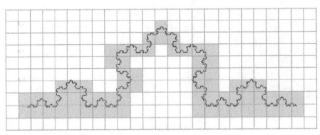

L_2 = the length of a side of a tile = 1/2
N_2 = the minimum number of tiles to cover the object = 60

FIGURE 8.33 Using a smaller size tile with a smaller side length L, the object intersects with a greater number of tiles N.

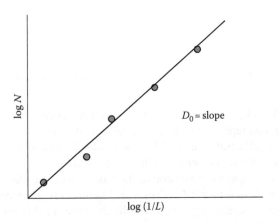

FIGURE 8.34 Capacity dimension is determined by the slope of N versus $1/L$ on a log–log plot.

and $N = 60$. We repeat this process for a range of grid sizes and plot N versus $1/L$ on a log–log plot. The dimension of the object is given by the slope of this line (Figure 8.34).

There are difficulties calculating the capacity dimension. First, even simple low-dimensional objects give a dimension that differs by about 10% from the true dimension. Second, this algorithm requires high resolution of the grid size, which can be computationally expensive. Third, the method is impractical for dimensions greater than 3 (Grassberger and Procaccia 1983).

In 1983, Grassberger and Procaccia introduced an accurate and efficient algorithm for calculating the dimension of an attractor, called the correlation dimension (Grassberger and Procaccia 1983). This algorithm uses time series generated by discretely sampling a trajectory on the attractor and reconstructing the attractor with state space reconstruction. In short, state space reconstruction of a time series of length N with embedding dimension m, and time lag k produces a vector time series of length $M = N - (m - 1)k$ (for a more detailed description of state space reconstruction see Chapter 3).

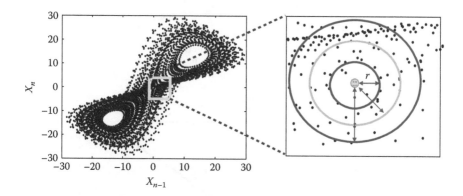

FIGURE 8.35 On the left is a series of points from the Lorenz attractor. On the right is an arbitrarily chosen point circumscribed by multiple circles of radius *r*. Counting the number of points within these circles is the first step in calculating the correlation sum.

After reconstructing the state space, we calculate the correlation sum. We pick one of your *M* vectors and we plot it as a point in m dimensional space. We draw an *m*-dimensional sphere around this point of radius *r*, and count the number of points that lie within the sphere (Figure 8.35). We do this for a range of different radii *r* and for each vector in the reconstructed attractor.

We can also calculate the correlation sum for each radius *r* as the sum, over all points on the attractor, of the count of the points within radius *r*, normalized by the number of points *M* in the attractor:

$$C(r) = \frac{2}{M(M-1)} \sum_{i,j}^{M} \theta\left(r - |x_i - x_j|\right) \qquad (8.10)$$

Where θ is the Heaviside function

$$\theta(d) = \begin{cases} 0 & \text{for } d < 0 \\ 1 & \text{for } d \geq 0 \end{cases} \qquad (8.11)$$

The term in front of the summation is the reciprocal of the total number of possible vector pairs that could be created. Thus, we can interpret the correlation sum as the probability that a randomly chosen vector pair will be closer than *r*.

After we calculate the correlation sum with various *r* values, the correlation dimension is simply the slope of a log–log plot of the correlation sum against the radii *r* (Figure 8.36).

When determining the slope, it is important to choose the correct scaling region. If we see a knee in the curve, this indicates the noise level. The scaling region should be evident by a region with constant slope. We can numerically differentiate our log–log plot to get a plot of the instantaneous slope versus the radii *r* (Figure 8.37). The scaling region is then indicated by a plateau.

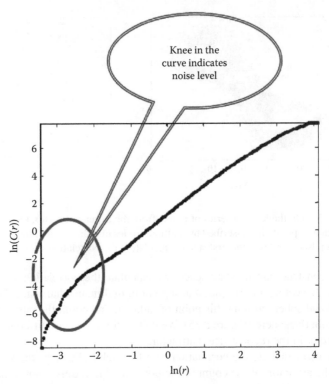

FIGURE 8.36 Correlation dimension is determined by calculating the slope of the plot of the correlation sum versus radii on a log–log plot. The slope should be taken from the region of constant slope following the knee in the curve.

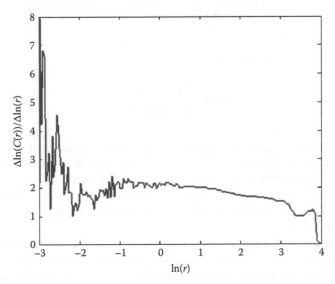

FIGURE 8.37 A region of constant slope can be determined by plotting the slope of the curve versus r and finding a plateau region.

TABLE 8.3

Suggested Data Lengths for Correlation Dimension Depend on the Dimension of the Attractor (D) and Vary Widely

Data Points Required (e.g., Dimension = 5)	Author	Year
$42^D \sim 1.3 \times 10^8$	Smith	1988
$10^D - 30^D \sim 1 \times 10^5 - 2.4 \times 10^7$	Wolf et al.	1985
$10^{D/2} \sim 317$	Ding et al.	1993
$10^{2+0.4D} \sim 1 \times 10^4$	Tsonis	1992

This table shows formulas for the dependence of data length on dimension D by various authors, as well as example data lengths for $D = 5$.

One possible pitfall of using correlation dimension is misidentifying colored noise. Colored noise can generate narrow scaling regions. To make sure that the data come from a strange attractor, and not colored noise, we can test whether the correlation dimension depends on the length of the time series. If so, this indicates nonstationarity and that the data are coming from colored noise.

Another issue with correlation dimension is the number of points in the time series needed to accurately quantify the dimension of the attractor. In the scientific literature, there are widely different opinions on this. In general, the number of points needed increases with the dimension of the attractor (Table 8.3; Ding et al. 1993; Smith 1988; Tsonis 1992; Wolf et al. 1985).

PRACTICAL APPLICATIONS

A method to evaluate the number of degrees of freedom during posture is to determine the dimensionality of the center of pressure (COP) time series (Newell 1997). The correlation dimension is a measure of the dimensionality of a dynamical system. It measures how the data points in a time series from a dynamical system (e.g., COP time series from a swaying body during posture) are organized within a state space (Sprott and Rowlands 1995; Stergiou et al. 2004). The correlation dimension approximates the actual area that the dynamical system occupies in the state space. Small correlation dimension values can indicate a smaller number of the available degrees of freedom. In addition, small values (between 1.5 and 2.5) generally coincide with data that are deterministic in nature. Large correlation dimension values will characterize completely random data (between 4 and 6; Longstaff and Heath 1999; Sprott and Rowlands 1995; Stergiou et al. 2004). Cignetti et al. (2011) examined the difference in COP sitting data for infants at three stages of development (from the initial onset of sitting until completely independent sitting). Across the initial to the later developmental stages, the infants exhibited a reduction in correlation dimension in their COP data in the anterior/posterior direction, but not so in the medial/lateral direction. This indicated that the infants were increasing control of anterior/posterior sway by reducing the degrees of freedom involved.

In summary, we presented a more detailed discussion of the autocorrelation function and mutual information. The autocorrelation function is a measure of average strength of each data point that is certain time steps away. Mutual information measures more general dependencies, including nonlinear dependencies among data points. Both methods could be used for the reconstruction of the state space. We also presented the correlation dimension which is a measure of the dimensionality of a dynamical system. It measures how the data points in a time series are organized within the state space. The correlation dimension approximates the actual area that the dynamical system occupies in the state space.

EXERCISES

1. State the advantage of autocorrelation over autocovariance.
2. Use a sequence, $x_i = 4, 3, 2, 1, 4, 3, 2, 1, 4, 3, 2, 1, i = 1, 2,\ldots, 12$ and calculate $r(k)$ for $k = 3$ and $k = 4$.
3. Use a computer program to make an autocorrelation plot of a sine wave.
4. Use a computer program to make an autocorrelation plot of biological data.
5. What was the time lag value found in Exercise 4? State how you find the time lag using an autocorrelation plot.
6. Explain how you would find a time lag for the reconstruction of the state space by using mutual information.
7. What are some drawbacks of the correlation dimension?

REFERENCES

Abarbanel, H.D.I. (1996). *Analysis of Observed Chaotic Data*. New York: Springer-Verlag.

Box, G.E.P., Jenkins, G.M., and G.C. Reinsel. (1994). *Time Series Analysis: Forecasting and Control,* 3rd edn., Englewood Cliffs, NJ: Prentice Hall.

Cignetti, F., Kyvelidou, A., Harbourne, R.T., and N. Stergiou. (2011). Anterior-posterior and medial-lateral control of sway in infants during sitting acquisition does not become adult-like. *Gait Posture*, 33(1):88–92.

Ding, M., Grebogi, C., Ott, E., Sauer, T., and J.A. Yorke. (1993). Plateau onset for correlation dimensions: When does it occur? *Physical Review Letters*, 70:3872.

Fraser, A.M. (1989). Reconstructing attractors from scalar time series: A comparison of singular system and redundancy criteria. *Physica D*, 34(3):391–404.

Fraser, A.M. and H.L. Swinney. (1986). Independent coordinates for strange attractors from mutual information. *Physical Review A*, 33(2):1134–1140.

Grassberger, P. and I. Procaccia. (1983). Measuring the strangeness of strange attractors. *Physica D: Nonlinear Phenomena*, 9(1–2):189–208.

Longstaff, M.G. and R.A. Heath. (1999). A nonlinear analysis of the temporal characteristics of handwriting. *Human Movement Science*, 18:485–524.

Makridakis, S., Wheelwright, S.C., and V.E. McGee. (1983). *Forecasting: Methods and Applications*, 2nd edn., New York: John Wiley & Sons.

Mandelbrot, B.B. (1977). *Fractals: Form, Chance, and Dimension*. San Francisco, CA: W.H. Freeman and Company.

Newell, K.M. (1997). Degrees of freedom and the development of center of pressure profiles. In: K.M. Newell and P.M.C. Molenaar (eds.), *Applications of Nonlinear Dynamics to Developmental Process Modeling* (pp. 63–84). Hillsdale, NJ: Erlbaum.

Smith, L.A. (1988). Intrinsic limits on dimension calculations. *Physics Letters A*, 133(6):283–288.

Sprott, J.C. (2003). *Chaos and Time Series Analysis*. New York, NY: American Institute of Physics, Oxford University Press.

Sprott, J.C. and G. Rowlands. (1995). *Chaos Data Analyzer: The Professional Version*. New York: American Institute of Physics.

Stergiou, N., Buzzi, U.H., Kurz, M.J., and J. Heidel. (2004). Nonlinear tools in human movement. In: N. Stergiou (ed.), *Innovative Analyses of Human Movement* (pp. 63–90). Champaign, IL: Human Kinetics.

Tsonis, A.A. (1992). *Chaos: From Theory to Applications*. New York: Plenum Press.

Wolf, A., Swift, J.B., Swinney, H.L., and J.A. Vostano. (1985). Determining Lyapunov exponents from a time series. *Physica D*, 16:285–317.

9 Case Studies

Anastasia Kyvelidou and Leslie M. Decker

CONTENTS

Introduction 344
Postural Control 344
    Sitting Posture in Infants 345
        Case Study of Infant Sitting Postural Control 345
    Multiple Sclerosis 349
        Case Study of Standing Postural Control in MS 350
    Standing Postural Control in Children with Autism Spectrum Disorders 350
        Case Study of Postural Control in Children with ASD 352
    Standing Postural Control in Aging 354
        Case Study of Postural Control in Elderly Participants 355
Gait 355
    Peripheral Arterial Disease 357
        Case Study of Gait in Peripheral Arterial Disease 357
    Chronic Obstructive Pulmonary Disease 358
        Case Study of Gait in Chronic Obstructive Pulmonary Disease 359
    Amputation 361
        Case Study of a Patient with Lower Limb Amputation 362
Motor Control 362
    Gait Variability in Stroke 362
        Case Study of Gait Variability from a Stroke Survivor 364
    Perception of Complex Motion in Children with Autism 365
        Case Study of Perception of Biological Motion in Autism 366
    Robotic Surgical Skills Training 366
Chaos in Animal Locomotion 372
    Mouse Model 372
    Duck Model 374
    Dog Model 378
Summary 382
Acknowledgments 382
References 382

And if you find her poor, Ithaka won't have fooled you.
Wise as you will have become, so full of experience,
you will have understood by then what these Ithakas mean.

Constantine P. Cavafy (1863–1933)

INTRODUCTION

This chapter presents a variety of case studies in which nonlinear analysis will be used to better clarify its usage in order to answer complex problems in human movement variability. In order to illustrate the generalizability of this approach, the studies used are from different areas of movement.

POSTURAL CONTROL

Human posture control involves controlling the body's position in space for two purposes: stability and orientation. Stability, also broadly referred to as balance, is the ability to control the center of mass in relationship to the base of support. Orientation is defined as the ability to maintain an appropriate relationship between the body segments and between the body and the environment (Shumway-Cook and Woollacott 2012). The center of pressure (COP) at the base of support in standing has traditionally been considered a reflection of the organization of posture (Massion 1992). Researchers have utilized the COP in the studies of postural control in adults (Buchanan and Horak 2001; Horak and Macpherson 1996; Newell et al. 1993; Winstein et al. 1989) and children (Horak et al. 1988; Nashner et al. 1983; Odenrick and Sandstedt 1984; Riach and Hayes 1987) developing standing skills. However, there have been conflicting interpretations of the COP data using the standard variables of length of path, excursion in the sagittal or frontal directions, and the area of the path of the COP during stable standing. For example, different researchers have interpreted an increased COP area to suggest greater motor control because the individual can recover from disruptions to posture (Hughes et al. 1996), while others interpret an increased area as a lack of postural control (Riach and Hayes 1987).

Common measures that have been used to analyze the COP trajectory are the average and the standard deviation, which are typical linear measures, to evaluate the postural sway while standing or sitting. However, a growing number of research studies suggests that linear measures only capture the "quantity" of movement, such as how much COP moves, but these measures do not give any information about how well controlled the movement is ("quality" of movement). For example, one infant may have a large amount of postural sway due to poor control of movement, whereas another infant may have a large amount of postural sway due to exploration of the environment after good posture control skills have been learned. Thus, measures of the "quantity" or amount of movement do not necessarily indicate the progress that an infant has made in the control of movement.

Our research group has been using nonlinear tools to study postural control by evaluating the dynamics of the COP. For example, the largest Lyapunov exponent

(LyE) is a measure of the average exponential rate of divergence or convergence of nearby COP trajectories in state space (Wurdeman et al. 2014a) and approximate entropy (ApEn) is a method to determine the unpredictability or irregularity of the COP time series (Yentes et al. 2013). Because these nonlinear analysis techniques are sensitive to patterns in the COP data, rather than the overall magnitude of the fluctuations, they could be ideal tools for quantifying the "quality" or temporal structure of postural sway, thus making them potentially clinically useful for studying both the healthy and pathological populations of motor control in human movement.

SITTING POSTURE IN INFANTS

Learning how to maintain upright sitting is an important motor developmental milestone. Upright sitting allows visual exploration of the environment and serves as a stable platform for reaching nearby objects. Once an infant can control the head and trunk in sitting, the arms are free for exploration and functional activities. However, independent sitting requires dynamic stabilization of all the linked segments of the body and is a complex process of learning and adaptation to various forces in the environment. Standard assessment tools used by clinicians to evaluate the progression of infant motor milestones, such as sitting, provide a measure of delay or abnormality but no information that can be easily transferred to direct intervention. Thus, clinicians do not have a precise and quantitative method to evaluate early postural movement or to describe how these early attempts to control postural sway may be changing over time or as a result of intervention. In contrast, the measures of postural sway variability have been found to be very valuable for various populations with motor and sensory disabilities (Cherng et al. 1999; Huisinga et al. 2012b; Rocchi et al. 2002). Examination of the temporal structure of the variability present in the early postural sway movement patterns during sitting posture was able to discriminate typically developing infants from infants with motor developmental delays and most importantly to reveal different postural sway strategies between infants with motor developmental delays and infants with motor developmental delays that were later diagnosed with cerebral palsy (Deffeyes et al. 2009; Harbourne and Stergiou 2003; Harbourne et al. 2009; Kyvelidou et al. 2013). Overall, the measures that investigate the temporal structure of the postural sway variability appear to be sensitive for the assessment of infant posture control and quantifying intervention response (Harbourne et al. 2010).

Case Study of Infant Sitting Postural Control

One typically developing infant (TD, 147 days old at first data collection) and one infant with developmental delays (DD, 296 days old at first data collection) participated in this study. Infants were screened for entry into the study using the Peabody Developmental Motor Scale-2 (Folio and Fewell 2000). Inclusion criteria for entry into the study for the infant with typical development were as follows: a score on the Peabody Gross Motor Quotient of greater than 0.5 standard deviation below the mean, age of 5 months at the time of initial data collection, and beginning sitting skills. The infant with developmental delay had the following inclusion criteria: age from

5 months to 2 years, a score on the Peabody Gross Motor Quotient of less than 1.5 deviations below the mean for their corrected age, and sitting skills described in the following section for beginning sitting.

Each infant participated in nine sessions. The first session was used to perform the Peabody Gross Motor Scale (Folio and Fewell 2000), which is a standardized clinical test. In addition, the child was tested to determine adequate prop sitting skills to begin the study and to familiarize the family with the procedures used in the study. The other eight sessions were dispersed over a time period of 4 months. The infants were tested twice in 1 week at each of the 4 months of the study. A physical therapist ranked each infant's sitting behavior at each session according to three stages of sitting: (1) prop sitting, (2) variable, approximately 10 s of sitting, and (3) sits upright all the time without the help of hands. Stage identification was always performed by the same physical therapist.

After the parent undressed the child, the infant was placed by the parent on a force platform that was covered with a pad, securely adhered with tape to the force platform. The baby was placed in the sitting position in the middle of the platform when calm and happy. The investigator and the parent remained at one side and in front of the infant, respectively, during all data collection times to ensure that the infant did not fall or become insecure. Trials were performed until we had collected three trials that were acceptable for our criteria or until the infants were no longer cooperative. For data acquisition, infants sat on an AMTI force platform (Advanced Mechanical Technology Inc., Oxford, England) interfaced to a computer system running Vicon data acquisition software. COP data in both the anterior–posterior (AP) and the medial–lateral (ML) directions were acquired through the Vicon software at 240 Hz. The sampling frequency was established based on pilot work, which indicated that the range of signal frequencies that contain 99.99% of the overall signal power was between 1 and 29 Hz. No filtering was performed on the data because such a procedure can affect the variability present in the signal and especially the nonlinear analysis. Video of each trial was collected, and the cameras were positioned to record a sagittal (AP) and a frontal (ML) view of the subject. The three segments of acceptable data (8.3 s each) were selected from the videotaped record at each session. The COP time series was subjected to both linear and nonlinear analysis. Specifically, we used root-mean-square (RMS) and ApEn (Chapter 6) to identify postural control differences across sitting acquisition between an infant with developmental delays and a typically developing infant. For the purpose of this case study, we are presenting only the RMS and ApEn values from the AP direction.

The results (Figure 9.1) showed that the infant with DD exhibited very irregular sway at Stage 1 of sitting, but as sitting progressed, regularity increased, and the infant was able to control sitting posture much more efficiently (decreased ApEn values from Stage 1 to Stage 3) and possibly allowing exploration to occur. This is also evident by the increase in RMS in the same direction across the stages of sitting of the infant with DD (Table 9.1). In contrast, the infant with TD employed a different strategy to acquire sitting. The infant with TD presented decreased regularity from Stage 1 and at the same time explored possible avenues of self-organization for successful sitting (increased RMS values).

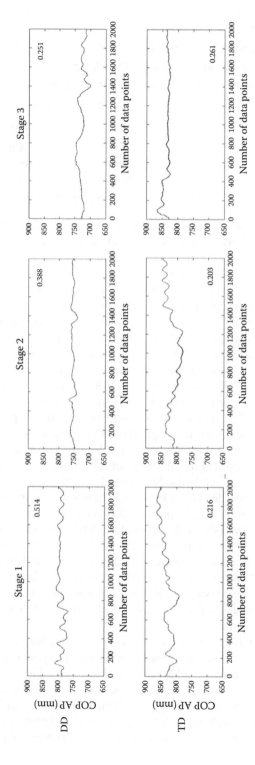

FIGURE 9.1 Postural sway time series for a typically developing (TD) infant and an infant with developmental delays (DD) across the three stages of sitting. Values on the graphs represent the approximate entropy (ApEn) values for each time series in bits.

TABLE 9.1

Root-Mean-Square Values for a Typically Developing (TD) Infant and an Infant with Developmental Delays (DD) across the Three Stages of Sitting

	RMS in AP (mm)	
	DD	TD
Stage 1	8.87	18.56
Stage 2	4.94	19.33
Stage 3	10.41	8.77

Another nonlinear tool that has been used to investigate infant sitting postural control was the largest LyE (Chapter 4). Deffeyes et al. (2009) investigated how sitting postural sway in typically developing infants differs from developmentally delayed infants. Infants in the developmentally delayed group were either diagnosed later with cerebral palsy, or they were developmentally delayed at the risk of cerebral palsy. Motor development in infants with cerebral palsy is delayed, meaning that developmental milestones such as sitting, standing, or walking may occur later for them than in infants with typical development, and in severe cases, these milestones may never be met (Fedrizzi et al. 2000; Wu et al. 2004). The results from Deffeyes et al. (2009) showed that the LyE was the only parameter of COP time series that revealed significant differences ($p < 0.000$) between infants with typical versus delayed development. This study suggested that the infants with delayed development appear to further minimize the fluctuations that are present in their postural sway patterns indicating more rigid control than infants with typical development. If it is assumed that the infants with typical development have better motor control, then it can be suggested that these infants are exploring a wider variety of solutions to postural control. It can also be assumed that infants with delayed development are further freezing degrees of freedom to have fewer control parameters to manipulate as they maintain upright posture. Based on the theoretical framework of optimal movement of variability (Stergiou et al. 2006), the infants with delayed development behave in a more robotic and periodic fashion than healthy typically developing infants. Furthermore, the healthy infants seem to move between randomness and optimal variability as they explore effective strategies for postural control. Importantly, the nonlinear measure of LyE has the potential to add the specificity of diagnosis in the early months of life, when most standardized tests of infant development have little predictive value.

For the purpose of this case study, we are also presenting here the results from LyE in the AP direction. It is apparent that the infant with DD performs with greater divergence of the COP trajectories at the onset of sitting (Stage 1, Figure 9.2). However, as sitting progresses, the infant with DD is able to hone in to the appropriate sitting patterns and eventually reach the postural control behavior of the typically developing infant. This is in agreement with the study by Deffeyes et al. (2009). It is also important to state here that both linear and nonlinear measures of variability of postural sway

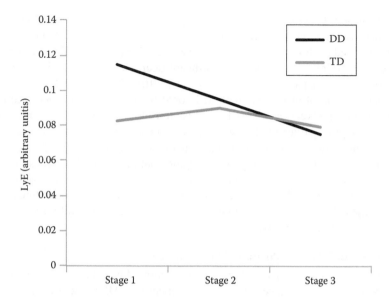

FIGURE 9.2 Lyapunov exponent (LyE) values for a typically developing (TD) infant and an infant with developmental delays (DD) across the three stages of sitting.

have been found intra- and intersession reliable to examine infants sitting postural control as expressed with intra-class correlations coefficients in both typically developing infants and infants with developmental delays (Kyvelidou et al. 2009, 2010). In addition, we have checked stationarity of our time series and they were found to be stationary using the difference method (Chapter 2 for more details).

MULTIPLE SCLEROSIS

Multiple sclerosis (MS) is the most prevalent progressive neurological disease among young people and is associated with a wide range of physical symptoms that include increased falls, exaggerated fatigue, motor weakness, poor balance, spasticity, and decreased physical activity (White and Dressendorfer 2004). Despite the fact that disturbances in postural control are often reported of patients with MS due to declined muscle strength and poor physical capacity, previous studies were not able to differentiate between patients with MS and controls on their ability to maintain balance using subjective clinical tests (Frzovic et al. 2000; Soyuer et al. 2006). However, recent studies (Cattaneo and Jonsdottir 2009; Van Emmerik et al. 2010) utilizing the COP data were able to detect postural abnormality in patients with MS, for example, decreased COP displacement during reading. These studies suggested that the objective COP measurements could distinguish patients with MS from healthy controls in terms of postural sway.

Huisinga et al. (2011) further used COP data to investigate the effect of supervised resistance training on postural control in patients with MS. Postural control was assessed using the linear RMS, a measure of the amount of postural sway variability, and the nonlinear LyE from 15 patients with MS. Surrogation analysis was also performed. Posture was evaluated before and after completion of 3 months of resistance training. There were significant differences between patients with MS pretraining and healthy controls for both LyE and RMS, but no differences between groups after training. There was a significant decrease in RMS and a significant increase in LyE for patients with MS pre- to posttraining. The findings suggested that postural control of patients with MS could be affected by a supervised resistance training intervention. Using LyE, this study found that before training these MS patients had significantly less variability in the temporal structure of their COP displacement. After resistance training, 15 patients with MS significantly increased the complexity of the COP sway, which suggests that the postural control system has more degrees of freedom and is more adaptable to the task or the environment. In this study, Huisinga et al. (2012a) acknowledged that the combination of linear RMS and nonlinear LyE allows for a more holistic view of the variability present in the postural control in patients with MS.

Case Study of Standing Postural Control in MS

One healthy control participant, 31 years of age (mass: 64.6 kg, height: 170.2 cm), and a 53-year-old (mass: 99.3 kg, height: 170.2 cm) patient with MS participated in this case study. Subjects stood quietly for 5 min with eyes open approximately 10 m from a wall, while COP data were collected. Feet were placed at approximately hip width apart, toes facing forward. Kinetic data were collected using a force platform (Kistler Model: 9281-B11; Amherst, NY; 10 Hz that was established based on pilot work). Unfiltered data were cropped to 2000 data points. Data were collected and analyzed unfiltered so as not to mask or remove any dynamical properties or variability present within the system.

The coordinates of the COP in the ML and AP directions were calculated for each trial. Temporal structure of sway variability was quantified from both directions using LyE and ApEn. The LyE was calculated using an embedding dimension of six which was calculated using the global false nearest neighbor analysis (Stergiou et al. 2004). ApEn was calculated using lag = 6, m = 2, and r = 0.2 as default parameters. The results suggest that the patient with MS has altered temporal structure of variability in comparison to the control participant. Both LyE and ApEn values were lower for the patient with MS (Figures 9.3 and 9.4), which may be indicative of reduced ability to control posture. The lower LyE and ApEn values in the patient with MS suggest that possibly the individual lacks the ability of adapting to external and internal perturbations. This is especially evident when we take into consideration that, in general, patients with MS have an increased amount of variability in their postural sway (Huisinga et al. 2012b).

STANDING POSTURAL CONTROL IN CHILDREN WITH AUTISM SPECTRUM DISORDERS

Children with autism spectrum disorders (ASD) seem to exhibit more rigid and less adaptive behavior, including posture, under most conditions (Kohen-Raz et al. 1992). It is plausible that children with ASD fixate on repetitive aspects of motion (i.e., watching wheels spin) and engage in repetitive motor responses (rocking). This perceptual and motor rigidity interferes with their attention to and perception of the complex variability found in the motion of others and thus their ability to

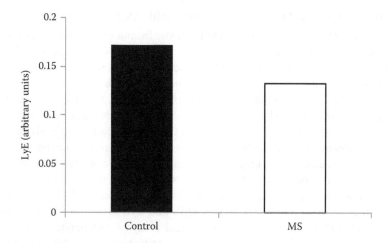

FIGURE 9.3 Lyapunov exponent (LyE) values for a patient with multiple sclerosis (MS) and a control participant.

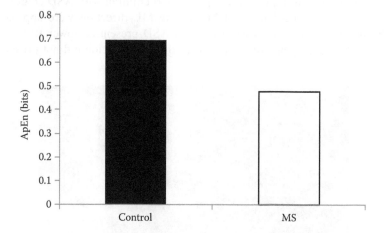

FIGURE 9.4 Approximate entropy (ApEn) values for a patient with multiple sclerosis (MS) and a control participant.

discriminate biological from nonbiological motion. Gepner and Feron (2009) suggested that the phenotypic expressions of ASD are directly related to a neurophysiologic base stemming from temporospatial processing disorder. Under this theoretical approach, it is entirely reasonable that posture (a continuous gross motor behavior which relies heavily on the online incorporation of sensory information) would suffer in persons with ASD. This has been shown to be the case by Molloy et al. (2003), who report drastic effects on posture under the conditions of modified sensory input. Minshew et al. (1997) have also shown that children with autism are less able to adapt to manipulations of somatosensory information and continue throughout life to express developmentally delayed postural control.

Case Study of Postural Control in Children with ASD

COP was recorded via force plate (AMTI, OR6) from a group of 10 children, age 4–6 years old. Four of these children have been diagnosed with ASD, while six have not. The children were provided a static point target on a television monitor, 1.5 m from where they stood (Figure 9.5). The height of the monitor was adjusted, so the target was positioned at the eye level of each child. Eye tracking equipment (Seeing Machines, faceLAB) was used to verify the maintenance of attention during collection. Trials lasted for 3½ min with COP data recorded at 50 Hz based on pilot work. Postprocessing included identification of segments during which the child was not speaking or making overt motions with his or her head or arms (none of the children moved their feet during the trial). The longest common segment across all children was 750 data points, or 15 s of continuous COP. These segments were further processed to generate the RMS and LyE measures of variability in both the AP and ML direction. For statistical analysis, independent t-tests were performed to identify differences between typically developing children and children with ASD.

RMS in the AP and the ML direction did not present any significant differences between children with typical development and children with ASD (Figure 9.6). However, the differences in the RMS in the ML direction were approaching significance ($p = 0.07$), with children with ASD presenting lower RMS values than typically developing children. LyE in the AP direction did not present any

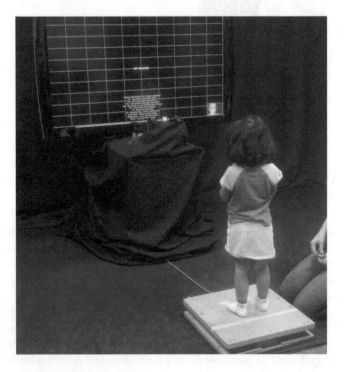

FIGURE 9.5 Experimental setup.

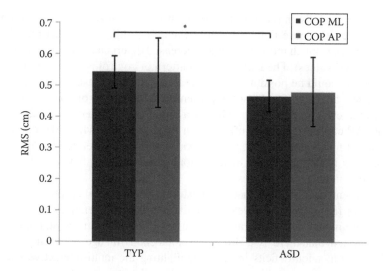

FIGURE 9.6 Root-mean-square (RMS) values for the center of pressure data in the medial–lateral (ML) and anterior–posterior (AP) direction in typically developing (TYP) children and children diagnosed with autism spectrum disorders (ASD).

significant differences between children with typical development and children with ASD (Figure 9.7). However, children with ASD presented statistically significant higher LyE values in the ML direction than typically developing children. Overall, children with ASD appear to have reduced amount of COP variability (RMS), and redundant use of postural strategies in the ML direction (LyE).

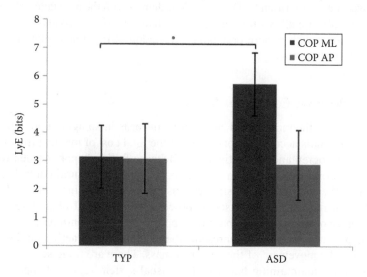

FIGURE 9.7 Lyapunov exponent (LyE) values for the center of pressure data in the medial–lateral (ML) and anterior–posterior (AP) direction in typically developing (TYP) children and children diagnosed with autism spectrum disorders (ASD).

Therefore, especially in the ML direction, children with ASD appear not only to sway significantly more than typically developing children (RMS) but also the way they move is much more noisy with increased divergence in the COP trajectories (high LyE values). The fact that this pattern of control is apparent only in the ML direction could be possibly due to the following two reasons: (a) the postural control trials analyzed for the study presented here are part of a larger study that involved the eye and posture tracking of a target moving medio-laterally and (b) possibly AP control is already effective in these children, while ML control that is important for dynamic tasks, such as walking, is not as refined as AP postural control. This is also indicative of less cooperative behavior between the components of the underlying control system.

The present data suggest that the postural sway variability of children with ASD differs from typically developing children. These differences are noticeable in both the amount and temporal variations of COP sway during standing. It has been suggested that there is a direct developmental linkage between motor and social communication deficits in ASD highlighting the multi-interactive nature of the perception–action–cognition cycle, and thus, the importance of motor deficits in children with ASD. These results have further implications for assessing motor development behavior in children with ASD and the development of future therapeutic protocols.

Note: The LyE values in this case study are much higher than other case studies. The difference is not due to the algorithm as always the same algorithm is used (Wolf et al. 1985). However, the difference is due to different types of software used. Earlier software used by our research team was commercially available (Chaos Data Analyzer Professional software). However, more recent software, which is available on our website, was written by Dr. Shane Wurdeman with the assistance of Dr. Alan Wolf. This software allows for the input of actual time (i.e., seconds) between data points providing with a more pragmatic calculation of the time evolution between data points in state space.

STANDING POSTURAL CONTROL IN AGING

Falls are among the most significant health concerns in an aging population. It is estimated that falls account for one-third of the total cost of medical treatment for all injuries (Sjögren and Björnstig 1991). Because falling happens when the center of mass moves outside the base of support, studying postural control can give insight into the control mechanisms responsible for maintaining balance. Postural control is an intricate neuromuscular process with the goal of maintaining the body's center of mass over the base of support. COP is a common measure used to assess postural control and represents the resultant forces acting on the ground and reflects the movement of the center of mass. There are three sensory systems responsible for maintaining balance: The visual system senses changes in body position through visual input, the somatosensory system senses changes in body position through mechanisms such as proprioception in the feet, limb position, and muscle length, and the vestibular system senses changes in head position and movement. When measuring postural control, there will be an inherent variability present since an individual cannot stand perfectly still. Previously, it was thought that by reducing variability in standing posture a reduction in fall risk would occur. However, it is now known that a healthy biological system requires variability, and this variability has a temporal structure that exhibits nonlinearities (Stergiou et al. 2006). Thus, nonlinear methods have been used to explore the temporal structure of variability and have provided a better picture of the overall health of the neuromuscular system.

Case Study of Postural Control in Elderly Participants

One healthy young (age: 25 years; height: 179 cm; mass: 81.4 kg) and one healthy older adult (age: 84 years; height: 157 cm; mass: 66 kg) were screened and consented for participation in this study. COP was recorded for all participants using the Neurocom® Balance Manager™ System (Neurocom International Inc., Clackamas, OR; 100 Hz). Each participant completed one trial of natural standing, each lasting 90 s. Subjects were instructed to stand with feet shoulder width apart and even weight distribution. The COP signal was analyzed in the AP and ML. The nonlinear dependent variable that we used was detrended fluctuation analysis (DFA, Chapter 7) to evaluate the temporal structure of the COP. DFA was used in the present case study due to the presence of possible trends introduced due to utilization of the Neurocom. DFA is a technique used to measure long-range correlations in nonstationary time series. Analyzing long-range correlations allows exploration of how movements on different time scales are related to each other. Stronger long-range correlations indicate that future movements rely more heavily on previous movements. Weaker long-range correlations indicate that movements rely less heavily on the memory of past events.

Even though DFA values in the AP direction do not seem to be different between the healthy young and the healthy older participant, DFA values in the ML direction are much greater for the healthy elderly participant (Figure 9.8). Typically, a DFA value of 0.5 is characteristic of uncorrelated white noise, 1.0 of pink noise, and 1.5 of brown noise. Evidently (Figure 9.8), the DFA value in the ML direction of the healthy elderly participant is very close to brown noise. This finding could be indicative of greater reliance of the healthy elderly participant to the past postural control states and therefore inability to adapt to new and unforeseen situations. Postural sway is a multifactorial component that has a strong neuromuscular basis. Typically, aging is associated with decline of the neuromuscular system; however, it appears that nonlinear measures provide a different view of neuromuscular control. Another interesting result that the older individual is closer to brown noise while during walking older individuals are usually closer to white noise. Thus, it is possible that the way aging affects the exponent from DFA is task specific.

GAIT

Walking is a fundamental movement skill that enables humans to carry out daily activities. This most fundamental skill is extensively studied for the purposes of understanding development across the life span, identifying adaptations due to

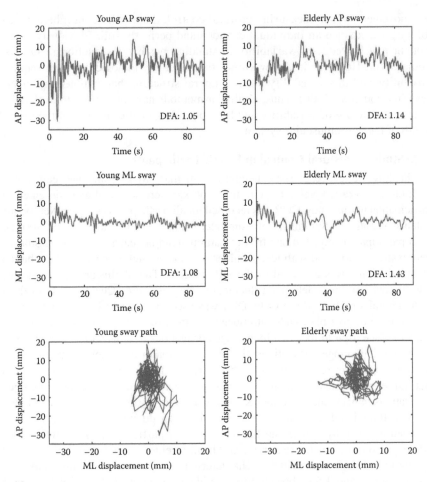

FIGURE 9.8 Anterior–posterior (AP, top row) and medial–lateral (ML, second row) postural sway time series and postural sway paths (bottom row) for a young and an elderly participant.

injury and pathology, and seeking rehabilitation methods to restore walking abilities. Investigating the variability in gait for these purposes is ideal, as variability analyses are thought to provide insight into multiple levels of movement organization (Newell and Corcos 1993). Variability in gait is demonstrated through differences that occur from one step to the next. Specifically, investigators have examined variability in step timing and the way the leg joints flex and extend throughout multiple steps. Analysis of gait patterns has provided insight into strategies used by different populations to control movement and has shown potential as a prognostic tool. In the following section, several examples are presented that have examined the variability of gait patterns using different measures. An important note is that for each of these studies, variability seen in healthy individuals is considered as the optimal state/level of variability. This allows us to make inferences regarding the effects of malfunction and/or disease.

PERIPHERAL ARTERIAL DISEASE

Peripheral arterial disease (PAD) is a result of atherosclerosis that leads to blockages in lower extremity arteries. In these patients, blood flow to the leg is inadequate and typically results in pain during walking known as intermittent claudication. Claudicating patients have reduced mobility, which led to multiple biomechanical studies to clearly identify the signature of gait in these individuals (Celis et al. 2009; Koutakis et al. 2010; McGrath et al. 2012; Myers et al. 2009, 2011; Wurdeman et al. 2012a,b). In these studies with PAD patients, gait was assessed through kinematics, specifically investigating the limit cycle that is evident in the relative angle range of motion time series for the ankle, knee, and hip joints.

Case Study of Gait in Peripheral Arterial Disease

Lower extremity kinematics were acquired at a rate of 60 Hz, while the patient and control subjects, both 68 years old, walked at their self-selected speed on a treadmill. The patient completed 3 min of walking prior to the onset of claudication (pain-free) and after the onset of claudication (pain), while the healthy control subject walked for 3 min as a control condition. Nonlinear analysis included calculation of the largest LyE and pseudoperiodic surrogation analysis (Miller et al. 2006; Small et al. 2001). One important consideration for utilizing nonlinear measures in patients with PAD is that they can walk for a limited amount of time before the onset of pain and after the onset of pain. To include the maximum number of patients possible, we wanted to perform analysis on the shortest necessary amount of data. It was previously determined by different research groups (Stergiou and colleagues, Dingwell and colleagues, Bates classic work on single subject analysis, see also discussion on this topic in Chapter 4) that 30 gait cycles per trial is adequate for evaluating the LyE from gait data calculated at 60 Hz. To determine the length of data needed to include 30 gait cycles, all joint angle time series were graphed and the number of data points required to reach 30 gait cycles was counted. After the minimum number of data points for 30 gait cycles was determined for both subjects, all data were cropped to that length, ensuring that all time series included at least 30 gait cycles. The relative joint angle time series, the embedding dimension, and time lag were calculated using custom software in MATLAB® to be used for the surrogation analysis. Gait has inherent periodicity, with a cycle occurring with each step. Therefore, the pseudoperiodic algorithm was used. Surrogated data sets were calculated for each original joint angle time series for each subject. Next, the largest LyE was calculated for both the original and surrogated time series and compared using dependent t-tests ($p = 0.05$). Significant differences between data sets indicate that the variations present in the original data set are not random but they exhibit a structure. For the purpose of this case study, we compared the pain-free condition of the patient with PAD and a healthy, age-matched control subject. The results indicated that the patient with PAD had higher LyE values than the control subject for the ankle, knee, and hip joint. A representative ankle joint angle time series and a phase portrait are shown in Figures 9.9 and 9.10. The value of LyE for the PAD time series was 0.116 and for the control subject was 0.094. While visually minimal differences in variability of the time series are evident, the phase portrait illustrates a less organized signal, with more divergence with each cycle in the

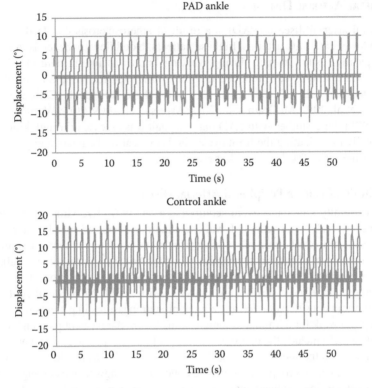

FIGURE 9.9 Ankle joint angle time series of a patient with peripheral arterial disease (PAD) and a control participant.

PAD patient compared with the healthy control. This is clearly evident, especially in the lower left quadrant of the phase portraits. In the phase portrait of the patient with PAD, we observe little overlap of the ankle trajectories, while in the phase portrait of the control subject, we see greater overlap and a very "dense" phase portrait. A patient with PAD presents with increased noise and randomness of the locomotor system, which may result in an inability to correctly select the appropriate response under challenging conditions. This may be directly linked to the increased risk of falling of patients with PAD. Additional studies have utilized gait variability analysis to further investigate mechanisms contributing to mobility problems in PAD (Myers et al. 2010, 2013). Future studies will continue to investigate the effect of myopathic and neuropathic changes on gait variability, and nonlinear tools will be utilized to evaluate the effectiveness of current treatments in improving mobility.

CHRONIC OBSTRUCTIVE PULMONARY DISEASE

While chronic obstructive pulmonary disease (COPD) is a pulmonary disease that leads to narrowing of the airways, destruction of lung tissue, and dynamic hyperinflation, COPD also affects the structure and function of skeletal muscle tissue (Gosker et al. 2002, 2007; Puente-Maestu et al. 2009). It is well established that these

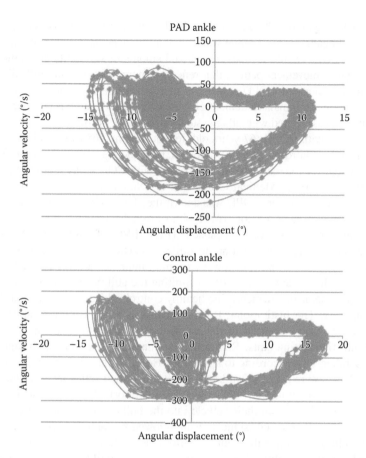

FIGURE 9.10 Phase portraits of a patient with peripheral arterial disease (PAD) and a control participant.

abnormalities in the muscular system of patients with COPD are present, and the next logical question becomes as follows: does this have any effect on their overall function? Assessment of the overall function and functional limitations of patients with COPD may provide insight into the auxiliary "systemic and complex abnormalities" affecting peripheral systems in patients with COPD (Fabbri and Rabe 2007). Recent research has led to findings of functional limitations being documented in this population. Patients with COPD demonstrate muscle fatigue (Baghai-Ravary et al. 2009; Saey et al. 2003), muscle weakness (Seymour et al. 2010), gait abnormalities (Marquis et al. 2009; Yentes et al. 2011), and increased risk of falls (Roig et al. 2009, 2011).

Case Study of Gait in Chronic Obstructive Pulmonary Disease

The current case study proposes that through the analyses of both amount and temporal structure of variability while walking, limitations in overall functional mobility in this population would be uncovered. It was hypothesized that the patient with COPD would demonstrate adaptations in both the amount and temporal structure (i.e., as calculated through sample entropy, Chapter 6) of variability in walking patterns as compared to age-matched healthy control while walking at a self-selected speed. Specifically, the patient with COPD would demonstrate altered amount of variability and a more predictable/regular movement pattern that reflects a more restricted and inflexible, gait. The pathophysiology of COPD appears to increase regularity in autonomic nervous system functions (Iranmanesh et al. 2011; Veiga et al. 2011), and it is possible that this same pattern is associated with other systems affected by the disease.

One patient with COPD (67 years old, female, height: 165.1 cm, weight: 54.4 kg) and one healthy control subject (70 years old, male, height: 193 cm, weight: 95.5 kg) were evaluated for this case study. The patient with COPD was recruited from the University of Nebraska Medical Center and the Nebraska-Western Iowa Veterans' Affairs Healthcare Center. COPD was determined based on the previously reported diagnosis of the disease and confirmed with spirometry testing ratio of forced expiratory volume in 1 s to forced vital capacity (FEV_1/FVC) of less than 0.7. Spirometry testing was completed without a bronchodilator. Participants were excluded if they presented the history of back or lower extremity injury or surgery that affected the subject's mobility or any other process limiting the ability to walk, including neurological disease or impairment. The healthy control subject was recruited through the community. The Institutional Review Boards at both institutions approved all procedures. Subjects reported to the biomechanics laboratory and were asked to change into tight-fitting suits. Retroreflective markers were placed on anatomical locations, bilaterally, according to a modified Helen Hayes marker set (Houck et al. 2005). Subjects were asked to walk on a treadmill at their self-selected pace. A self-selected pace was defined for the subjects as a comfortable walking speed, a pace that they would walk from their vehicle into the building or across the campus. In order to choose their speed, subjects were allowed to control their walking speed on the treadmill and once they felt a comfortable walking speed, the investigators increased the speed slightly. The speed was increased until the subject said that the treadmill was moving faster than they were comfortable walking. The treadmill was then slowed again in phases until subjects mentioned that it felt too slow. These steps were repeated until a speed, that was a comfortable walking pace for the subject, was found. This process took anywhere between 5 and 10 min for most subjects.

Once a comfortable walking speed was chosen, subjects were allowed to rest for a minimum of 2 min. After they were well rested, they returned to the treadmill to complete 3½ min of walking on the treadmill at their self-selected pace. Three-dimensional marker positions from the last 3 min of walking were recorded (Motion Analysis Corp., Santa Rosa, CA; 60 Hz). A custom MATLAB program (MATLAB 2007, Mathworks Inc., Concord, MA) was used to calculate the speed of the treadmill for each self-selected speed, and the healthy control subject was identified from our group of health controls to match for speed with the patient with COPD. The speed of the treadmill was calculated from the derivative of the heel marker in the AP direction during the foot's stance phase of gait. This speed was averaged for each step on the right and the left to provide the speed of the treadmill belt. Unfiltered three-dimensional marker data were used to calculate three spatiotemporal time series for each subject. Custom MATLAB programs were used to calculate step width for the walking trial. Step width was calculated

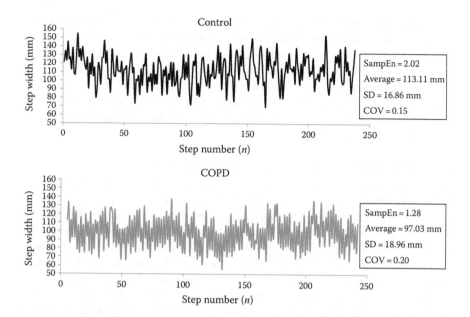

FIGURE 9.11 Step width time series of a patient with chronic obstructive pulmonary disease (COPD) and a control participant. On the right side of each time series, we can see the sample entropy (SampEn), average, standard deviation (SD), and coefficient of variation (COV) values of each step width time series.

as the ML distance from the heel strike of the right foot to the heel strike of the left foot and the same for continuing contralateral and ipsilateral steps. The following dependent variables were calculated for each 238-step time series of step width: mean, standard deviation (SD), coefficient of variation (COV), and sample entropy (SampEn, $m = 2$, $r = 0.25$, $N = 238$). Sample entropy is utilized here because this is what our hypothesis dictates based on the physiological questions we generated in this population. In addition, we have a quite short time series in comparison with what is required by other nonlinear tools.

The results (Figure 9.11) showed that the patient with COPD had more regular gait patterns (lower SampEn values) but presented with greater amount of variability (greater SD and COV values). These findings provide further evidence that amount of variability and structure of variability provide information regarding different processes and offer complementary information regarding the behavior of the system.

Amputation

Lower limb amputation presents a major change to the patient's neuromuscular system. The loss of peripheral structures and neural endpoints creates an obstacle for individuals as they potentially learn to walk again following prosthetic rehabilitation. The neuromuscular system must learn new strategies in order to fully integrate a foreign device into its natural movement pattern. Consider prior to amputation, during the common task of walking, the neuromuscular system had developed a movement strategy that encompassed an active, biological leg. Following amputation, major components of the anatomy that led to the solution that the neuromuscular system had settled on are no longer present, thereby leaving the neuromuscular system to learn a new solution if the person is to walk again with a prosthesis. The need for the neuromuscular system to learn a new solution is not unique to limb loss, but occurs under many different pathologies affecting the neuromusculoskeletal system.

Case Study of a Patient with Lower Limb Amputation

The participant is a 65-year-old male (weight 221.5 lb, height 188 cm) who has a unilateral, transtibial amputation of the right leg as a result of an accident that occurred on the job 8 years ago. The individual is a farmer by trade. The individual is considered a Medicare K3 level individual that typically ambulates on a Seattle Soleus prosthetic foot with a pin suspension. The subject underwent consecutive adaptation periods to two different prosthetic setups, one which is clinically considered more appropriate for the subject with a K3 level foot (Freedom Senator) and the second which is clinically considered less appropriate due to the K2 level foot that it had (Willow Wood SACH). Importantly, socket and suspension were not altered to mitigate confounding effects of fit and suspension. All prostheses were properly aligned by a certified prosthetist.

The time series plots for the prosthetic side ankle motion have similar looking gait patterns (Figure 9.12). However, calculation of the largest LyE reveals that the subject was able to ambulate with decreased stride-to-stride fluctuations with the more appropriate prosthesis (LyE = 2.09) compared to the less appropriate prosthesis (LyE = 2.63). Previous research has shown a strong relationship between the difference in LyE and prosthesis preference among amputees (Wurdeman et al. 2014a). Wurdeman et al. (2014a,b) have proposed that the LyE represents how well the two subsystems (biological person and mechanical prosthetic leg) are functioning together as a single system to accomplish the task of walking as opposed to two subsystems fighting to dominate the movement. Such antagonistic behavior would be believed to result in increased LyE values.

MOTOR CONTROL

GAIT VARIABILITY IN STROKE

Treating human movement variability as a source of noise and error in the motor system has led to ignorance of a very important source of clinical information. Especially, since altered human movement, variability is found increasingly in a variety of motor-related disorders indicating reduced adaptive capacity in the neuromuscular system. Such a source of information can help tremendously in the determination of the best approaches for therapies grounded on the restoration of movement capabilities in patients suffering from sensorimotor disorders like stroke. In the following case study, we present differences in gait variability from a stroke survivor and a healthy adult.

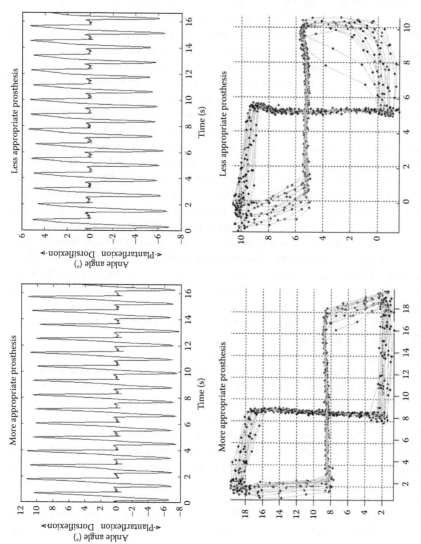

FIGURE 9.12 Ankle joint angle time series of a participant with lower limb amputation with the appropriate (top row, left) and less appropriate (top row, right) prosthesis. On the bottom row, you can observe the respective ankle time series embedded into two dimensions.

Case Study of Gait Variability from a Stroke Survivor

The stroke patient was recruited from the regular outpatient clinic of the Department of Neurological Sciences at the University of Nebraska Medical Center. The inclusion criteria for the stroke survivor included the following: (1) first time "diagnosed' carotid distribution ischemic, hemorrhagic, or brainstem stroke, at least 3 months after the incidence, (2) age >55 and <70, (3) lived in the community prior to stroke, (4) mild-to-moderate stroke based on the Orpington Prognostic Score >2.8 and <5, (5) Folstein Mini-Mental Score >25.64, and (6) free of major poststroke complications (e.g., recurrent stroke, hip fracture, and myocardial infarction). The stroke patient was screened to have a unilateral lesion; whose dominant side was affected; and who has at least 20/40 corrected vision (visual acuity testing). Subjects, who had a stroke due to subarachnoid hemorrhage, lesions in either temporal or in parietal lobe leading to asomatognosia or unilateral neglect, with progressing dementia, posterior circulation stroke, obtunded or comatose, a history of fractures or injuries in the lower limb of less than 6 months duration, apraxia (Florida Apraxia Score <27), more than one stroke episode, pain at the time of screening, neglect, poorly controlled diabetes, amputation, blind, progressive neurological diseases (e.g., Parkinson's disease), peripheral nerve pathology, and lived more than 60 miles from University of Nebraska Omaha, were excluded from this case study.

Subjects reported to the biomechanics laboratory and were asked to change into tight-fitting suits. Retroreflective markers were placed on anatomical locations, bilaterally and were asked to walk on a treadmill at their self-selected pace. After the self-selected pace was established, the subjects rested for 5 min and then resumed walking at their self-selected pace until we had collected a total of 200 strides. From the kinematics, we derived the time series of the stride times, which are the time intervals from one leg's heel contact to the same leg's heel contact. The following dependent variables were calculated for each 200 stride time intervals: mean, standard deviation (Std Dev), and sample entropy.

When comparing the stride times of a stroke patient to a healthy control, there are some clear differences (Figure 9.13). The linear measures of mean and standard deviation show a distinction between the healthy person and the stroke patient, and in this case, the stroke patient has a greater stride time and a greater amount of stride time variability. When comparing the stroke patients' affected leg to their unaffected leg, the linear measures do not provide any distinction. In this case, the mean and standard deviation between the two legs are almost identical. However, when utilizing sample entropy to quantify the temporal structure of stride time variability and specifically the regularity of the stride time series, we are able to see clear distinctions between not only the healthy control and the patient, but also between the patient's affected and unaffected leg (Figure 9.13). Because sample entropy measures the regularity of a time series, with lower values being more regular, we can see that the stride times of the stroke patient are less regular than a healthy control. In this case, the sample entropy is also able to distinguish between the affected and unaffected leg in the stroke patient, with the affected leg showing less regularity than the unaffected leg. In addition, it allowed us to make inferences about additional aspects of the control strategies used, which are not present if measures of the amount of variability are the only ones being considered.

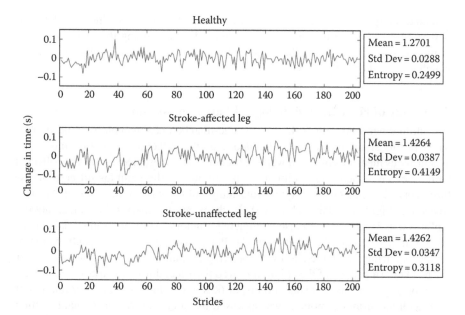

FIGURE 9.13 Stride-time series of a healthy participant, the affected leg of a stroke patient and the unaffected leg of a stroke patient. On the right side of each time series, we can see the mean, standard deviation (Std Dev), and the sample entropy (Entropy) values of each time series.

PERCEPTION OF COMPLEX MOTION IN CHILDREN WITH AUTISM

Typically, developing children recognize biological motion in point-light displays. Interestingly, they specifically prefer to watch locomotion coherent with their own mode of locomotion; that is, crawlers prefer to watch crawling, whereas walkers prefer to watch walking (Sanefuji et al. 2008). This observation provides insight into how children recognize and replicate movements of others in their social environment. The development of motor behavior relies, in part, on being able to incorporate the lessons learned from viewing others' attempts at similar motor performance. By watching others, we are able to multiply our own experience and knowledge of successful movement strategies. For individuals with autism, this is contingent, however, on whether or not the action of the model is perceptible, which unfortunately does not seem to be the case. Gepner and Feron (2009) suggest that the phenotypic expressions of ASD are directly related to a neurophysiologic base stemming from temporospatial processing disorder. Disordered processing provokes confusion and discomfort in environments that contain rich sources of temporally relevant sensory information. Gepner and Feron present examples of an inability to perceive and produce overt responses; however, even the observation of a more covert behavior, such as another person's eye movements, has been shown distracting to some with autism (Grandin 1995). In light of a vast amount of work in biomechanics, we suggest that the specific aversion to the complex temporospatial aspects of others' movements is related directly to the perception of chaotic motion of the observed individual. Chaos is pervasive in human movement, and a deficit in recognizing this particular type of motion structure could be the basis for the lack of attention to biological motion, which is typical of children with autism.

Case Study of Perception of Biological Motion in Autism

One child diagnosed with ASD and one age-matched healthy control child participated in this study. Participants attended a single collection session during which synchronous measures of eye movement (Seeing Machines, faceLAB) were collected while viewing a point-light stimulus. The motion of the stimulus differed across three conditions, determined by scaling temporal complexity in terms of ApEn; a sine wave (highly regular, ApEn = 0.032), chaos (approximate to biological motion, ApEn = 0.097), and brown noise (completely random, ApEn = 0.136). Trials lasted for 3½ min, with data recorded at 50 Hz. Postprocessing included identification of segments during which the child was speaking or making overt motions with his or her head or arms (none of the children moved their feet during the trial). The longest common segment was 3000 data points, or 60 s of continuous data. Coordination of gaze with the stimulus motions was assessed using cross recurrence quantification analysis, including rate and duration of bouts of coordination.

Results showed that the child with ASD did not express an affinity to chaotic motion of the stimulus in the same way as the child without ASD (Figure 9.14). The typically developing child showed increased rate and duration of coordination with the chaos stimulus, suggesting some interest or affinity to viewing this type of motion. It has been previously been shown that chaotic motion is an integral characteristic of human movement. We contend that this indifference to chaotic motion by children with ASD is related to, and possibly responsible for, the general disinterest in biological motion shown by these children.

ROBOTIC SURGICAL SKILLS TRAINING

Robot-assisted laparoscopy is a common minimally invasive surgery performed by a surgeon who controls a specialized robot. Similar to conventional laparoscopy, small incisions are made, and the robotic manipulators and endoscopic camera are inserted into the patient. Surgical robots, such as the da Vinci™ surgical system (dVSS, Intuitive Surgical Inc., Sunnyvale, CA), have specialized features such as an ergonomically designed surgeon's console, interactive robotic arms, high-resolution 3D endoscope, and wrist-like master controls (Moorthy et al. 2004). These features give the surgical robot distinct advantages over traditional laparoscopy, such as reduced surgeon fatigue, enhanced view, larger range of motion, tremor cancellation, and scaled motion (D'Annibale et al. 2004; Hernandez et al. 2004; Moorthy et al. 2004).

Most studies using the dVSS have found that medical students and residents reduced the time to complete simple surgical tasks after training (Narazaki et al. 2006, 2007; Prasad et al. 2002; Sarle et al. 2004). Skilled surgeons with robotic surgical experience also performed tasks faster than novice users (Judkins et al. 2009). Current

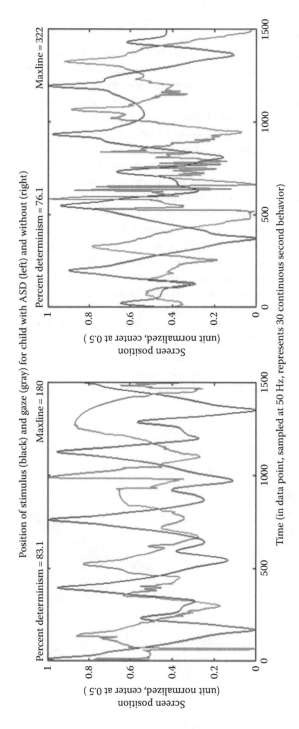

FIGURE 9.14 Time series of the position of stimulus (black) versus the gaze time series (gray) for a child with autism spectrum disorders (ASD, left) and a neurotypical child (right).

measures of evaluating surgical performance and skill acquisition in robot-assisted surgery focus on objective measures, including total traveled distance, number of errors occurred, and subjective evaluations by an expert using objective structured assessment of technical skill (OSATS, Hanly et al. 2004; Prasad et al. 2002; Sarle et al. 2004). Although these objective measures are able to quantify the robotic surgical performance, these measures do not evaluate any characteristics of movement in surgical skills such as consistency. One of the key components of being an expert surgeon is to maintain consistent skills performance. It is important to explore the measurement that can evaluate consistency of robotic surgical skills performance.

In our study, we evaluated the consistency of movement trajectory in robot-assisted surgery using objective measures that examine the amount and the structure of movement variability. Amount of variability is generally measured by the standard deviation, a measure of statistical dispersion, and coefficient of variation, which is a normalized measure of dispersion. The largest LyE, a measure of structure of variability, is used to examine consistency by evaluating the rate of change in movement trajectories; more diverged or less consistent movement is indicated as LyE increases (Stergiou et al. 2004). Thus, reduction in the LyE measure indicated increased consistency of movement trajectories. The structure of variability has been utilized in evaluating consistent patterns in human movement (Kay 1988).

Ten novice medical students (29.4 ± 7.0 years) with no prior experience using the dVSS, participated in this study. All participants were right handed. Each participant passed a 17-mm Polysorb™ surgical needle through 10 designated points along an inanimate material in the horizontal plane using the dVSS laparoscopic graspers (Figure 9.15). The task required the participant to control the robotic surgical instrument (grasper) and accurately pass a needle through each designated point along

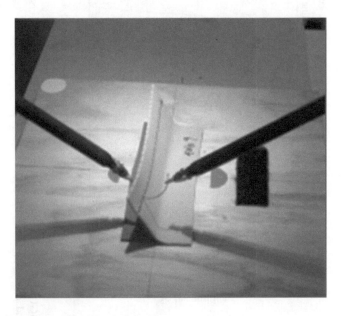

FIGURE 9.15 Surgical needle passing task.

the inanimate material using the dominant (right) hand and pull the needle out by controlling the other robotic arm with the nondominant (left) hand. Each participant performed the needle-passing task first as a pretraining test followed by training sessions and finally a posttraining test.

All objective measures of performance were based on the kinematic measures from the instrument tips of the dVSS collected at 100 Hz using the application programmer's interface (API) provided by Intuitive Surgical Inc. (Sunnyvale, CA). The sampling frequency was set by the manufacturer. The surgical movement paths of the horizontal and the vertical directions of both nondominant and dominant sides were calculated to evaluate the performance. From these time series, we derived the standard deviation, the coefficient of variation and the largest LyE (Figure 9.16). The data were down-sampled from 100 to 10 Hz in order to properly reconstruct the state space as we realized through our frequency analysis that the manufacturer's imposed sampling rate was quite high. Investigation of the characteristics of the state space is a powerful tool for examining a dynamic system because it provides information that is not apparent by just observing the data (Abarbanel et al. 1993; Baker et al. 1996; further details of state space reconstruction refer to Chapter 3).

Data set included 16 cycles of needle passing with a minimum of 896 data points that were used to generate the time series. This is, in fact, a limitation of this data as these numbers are lower than what is needed to utilize the LyE. The data were unfiltered so as to get a more accurate representation of the variations within the system (Mees and Judd 1993). It was assumed that since the same instrumentation (dVSS) was used for all subjects, the level of measurement noise would be consistent for all subjects, and thus, any differences could be attributed to changes within the system itself (Abarbanel et al. 1993; Mees and Judd 1993). The independent variables were laterality (dominant vs. nondominant), movement direction (vertical vs. horizontal), and training (pre- vs. posttraining).

No significant training effects were found for the standard deviation (SD) and the coefficient of variation (CV). However, significant movement directional effects were shown for both SD and CV, which were significantly smaller in the vertical direction than the horizontal. A significant laterality effect was also found for both SD and CV. These were significantly smaller in the nondominant hand than in the dominant. Although there was no three-way interaction among the three effects, a significant interaction was shown between direction and laterality. In the follow-up pairwise comparison, a significant difference in CV was found between the dominant and the nondominant hand in the horizontal direction but not in the vertical direction.

A significant effect of laterality revealed that the LyE was smaller in the nondominant hand. A significant effect of movement direction showed that the LyE was significantly smaller in the horizontal direction. Although there was no three-way interaction among three effects, two significant two-way interactions between training and laterality and between movement direction and laterality were found. In the follow-up pairwise comparisons, significantly smaller LyE was only found in the nondominant hand from pre- to posttraining tests (Figure 9.16). The dominant hand did not show differences across training. Moreover, there was a significant reduction in LyE from the dominant to the nondominant hand only in the horizontal but not in the vertical direction (Figure 9.17). We can also see these differences in Figure 9.16

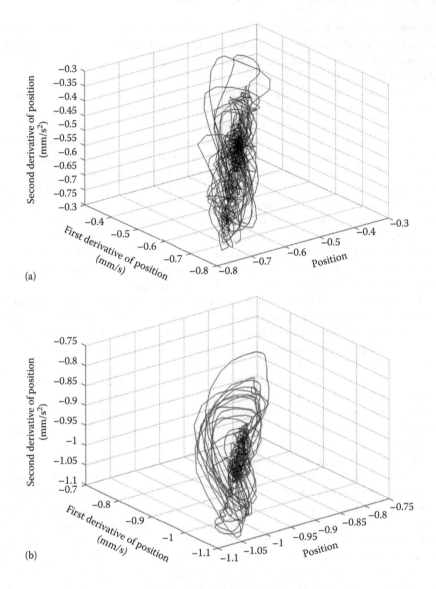

(a)

(b)

FIGURE 9.16 Pre- and posttraining three-dimensional reconstruction of the position of the needle. (a) Pretraining (LyE = 0.224) and (b) post training (LyE = 0.184).

where the horizontal movement paths from pre- to posttraining tests are in three-dimensional state-space plots. This three-dimensional state-space plot presents the movement path, where the second derivative is plotted versus the first derivative and the position of the movement. The trajectory of the movement path shows a more consistent, cleaner, and less divergent movement pattern after training.

The objective of this study was to determine variables that can be used to assess the complexity of surgical movement qualitatively and identify a better way to examine

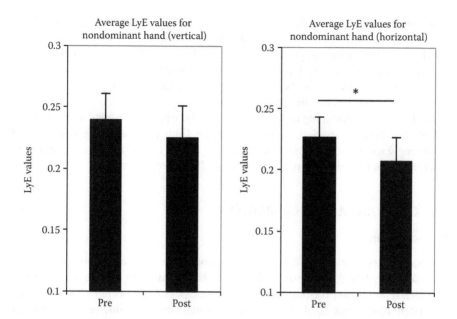

FIGURE 9.17 Lyapunov exponent (LyE) values from pre- and post training for the nondominant hand in the vertical and horizontal direction.

consistency of surgical performance using the amount of variability and structure of variability measure in robot-assisted surgery. We found that surgical skill improvement can be assessed through the investigation of the temporal structure of variability. As the LyE reduced after training, the surgical movement patterns became more consistent. In previous studies, the time to task completion and the total traveled distance have been used to describe surgical skills learning. However, they do not describe all aspects of robotic surgical performance. This is because a surgeon is more concerned with safety and accuracy during the actual surgery rather than time or longer trajectories of the surgical tools. A surgeon is expected to be cautious in order to prevent tissue damage or other complications in operating theater (Hernandez et al. 2004; Sarle et al. 2004; Smith et al. 2001). In addition, our previous studies (Narazaki et al. 2006, 2007) have suggested that traditional variables, such as the task completion time, may partially indicate the extent of proficiency of skill acquisition; they may not provide the whole picture as far as the consistency of performance is concerned.

In this study, to measure the consistency of surgical movement, both the amount and the structure of variability were measured and compared. Only the structure of variability measure detected the effect of training showing more consistent movement pattern after training. It is possible that the amount of variability measures of variability may not be sensitive enough to examine highly complex movement patterns that require unfolding of more degrees of freedom at higher dimensional state space to be evaluated. Thus, using the LyE, we found that the performance of the trainee did yield significant differences in the consistency of the nondominant hand of the surgical movements after training. Interestingly, there were no significant differences regarding the dominant hand for the LyE. Such findings have been reported in previous studies (Mettler et al. 2006; Ridding and Flavel 2006). Based on the dynamic-dominance hypothesis (Sainburg 2002; Shabbott and Sainburg 2008), interlimb dynamics for the dominant and nondominant hands are controlled differently by the cerebral hemispheres. The dynamic dominance hypothesis of motor lateralization suggests that the dominant hemisphere, with repeated use, has become specialized for coordinating movements efficiently, whereas the nondominant hemisphere has become specialized for controlling limb impedance, as required for achieving stable postures. Therefore, there is a "ceiling effect" for the dominant arm, whereas the nondominant arm has more room for improvement.

CHAOS IN ANIMAL LOCOMOTION

MOUSE MODEL

For many years, a lot of studies concerning locomotor activity and/or locomotor control used rodent models. These small mammals, of which the lineage is known and of which reproduction is controlled, are now indispensable tools in biology (Atchley and Fitch 1991; Beck et al. 2000). The high number of strains, of transgenic, or knock-out mice showing anomalies at various levels of the motor nervous control provides a useful model to investigate the complex motor behavior. It is necessary to define precisely the normal locomotor pattern of the different mice strains as reference models (Herbin et al. 2004; Leblond et al. 2003) to evaluate the level of impairment, or to evaluate the actual impact of a pharmacological treatment or the influence of the exercise in a possible locomotor recovery (Grondard et al. 2005; Kirkinezos et al. 2003; Mahoney et al. 2004). In this way, many kinematic studies use the motor-driven treadmill because it presents a good standardization of the experimental conditions, the convenience of obtaining measurements in moving animals, and to produce a consistent number of readily quantifiable homogeneous and continuous series of cycles over a large range of velocities (Herbin et al. 2007).

Mouse models of a neurodegenerative disease (e.g., Parkinson's disease and Huntington's disease) are used to understand the pathologies of the diseases and to accelerate the testing of new therapies to correct motor deficiencies. Several studies in mouse models of Parkinson's disease and Huntington's disease assessed gait by estimating stride length and stride width determined by painting the animals' paws (Carter et al. 1999; Fernagut et al. 2002). They reported that the stride length is a reliable index of motor disorders due to basal ganglia dysfunction in mice. However, gait assessment in humans extends beyond the measure of stride length by analyzing other spatial and temporal gait parameters and their variability over time during continuous treadmill walking (e.g., variability of lower extremity joint angles; Myers et al. 2009).

Recently, in addition to the study of various gait parameters, Amende et al. (2005) made an attempt to examine stride-to-stride variability in mouse models of Parkinson's disease and Huntington's disease. Measures of stride-to-stride variability were determined as the standard deviation and the coefficient of variation. The standard deviation reflects the dispersion about the average value for a parameter. The coefficient of variation was calculated from the equation: *100 × standard deviation/mean value.*

The motor speed was set to 34 cm/s for all mice. Approximately, 3 s of videography was collected for each walking mouse to provide more than seven sequential strides. Parkinson's mice demonstrated significant gait disturbances, including shortened stride length, increased stride frequency, and increased stride-to-stride variability, symptoms characteristic of patients with Parkinson's disease. Huntington's mice demonstrated an increased forelimb stride-to-stride variability and a more open paw placement angle of the hindlimbs. Gait failure in Huntington's mice resulted from an ability of the hindlimbs to engage in stepping while forelimb gait remained intact. Findings of Amende et al.'s study provide a basis for additional studies of gait measurements and their variability in mouse models of neurodegenerative diseases.

The present study examined gait variability in healthy mice and Parkinson's mice walking on the treadmill at two different treadmill speeds: 6.9 and 15.1 cm s⁻¹. We explored the following: (1) changes in gait variability in response to changes in gait speed; (2) differences in gait variability between the two groups of mice (i.e., healthy vs. Parkinson's mice); (3) at which gait speed (i.e., 6.9 or 15.1 cm s⁻¹), these inter-group differences in gait variability are the most evident.

Healthy and Parkinson's mice were filmed in the lateral view using cineradiography at 250 frames per second. Cineradiography is a technique that allows recording the successive positions of every bone segment of animals in motion. Markers (small radio-opaque balls) were placed at the right and left forelimb and hindlimb foot. All mice walked on the treadmill at two different treadmill speeds: 6.9 and 15.1 cm s⁻¹ (Figure 9.18). In total, three healthy mice and five Parkinson's mice walking at the speed of 6.9 cm s⁻¹, and four healthy mice and three Parkinson's mice walking at the speed of 15.1 cm s⁻¹ were analyzed. The y-coordinate (vertical displacement) for each marker was analyzed. All time series contained a minimum of 946 data points. Data were analyzed unfiltered so as to get a more accurate representation of the fluctuations within the time series. Furthermore, since the same instrumentation was used for all mice, it is assumed that the level of measurement noise was consistent for all mice. For the mice data set, a 2×3 (group by treadmill speed) analysis of variance (ANOVA) was performed on ApEn and largest LyE values for all the marker displacement data (Kaplan and Glass 1995; Wolf et al. 1985).

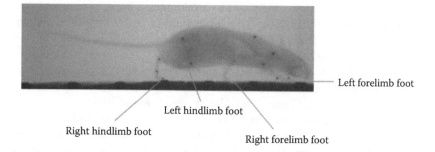

FIGURE 9.18 A mouse walking on the treadmill filmed in lateral view at 250 frames per second using cineradiography. Markers were placed at the right and left forelimb and hindlimb foot.

No significant interactions were found between the two factors (i.e., mouse group and treadmill speed). Even though not significant, ApEn values in Parkinson's mice were higher than those in healthy mice (Figure 9.19). Additionally, a significant main effect of the treadmill speed factor was found for the ApEn values of the left hindlimb. Even though not significant for the other limbs, it seems that a speed treadmill set at 6.9 cm s^{-1} better differentiates between healthy mice and Parkinson's mice.

Results from the largest LyE were similar to those of ApEn. No significant interactions were found between the two factors (i.e., mouse group and treadmill speed). Even though not significant, the largest LyE values in Parkinson's mice were higher than those in healthy mice when the treadmill speed was set at 6.9 cm s^{-1} (Figure 9.20). This tendency seems to be reversed with increased treadmill speed (i.e., 15.1 cm s^{-1}). As observed for ApEn values, a significant main effect of the treadmill speed factor was found for largest LyE values of the left hindlimb. Even though not significant for the other limbs, it seems that a treadmill set at speed 6.9 cm s^{-1} better differentiates between healthy mice and Parkinson's mice.

Taken together, these findings indicate differences in the temporal structure of the gait variability in Parkinson's mice compared to healthy mice. Specifically, higher ApEn and largest LyE values in the Parkinson's mice might indicate increased irregularities and randomness in their gait patterns, and an indication of loss of gait control mechanism. A mouse model that replicates disease symptoms could improve the understanding of its pathogenesis and treatment, while measures of gait variability are increasingly being recognized as important markers of neurological diseases (Harbourne and Stergiou 2009; Stergiou et al. 2004).

DUCK MODEL

Although the biology of flight has seen extensive study, terrestrial locomotion in birds has received comparatively less attention. Studies of the kinematics of terrestrial locomotion in birds included little quantitative analysis. While limb posture in birds clearly differs from humans, it is unclear how their limb segments move within a stride. Quantified kinematic profiles are limited. Muir et al. (1996) quantify hip, knee, and ankle profiles for slow walks in hatchling and 2-week-old chicks (speed not given), Jacobson and Hollyday (1982) present profiles for hip, knee, and ankle angles in the chicken, Gatesy (1999) provides kinematic profiles for the hip angle in guinea fowl moving at three speeds, and Dagg (1977) discusses ankle kinematics in a series of birds. Additional anecdotal data (primarily stick figures of single strides) are presented in the studies of stride characteristics, muscle function, or force dynamics (Cracraft 1971; Gatesy 1999; Gatesy and Biewener 1991).

In this study, we quantified variability of limb kinematics in ducks walking on a treadmill. Especially, we explored whether there exists a gradient of variability from the upper to the lower limb joints (as observed in humans). Four ducks were filmed in dorsoventral view and eight ducks in lateral view using cineradiography at 200 frames per second. Markers (small radio-opaque balls) were placed at the back of the head, the first thoracic vertebrae, the sacral vertebrae, the keel, the hip joint,

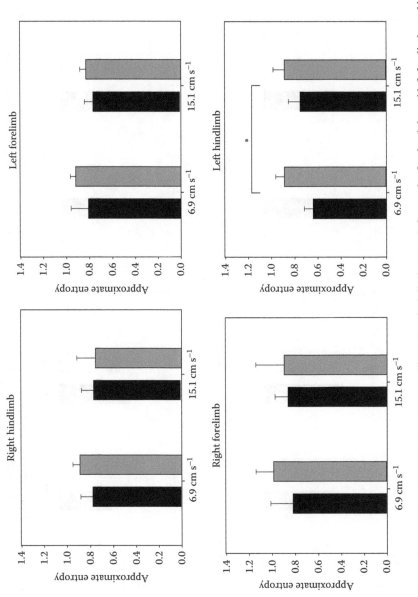

FIGURE 9.19 Approximate entropy (ApEn) values of y-coordinate (vertical displacement) time series for the right and left forelimbs and hindlimbs of healthy mice and Parkinson's mice at two different treadmill speeds: 6.9 and 15.1 cm s^{-1}. Black bar: healthy mice; gray bar: Parkinson's mice.

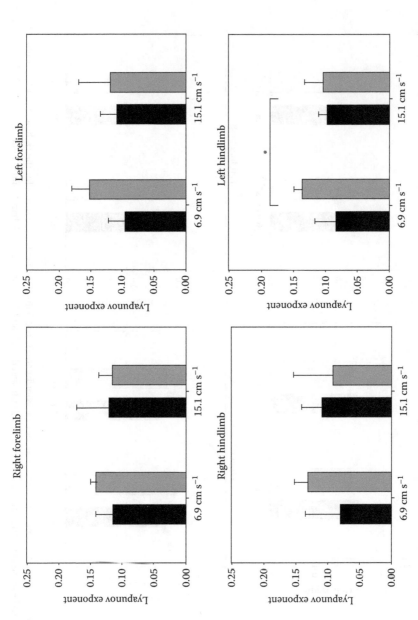

FIGURE 9.20 Lyapunov exponent values of y-coordinate (vertical displacement) time series for the right and left forelimbs and hindlimbs of healthy mice and Parkinson's mice at two different treadmill speeds: 6.9 and 15.1 cm s^{-1}. Black bar: healthy mice; gray bar: Parkinson's mice.

the knee joint, the intertarsal joint, and the metatarsal joint, and the ungual phalanx of the third toe. Markers were placed on the right limb only because it is difficult to distinguish between markers on the right and left limbs by cineradiography. All ducks walked on a treadmill at a comfortable speed of 1 km h⁻¹ (Figure 9.21). The y-coordinate (vertical displacement) for each marker was analyzed. All time series contained a minimum of 1023 data points.

ApEn (Figure 9.22) and largest LyE (Figure 9.23) results showed a decreasing gradient of variability from the upper to the lower limb joints in the lateral view,

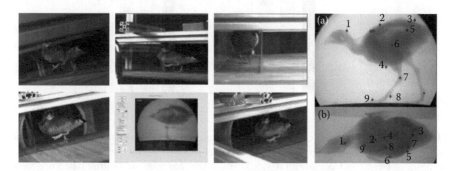

FIGURE 9.21 *Left picture*: a duck walking on the treadmill filmed in lateral view at 200 frames per second using cineradiography. *Right picture*: X-ray frames. (a) lateral view; (b) dorsoventral view. The black spots are the markers. 1, head; 2, vertebral column, thoracic level; 3, vertebral column, sacral level; 4, keel; 5, hip joint; 6, knee joint; 7, intertarsal joint; 8, metatarsophalangeal joint; 9, claw toe 3.

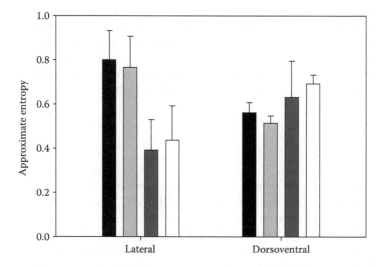

FIGURE 9.22 Approximate entropy values of y-coordinate (vertical displacement) time series for the hip, knee, intertarsal, and metatarsal joints of healthy ducks during treadmill walking in lateral and dorsoventral views. Black bar: hip joint; light gray bar: knee joint; dark gray bar: intertarsal joint; white bar: metatarsal joint.

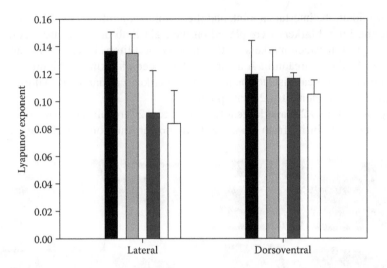

FIGURE 9.23 Lyapunov exponent values of y-coordinate (vertical displacement) time series for the hip, knee, intertarsal, and metatarsal joints of healthy ducks during treadmill walking in lateral and dorsoventral views. Black bar: hip joint; light gray bar: knee joint; dark gray bar: intertarsal joint; white bar: metatarsal joint.

but not in the dorsoventral view. Birds live in highly diverse biotypes and have very different lifestyles, but all have a similar skeletal geometry. All birds have the same basic skeletal features: compact, rigid trunk, long pliant neck, short tail, forelimbs converted into wings and hindlimbs with three long bones and toed feet. However, this basic morphological "avian model" may be adapted to allow different types of locomotor behavior. These morphological adjustments affect the kinematics of walking, and it is clear from simple observation that ducks do not walk like hens, for example. Further studies are needed to determine how the structural (e.g., size effects, morphological adjustments) and functional (e.g., energetic constraints) features of birds affect kinematic variability during walking.

DOG MODEL

Computer-assisted video kinematic gait analysis has become the most useful system for the analysis of movement in dogs (DeCamp 1997), but, despite the availability of gait analysis systems, few publications have described the normal gait of dogs during walking (Hottinger et al. 1996) or trotting (Allen et al. 1994; DeCamp et al. 1993; Gillette and Zebas 1999; Schaefer et al. 1998). Researchers have shown that in order for quantitative gait analysis to be comparable between dogs, within dogs, and between sides (i.e., left and right) of the dogs, they must be traveling at a constant velocity in a symmetrical gait such as the trot. One study found that there was no significant difference between the movements of the left and right sides of the body in a trot gait. It was concluded that the trot gait is symmetrical and that a two-dimensional system can be used to analyze gait in the dog (Gillette and Zebas 1999).

With the various morphological shapes between breeds, there is a clear need to study breed-specific kinematic differences. One study has already been conducted and found that apparent differences in the trotting gait between Labrador retrievers and greyhounds are mainly attributable to differences in size and that dogs of these two breeds move in a symmetrically similar manner during the trot (Bertram et al. 2000). However, Colborne et al. (2005) contradicted the outcome of the Bertram et al. (2000) study by stating that gross differences in pelvic limb kinematics are evident between greyhounds and Labrador retrievers. Thus, more research needs to be conducted in the area of different breed kinematics. In the present study, we quantified variability of the forelimb and hindlimb kinematics in a Labrador retriever trotting on a treadmill. Especially, we explored whether there exists a gradient of variability from the upper to the lower limb joints (as observed in humans).

One adult Labrador retriever was studied. The dog was filmed in lateral view using a video camera at 240 frames per second. Markers were placed on the right side of the dog at the iliac crest (pelvis), the greater trochanter of the femur (hip), the femorotibial joint (knee) between the lateral epicondyle of the femur and the fibular head, the lateral malleolus of the distal tibia (ankle), the distolateral aspect of the fifth metatarsus (hindlimb foot), the dorsal aspect of the scapular spine (shoulder), midway between the acromion and the greater tubercule of the humerus, the lateral epicondyle of the humerus (elbow), the ulna styloid process (wrist), and the caudal zygoma of the skull (forelimb foot) (Figure 9.24). The dog performed three trials trotting overground. The z-coordinate (vertical displacement) for each marker was analyzed. All time series contained a minimum of 2368 data points.

Similar to the duck model, ApEn (Figures 9.25 and 9.26) and largest LyE (Figures 9.27 and 9.28) results of the dog model showed a decreasing gradient of variability from the shoulder to the wrist joints for the forelimbs and from the hip to the ankle joints for the hindlimbs. Findings from both duck and dog models revealed

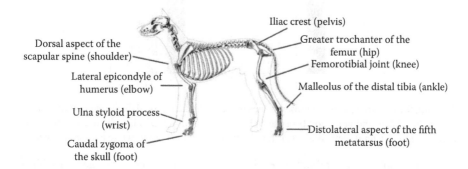

FIGURE 9.24 A dog trotting overground videotaped in lateral view at 240 frames per second using cineradiography. Markers were placed at the joints of the right and left hindlimb and forelimb.

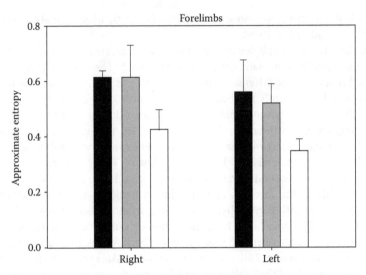

FIGURE 9.25 Approximate entropy values of z-coordinate (vertical displacement) time series for the shoulder, elbow, and wrist joints of the right and left forelimb of a healthy dog during treadmill trotting in lateral view. Black bar: shoulder joint; gray bar: elbow joint; white bar: wrist joint.

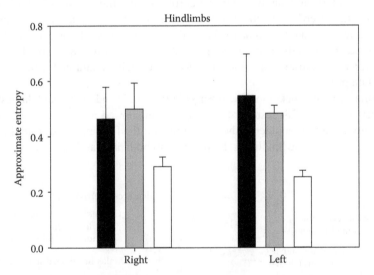

FIGURE 9.26 Approximate entropy values of z-coordinate (vertical displacement) time series for the hip, knee, and ankle joints of the right and left hindlimb of a healthy dog during tread-mill trotting in lateral view. Black bar: hip joint; gray bar: knee joint; white bar: ankle joint.

that nonlinear tools are reliable to evaluate the temporal structure of gait variability and undercover the underlying complexity in various animal models. As veterinary rehabilitation becomes more popular, locomotor analysis, and especially kinematic variability of overground and treadmill gait, will be utilized to a greater extent (Feeney et al. 2007; Weigel et al. 2005).

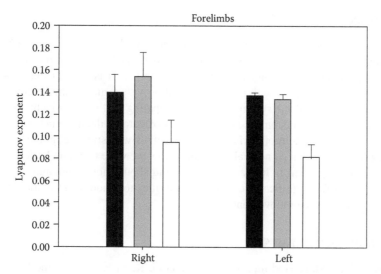

FIGURE 9.27 Lyapunov exponent values of z-coordinate (vertical displacement) time series for the shoulder, elbow, and wrist joints of the right and left forelimb of a healthy dog during treadmill trotting in lateral view. Black bar: shoulder joint; gray bar: elbow joint; white bar: wrist joint.

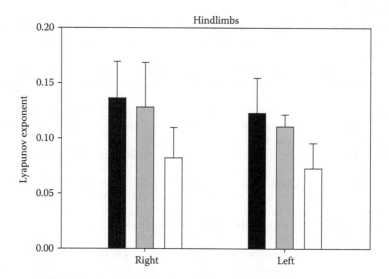

FIGURE 9.28 Lyapunov exponent values of z-coordinate (vertical displacement) time series for the hip, knee, and ankle joints of the right and left hindlimb of a healthy dog during treadmill trotting in lateral view. Black bar: hip joint; gray bar: knee joint; white bar: ankle joint.

SUMMARY

In this chapter, we were able to demonstrate how nonlinear measures can be used not only in a variety of different tasks and populations, but also with different species and provide a better understanding of variability. It is evident that nonlinear measures in combination with linear tools can provide a more complete evaluation of the organization of the system. We are anticipating that progressively these nonlinear measures will become a necessary part of data evaluation such as standard deviation and coefficient of variation, and scientists will start recognizing that not all data fit the bell-shaped normal distribution that we were taught in basic statistics. Nonlinearity is present in human movement and should not be ignored. Nonlinear methods will offer significant scientific possibilities to guide rehabilitation practice and research in human movement.

ACKNOWLEDGMENTS

We thank Drs. Marc Herbin, Anick Abourachid, Rémi Hackert of the UMR 7179 CNRS/National Museum of Natural History of Paris, and Paul-Antoine Libourel of the UMR 5292 CNRS/1028 INSERM of Lyon, for providing data from various animal models presented in this research study. We also thank the graduate students and postdocs of the biomechanics team at the University of Nebraska, Omaha, that provided data from the different studies presented in this chapter.

REFERENCES

Abarbanel, H.D.I., R. Brown, J.J. Sidorowich, and L.S. Tsimring, The analysis of observed chaotic data in physical systems, *Reviews of Modern Physics* 65, 4 (1993): 1331–1392.

Allen, K., C.E. DeCamp, and T.D. Braden, Kinematic gait analysis of the trot in healthy mixed breed dogs, *Veterinary and Comparative Orthopaedics and Traumatology* 7 (1994): 148–153.

Amende, I., A. Kale, S. McCue, S. Glazier, J.P. Morgan, and T.G. Hampton, Gait dynamics in mouse models of Parkinson's disease and Huntington's disease, *Journal of NeuroEngineering and Rehabilitation* 2 (2005): 20.

Atchley, W.R. and W.M. Fitch, Gene trees and the origins of inbred strains of mice, *Science* 254, 5031 (1991): 554–558.

Baghai-Ravary, R., J.K. Quint, J.J. Goldring, J.R. Hurst, G.C. Donaldson, and J.A. Wedzicha, Determinants and impact of fatigue in patients with chronic obstructive pulmonary disease, *Respiratory Medicine* 103, 2 (2009): 216–223.

Baker, G.L., J.P. Gollub, and J.A. Blackburn, Inverting chaos: Extracting system parameters from experimental data, *Chaos* 6, 4 (1996): 528–533.

Beck, J.A., S. Lloyd, M. Hafezparast, M. Lennon-Pierce, J.T. Eppig, M.F.W. Festing, and E.M.C. Fisher, Genealogies of mouse inbred strains, *Nature Genetics* 24, 1 (2000): 25.

Bertram, J.E., D.V. Lee, H.N. Case, and R.J. Todhunter, Comparison of the trotting gaits of Labrador retrievers and greyhounds, *American Journal of Veterinary Research* 61 (2000): 832–838.

Buchanan, J.J. and F.B. Horak, Transitions in a postural task: Do the recruitment and suppression of degrees of freedom stabilize posture? *Experimental Brain Research* 139, 4 (2001–8): 482–494.

Carter, R.J., L.A. Lione, T. Humby, L. Mangiarini, A. Mahal, G.P. Bates, S.B. Dunnett, and A.J. Morton, Characterization of progressive motor deficits in mice transgenic for the human Huntington's disease mutation, *Journal of Neuroscicence* 19 (1999): 3248–3257.

Cattaneo, D.D. and J. Jonsdottir, Sensory impairments in quiet standing in subjects with multiple sclerosis, *Multiple Sclerosis (13524585)* 15, 1 (2009): 59–67.

Celis, R., I.I. Pipinos, M.M. Scott-Pandorf, S.A. Myers, and N. Stergiou, Peripheral arterial disease affects kinematics during walking, *Journal of Vascular Surgery* 49, 1 (2009): 127–132.

Cherng, R.J., F.C. Su, J.J.J. Chen, and T.S. Kuan, Performance of static standing balance in children with spastic diplegic cerebral palsy under altered sensory environments, *American Journal of Physical Medicine Rehabilitation* 78, 4 (1999): 336–343.

Cracraft, J., The functional morphology of the hind limb of the domestic pigeon, *Columba livia, Bulletin of the American Museum of Natural History* 144, 3 (1971): 171–268.

Colborne, G.R., J.F. Innes, E.J. Comerford, M.R. Owen, and C.J. Fuller, Distribution of power across the hind limb joints in Labradors and greyhounds, *American Journal of Veterinary Research* 66 (2005): 1563–1571.

Dagg, A.I., The walk of the silver gull (*Larus novaehollandiae*) and of other birds, *Journal of Zoology London*, 182 (1977): 529–540.

D'Annibale, Annibale A., V. Fiscon, P. Trevisan, M. Pozzobon, and V. Gianfreda, The da Vinci robot in right adrenalectomy: Considerations on technique, *Surgical Laparoscopy Endoscopy Percutaneous Techniques* 14, 1 (2004): 38–41.

DeCamp, C.E., Kinetic and kinematic gait analysis and the assessment of lameness in the dog, *Veterinary Clinics of North America: Small Animal Practice* 27 (1997): 825–840.

DeCamp, C.E., R.W. Soutas-Little, J. Hauptman, B. Olivier, T. Braden, and A. Walton, Kinematic gait analysis of the trot in healthy greyhounds, *American Journal of Veterinary Research* 54, 4 (1993): 627–634.

Deffeyes, J.E., R.T. Harbourne, A. Kyvelidou, W.A. Stuberg, and N. Stergiou, Nonlinear analysis of sitting postural sway indicates developmental delay in infants, *Clinical Biomechanics* 24, 7 (2009): 564–570.

Fabbri, L.M. and K.F. Rabe, From COPD to chronic systemic inflammatory syndrome? *Lancet* 370, 9589 (2007): 797–799.

Fedrizzi, E.E., E. Pagliano, M. Marzaroli, E. Fazzi, and I. Maraucci, Developmental sequence of postural control in prone position in children with spastic diplegia, *Brain Development* 22, 7 (2000): 436–444.

Feeney, L.C., C.-F. Lin, D.J. Marcellin-Little, A.R. Tate, R.M. Queen, and B. Yu, Validation of two-dimensional kinematic analysis of walk and sit-to-stand motions in dogs, *American Journal of Veterinary Research* 68 (2007): 277–282.

Fernagut, P.O., E. Diguet, B. Labattu, and F. Tison, A simple method to measure stride length as an index of nigrostriatal dysfunction in mice, *Journal of Neuroscience Methods* 113 (2002): 123–130.

Folio, R. and R. Fewell, *Peabody Developmental Motor Scales*, 2nd edn. Austin, TX: Pro-Ed, 2000.

Frzovic, D.D., M.E. Morris, and L. Vowels, Clinical tests of standing balance: Performance of persons with multiple sclerosis, *Archives of Physical Medicine and Rehabilitation* 81, 2 (2000): 215–221.

Gatesy, S.M., Guineafowl hind limb function. I. Cineradiographic analysis and speed effects, *Journal of Morphology* 240 (1999): 115–125.

Gatesy, S.M. and A.A. Biewener, Bipedal locomotion: Effects of speed, size and limb posture in birds and humans, *Journal of Zoology London* 224 (1991): 127–147.

Gepner, B.B. and F. Feron, Autism: A world changing too fast for a mis-wired brain? *Neuroscience and Biobehavioral Reviews* 33, 8 (2009): 1227–1242.

Gillette, R.L. and C.J. Zebas, A two-dimensional analysis of limb symmetry in the trot of Labrador retrievers, *Journal of the American Animal Hospital Association* 35 (1999): 515–520.

Gosker, H.R., M.K.C. Hesselink, H. Duimel, K.A. Ward, and A.M.W.J. Schols, Reduced mitochondrial density in the vastus lateralis muscle of patients with COPD, *European Respiratory Journal* 30, 1 (2007): 73–79.

Gosker, H.R., H. van Mameren, P.J. van Dijk, M.P.K.J. Engelen, and G.J. van der Vusse, Skeletal muscle fibre-type shifting and metabolic profile in patients with chronic obstructive pulmonary disease, *European Respiratory Journal* 19, 4 (2002): 617–625.

Grandin, T., *Thinking in Pictures*. New York, NY: Vintage Press Random House, 1995.

Grondard, C., O. Biondi, A.-S. Armand, S. Lecolle, B.D. Gaspera, and C. Pariset, Regular exercise prolongs survival in a type 2 spinal muscular atrophy model mouse, *Journal of Neuroscience* 25, 33 (2005): 7615–7622.

Hanly, E.J., M.R. Marohn, S.L. Bachman, M.A. Talamini, S.O. Hacker, R.S. Howard, and N.S. Schenkman, Multiservice laparoscopic surgical training using the daVinci surgical system, *American Journal of Surgery* 187, 2 (2004): 309–315.

Harbourne, R.T., J.E. Deffeyes, A. Kyvelidou, and N. Stergiou, Complexity of postural control in infants: Linear and nonlinear features revealed by principal component analysis, *Nonlinear Dynamics Psychology Life Sciences* 13, 1 (2009): 123–144.

Harbourne, R.T. and N. Stergiou, Movement variability and the use of nonlinear tools: Principles to guide physical therapist practice, *Physical Therapy* 89, 3 (2009):267–282.

Harbourne, R.T. and N. Stergiou, Nonlinear analysis of the development of sitting postural control, *Developmental Psychobiology* 42, 4 (2003): 368–377.

Harbourne, R.T., S. Willett, A. Kyvelidou, J. Deffeyes, and N. Stergiou, A comparison of interventions for children with cerebral palsy to improve sitting postural control: A clinical trial, *Physical Therapy* 90, 12 (2010): 1881–1898.

Herbin, M., J.P. Gasc, and S. Renous, Symmetrical and asymmetrical gaits in the mouse: Patterns to increase velocity, *Journal of Comparative Physiology A, Neuroethology, Sensory, Neural, and Behavioral Physiology* 190, 11 (2004): 895–906.

Herbin, M., R., Hackert, J.P. Gasc, S. Renous, Gait parameters of treadmill versus overground locomotion in mouse, *Behavioural Brain Research* 181, 2 (2007):173-179.

Hernandez, J.D., S.D. Bann, Y. Munz, K. Moorthy, and V. Datta, Qualitative and quantitative analysis of the learning curve of a simulated surgical task on the Da Vinci system, *Surgical Endoscopy and Other Interventional Techniques* 18, 3 (2004): 372–378.

Horak, F.B. and J.M. Macpherson, Postural orientation and equilibrium, In: Rowell, L.B., Shepard, J.T., eds. *Handbook of Physiology*: Section 12, *Exercise Regulation and Integration of Multiple Systems*. New York: Oxford University Press, pp. 255–292, 1996.

Horak, F.B., A. Shumwaycook, T.K. Crowe, and F.O. Black, Vestibular function and motor proficiency of children with impaired hearing, or with learning disability and motor impairments, *Developmental Medicine and Child Neurology* 30, 1 (1988): 64–79.

Hottinger, H.A., C.E. DeCamp, N.B. Olivier, J.G. Hauptman, and R.W. Soutas-Little, Noninvasive kinematic analysis of the walk in healthy large-breed dogs. *American Journal of Veterinary Research*, 57, 3 (1996):381–388.

Houck, J.R., A. Duncan, and K.E. De Haven, Knee and hip angle and moment adaptations during cutting tasks in subjects with anterior cruciate ligament deficiency classified as noncopers, *Journal of Orthopaedic and Sports Physical Therapy* 35, 8 (2005): 531–540.

Hughes, M.A., P.W. Duncan, D.K. Rose, J.M. Chandler, and S.A. Studenski, The relationship of postural sway to sensorimotor function, functional performance, and disability in the elderly, *Archives of Physical Medicine and Rehabilitation* 77, 6 (1996): 567–572.

Huisinga, J.M., M.L. Filipi, and N. Stergiou, Elliptical exercise improves fatigue ratings and quality of life in patients with multiple sclerosis, *Journal of Rehabilitation Research Development* 48, 7 (2011): 881–890.

Huisinga, J.M., M.L. Filipi, and N. Stergiou, Supervised resistance training results in changes in postural control in patients with multiple sclerosis, *Motor Control* 16, 1 (2012a): 50–63.

Huisinga, J.M., J.M. Yentes, M.L. Filipi, and N. Stergiou, Postural control strategy during standing is altered in patients with multiple sclerosis, *Neuroscience Letters* 524, 2 (2012b): 124–128.

Iranmanesh, A.A., D.F. Rochester, J. Liu, and J.D. Veldhuis, Impaired adrenergic- and corticotropic-axis outflow during exercise in chronic obstructive pulmonary disease, *Metabolism—Clinical and Experimental* 60, 11 (2011): 1521–1529.

Jacobson, R.D. and M. Hollyday, A behavioral and electromyographic study of walking in the chick, *Journal of Neurophysiology* 48 (1982): 238–256.

Judkins, T.N., D. Oleynikov, and N. Stergiou, Objective evaluation of expert and novice performance during robotic surgical training tasks, *Surgical Endoscopy and Other Interventional Techniques* 23, 3 (2009): 590–597.

Kaplan, D.T. and L. Glass, *Understanding Nonlinear Dynamics*. New York: Springer-Verlag, 1995.

Kay, B.A., The dimensionality of movement trajectories and the degrees of freedom problem—A tutorial, *Human Movement Science* 7, 2–4 (1988): 343–364.

Kirkinezos, I.G., D. Hernandez, W.G. Bradley, and C.T. Moraes, Regular exercise is beneficial to a mouse model of amyotrophic lateral sclerosis, *Annals of Neurology* 53, 6 (2003): 804–807.

Kohen-Raz, R.R., F.R. Volkmar, and D.J. Cohen, Postural control in children with autism, *Journal of Autism and Developmental Disorders* 22, 3 (1992): 419–432.

Koutakis, P.P., J.M. Johanning, G.R. Haynatzki, S.A. Myers, and N. Stergiou, Abnormal joint powers before and after the onset of claudication symptoms, *Journal of Vascular Surgery* 52, 2 (2010): 340–347.

Kyvelidou, A., R.T. Harbourne, V.K. Shostrom, and N. Stergiou, Reliability of center of pressure measures for assessing the development of sitting postural control in infants with or at risk of cerebral palsy, *Archives in Physical Medicine and Rehabilitation* 91, 10 (2010): 1593–1601.

Kyvelidou, A., R.T. Harbourne, W.A. Stuberg, J. Sun, and N. Stergiou, Reliability of center of pressure measures for assessing the development of sitting postural control, *Archives in Physical Medicine and Rehabilitation* 90, 7 (2009): 1176–1184.

Kyvelidou, A.A., R.T. Harbourne, S.L. Willett, and N. Stergiou, Sitting postural control in infants with typical development, motor delay, or cerebral palsy, *Pediatric Physical Therapy* 25, 1 (2013): 46–51.

Leblond, H., M. L'Esperance, D. Orsal, and S. Rossignol, Treadmill locomotion in the intact and spinal mouse, *Journal of Neuroscience* 23, 36 (2003): 11411–11419.

Mahoney, D.J., C. Rodriquez, M. Devries, N. Yasuda, and M.A. Tarnopolosky, Effects of high-intensity endurance exercise training in the G93A mouse model of amyotrophic lateral sclerosis, *Muscle Nerve* 29, 5 (2004): 656–662.

Marquis, N.N., R. Debigare, L. Bouyer, D. Saey, and L. Laviolette, Physiology of walking in patients with moderate to severe chronic obstructive pulmonary disease, *Medicine and Science in Sports and Exercise* 41, 8 (2009): 1540–1548.

Massion, J., Movement, posture and equilibrium: Interaction and coordination, *Progress in Neurobiology* 38, 1 (1992): 35–56.

McGrath, D.D., T.N. Judkins, I.I. Pipinos, J.M. Johanning, and S.A. Myers, Peripheral arterial disease affects the frequency response of ground reaction forces during walking, *Clinical Biomechanics* 27, 10 (2012): 1058–1063.

Mees, A.I. and K. Judd, Dangers of geometric filtering, *Physica D* 68, 3–4 (1993): 427–436.

Mettler, L., N.F. Zuberi, P. Rastogi, and T. Schollmeyer, Role and value of laparoscopic training devices in assessing nondominant and two-handed dexterity, *Gynecological Surgery* 3, 2 (2006): 110–114.

Miller, D.J., N. Stergiou, and M.J. Kurz, An improved surrogate method for detecting the presence of chaos in gait, *Journal of Biomechanics* 39, 15 (2006): 2873–2876.

Minshew, N.J., G. Goldstein, and D.J. Siegel, Neuropsychologic functioning in autism: Profile of a complex information processing disorder, *Journal of the International Neuropsychological Society* 3, 4 (1997): 303–316.

Molloy, C.A., K.N. Dietrich, and A. Bhattacharya, Postural stability in children with autism spectrum disorder, *Journal of Autism Developmental Disorders* 33, 6 (2003): 643–652.

Moorthy, K., Y. Munz, A. Dosis, J. Hernandez, and S. Martin, Dexterity enhancement with robotic surgery, *Surgical Endoscopy and Other Interventional Techniques* 18, 5 (2004): 790–795.

Muir, G.D., J.M. Gosline, and J.D. Steeves, Ontogeny of bipedal locomotion: Walking and running in the chick, *Journal of Physiology London* 493 (1996): 589–601.

Myers, S.A., J.M. Johanning, I.I. Pipinos, K.K. Schmid, and N. Stergiou, Vascular occlusion affects gait variability patterns of healthy younger and older individuals, *Annals of Biomedical Engineering* 41, 8 (2013): 1692–1702.

Myers, S.A., J.M. Johanning, N. Stergiou, R.I. Celis, and L. Robinson, Gait variability is altered in patients with peripheral arterial disease, *Journal of Vascular Surgery* 49, 4 (2009): 924–931.

Myers, S.A., I.I. Pipinos, J.M. Johanning, and N. Stergiou, Gait variability of patients with intermittent claudication is similar before and after the onset of claudication pain, *Clinical Biomechanics* 26, 7 (2011): 729–734.

Myers, S.A., N. Stergiou, I.I. Pipinos, and J.M. Johanning, Gait variability patterns are altered in healthy young individuals during the acute reperfusion phase of ischemia-reperfusion, *Journal of Surgical Research* 164, 1 (2010): 6–12.

Narazaki, K., D. Oleynikov, and N. Stergiou, Robotic surgery training and performance: Identifying objective variables for quantifying the extent of proficiency, *Surgical Endoscopy and Other Interventional Techniques* 20, 1 (2006): 96–103.

Narazaki, K.K., D. Oleynikov, and N. Stergiou, Objective assessment of proficiency with bimanual inanimate tasks in robotic laparoscopy, *Journal of Laparoendoscopic Advanced Surgical Techniques* 17, 1 (2007): 47–52.

Nashner, L.M., A. Shumwaycook, and O. Marin, Stance posture control in select groups of children with cerebral palsy: Deficits in sensory organization and muscular coordination, *Experimental Brain Research* 49, 3 (1983): 393–409.

Newell, K.M. and D.M. Corcos, *Variability and Motor Control*. Champaign, IL: Human Kinetics, 1993.

Newell, K.M., R.E.A. VanEmmerik, D. Lee, and R.L. Sprague, On postural stability and variability, *Gait and Posture* 1, 4 (1993): 225–230.

Odenrick, P.P. and P. Sandstedt, Development of postural sway in the normal child, *Human Neurobiology* 3, 4 (1984): 241–244.

Prasad, S.M., H.S. Maniar, N.J. Soper, R.J. Damiano, and M.E. Klingensmith, The effect of robotic assistance on learning curves for basic laparoscopic skills, *American Journal of Surgery* 183, 6 (2002): 702–707.

Puente-Maestu, L., J. Pérez-Parra, R. Godoy, N. Moreno, A. Tejedor, F. González-Aragoneses, J.L. Bravo, F.V. Alvarez, S. Camaño, and A. Agustí, Abnormal mitochondrial function in locomotor and respiratory muscles of COPD patients, *European Respiration Journal* 33, 5 (2009): 1045–1052.

Riach, C.L. and K.C. Hayes, Maturation of postural sway in young children, *Developmental Medicine and Child Neurology* 29, 5 (1987): 650–658.

Ridding, M.C. and S.C. Flavel, Induction of plasticity in the dominant and non-dominant motor cortices of humans, *Experimental Brain Research* 171, 4 (2006): 551–557.

Rocchi, L., L. Chiari, and F.B. Horak, Effects of deep brain stimulation and levodopa on postural sway in Parkinson's disease, *Journal of Neurology Neurosurgery and Psychiatry* 73, 3 (2002): 267–274.

Roig, M.M., J.J. Eng, D.L. MacIntyre, J.D. Road, and W.D. Reid, Postural control is impaired in people with COPD: An observational study, *Physiotherapy Canada* 63, 4 (2011): 423–431.

Roig, M.M., J.J. Eng, J.D. Road, and W. Darlene Reid, Falls in patients with chronic obstructive pulmonary disease: A call for further research, *Respiratory Medicine* 103, 9 (2009): 1257–1269.

Saey, D.D., R. Debigare, P. LeBlanc, M.J. Mador, and C.H. Cote, Contractile leg fatigue after cycle exercise: A factor limiting exercise in patients with chronic obstructive pulmonary disease, *American Journal of Respiratory and Critical Care Medicine* 168, 4 (2003): 425–430.

Sainburg, R.L., Evidence for a dynamic-dominance hypothesis of handedness, *Experimental Brain Research* 142, 2 (2002): 241–258.

Sanefuji, W., H. Ohgami, and K. Hashiya, Detection of the relevant type of locomotion in infancy: Crawlers versus walkers, *Infant Behavior and Development* 31, 4 (2008): 624–628.

Sarle, R.R., A. Tewari, A. Shrivastava, J. Peabody, and M. Menon, Surgical robotics and laparoscopic training drills, *Journal of Endourology* 18, 1 (2004): 63–66.

Schaefer, S.L., C.E. DeCamp, J.G. Hauptman, and A. Walton, Kinematic gait analysis of hind limb symmetry in dogs at the trot, *American Journal of Veterinary Research* 59, 6 (1998): 680–685.

Seymour, J.M., M.A. Spruit, N.S. Hopkinson, S.A. Natanek, W.D. Man, A. Jackson, H.R. Gosker, A.M. Schols, J. Moxham, M.I. Polkey, and E.F. Wouters, The prevalence of quadriceps weakness in COPD and the relationship with disease severity, *European Respiratory Journal* 36, 1 (2010): 81–88.

Shabbott, B.A. and R.L. Sainburg, Differentiating between two models of motor lateralization, *Journal of Neurophysiology* 100, 2 (2008): 565–575.

Shumway-Cook, A. and M.H. Woollacott, *Motor Control: Translating Research into Clinical Practice*, 4th edn. Philadelphia, PA: Lippincott, Williams & Wilkins, 2012.

Sjögren, H. and U. Björnstig, Trauma in the elderly: The impact on the health care system, *Scandinavian Journal of Primary Health Care* 9, 3 (1991): 203–207.

Small, M., D. Yu, and R.G. Harrison, Surrogate test for pseudoperiodic time series data, *Physical Review Letters* 87, 18 (2001): 188101–188104.

Smith, C.D., T.M. Farrell, S.S. McNatt, and R.E. Metreveli, Assessing laparoscopic manipulative skills, *American Journal of Surgery* 181, 6 (2001): 547–550.

Soyuer, F.F., M. Mirza, and U. Erkorkmaz, Balance performance in three forms of multiple sclerosis, *Neurological Research* 28, 5 (2006): 555–562.

Stergiou, N., U.H. Buzzi, M.J. Kurz, and J. Heidel, Nonlinear tools in human movement, In: Stergiou, N., ed. *Innovative Analyses of Human Movement*. Champaign, IL: Human Kinetics, pp. 63–90, 2004.

Stergiou, N.N., R. Harbourne, and J. Cavanaugh, Optimal movement variability: A new theoretical perspective for neurologic physical therapy, *Journal of Neurologic Physical Therapy* 30, 3 (2006): 120–129.

Van Emmerik, R.E.A., J.G. Remelius, M.B. Johnson, L.H. Chung, and J.A. Kent-Braun, Postural control in women with multiple sclerosis: Effects of task, vision and symptomatic fatigue, *Gait and Posture* 32, 4 (2010): 608–614.

Veiga, J.J., A.J. Lopes, J.M. Jansen, and P.L. Melo, Airflow pattern complexity and airway obstruction in asthma, *Journal of Applied Physiology* 111, 2 (2011): 412–419.

Weigel, J.P., G. Arnold, D.A. Hicks, and D.L. Millis, Biomechanics of rehabilitation, *Veterinary Clinics of North America: Small Animal Practice* 35 (2005): 1255–1287.

White, L.J. and R.H. Dressendorfer, Exercise and multiple sclerosis, *Sports Medicine* 34, 15 (2004): 1077–1100.

Winstein, C.J, E.R. Gardner, D.R. McNeal, P.S. Barto, and D.E. Nicholson, Standing balance training: Effect on balance and locomotion in hemiparetic adults, *Archives of Physical Medicine and Rehabilitation* 70, 10 (1989): 755–762.

Wolf, A., J.B. Swift, H.L. Swinney, and J.A. Vastano, Determining Lyapunov exponents from a time series, *Physica D: Nonlinear Phenomena* 16 (1985): 285–317.

Wu, Y.W., S.M. Day, D.J. Strauss, and R.M. Shavelle, Prognosis for ambulation in cerebral palsy: A population-based study, *Pediatrics* 114, 5 (2004): 1264–1271.

Wurdeman, S.R., P. Koutakis, S.A. Myers, J.M. Johanning, I.I. Pipinos, and N. Stergiou, Patients with peripheral arterial disease exhibit reduced joint powers compared to velocity-matched controls, *Gait and Posture* 36, 3 (2012a): 506–509.

Wurdeman, S.R., S.A. Myers, A.L. Jacobsen, and N. Stergiou, Adaptation and prosthesis effects on stride-to-stride fluctuations in amputee gait, *Plos One* 9, 6 (2014a): e100125.

Wurdeman, S.R., S.A. Myers, J.M. Johanning, I.I. Pipinos, and N. Stergiou, External work is deficient in both limbs of patients with unilateral PAD, *Medical Engineering and Physics* 34, 10 (2012b): 1421–1426.

Wurdeman, S.R., S.A. Myers, and N. Stergiou, Amputation effects on the underlying complexity within transtibial amputee ankle motion, *Chaos*, 24, 1 (2014b): 013140.

Yentes, J.M., N. Hunt, K.K. Schmid, J.P. Kaipust, D. McGrath, and N. Stergiou, The appropriate use of approximate entropy and sample entropy with short data sets, *Annals of Biomedical Engineering* 41, 2 (2013): 349–365.

Yentes, J.M., H. Sayles, J. Meza, D.M. Mannino, and S.I. Rennard, Walking abnormalities are associated with COPD: An investigation of the NHANES III dataset, *Respiratory Medicine* 105, 1 (2011): 80–87.

Index

A

Algorithm 1
  AR2, 129–130
  autoregressive time series, 129
  Fourier transform, 124
  frequency distribution preservation, 129, 132
  inverse Fourier transform, 126
  linear correlation preservation, 126
  numerical example, 124, 127–128
  phase randomization, 126
  phases shuffling, 124
  probability distribution, 129, 133
  SampEn, 129, 131
  unique values, 129
Analysis of variance (ANOVA), 373
ApEn, *see* Approximate entropy (ApEn)
Application programmer's interface (API), 369
Approximate entropy
  calculation of
    comparison vector, 180
    data sets, 185
    lag parameter, 179
    numerical example, 181–184
    Φ function calculation, 184
    time-ordered list of numbers, 180
    vectors of length, 180
  infinite time series, 179
  in life sciences, 178
  normalization, 186–187
  parameter selection, 185–186
  publications, 178–179
  vs. sample entropy, 191, 197–198
  sample step width time series, 214–219
  sample time series, 219
  uses of
    body temperature, 190
    cardiology, 188
    endocrinology, 188–189
    gait and posture biomechanics, 189–190
    menopause, 190
    pathology, 187
    physiological control system, 187
    psychology/neuroscience, 189
    respiration, 188
  values of, 185
Approximate entropy (ApEn)
  chaos, 379–380
  COP time series unpredictability/irregularity
    determination, 345

  MS, 350–351
  Parkinson's mice, 374–375
  postural control, 346
Autism spectrum disorders (ASD)
  biological motion, 366–367
  COP, 352, 354
  experimental setup, 352
  LyE, 352–353
  phenotypic expressions, 351
  RMS values, 352–353
Autocorrelation function
  ARIMA model, 313
  covariance
    definition, 301
    height and weight,
      303–304
    limitation, 303
    N observations pairs, 301–302
    variable calculation, 302–303,
      305–306
  Lorenz attractors, 72, 75
  time lag calculation, 71–72
  time series
    data points, 310, 312
    joint angles for ankle, 308, 310
    lag k, 305
    logistic map, 312–313, 315
    Lorenz system, 313–314, 316
    periodic, 306–309
    random, 308–309, 311
    Rossler system, 313–314
Autocovariance function
  definition, 301
  height and weight, 303–304
  limitation, 303
  N observations pairs, 301–302
  variable calculation, 302–303, 305–306
Autoregressive fractionally integrated moving
    average (ARFIMA), 288
Autoregressive integrated moving average
    (ARIMA) model, 313

B

Band pass/notch pass filter, 43
Boids model, 15–16
Boltzmann entropy, 174
Butterfly effect, 13, 84
Butterworth filter, 43, 45

C

Cellular automata models, 16–18
Center of pressure (COP), 147, 287, 339,
    344–345, 353
Chaos, animal locomotion
    dog model
        ApEn, 379–380
        Labrador retrievers, 379
        LyE, 379, 381
    duck model, 374, 377–378
    mouse model
        ANOVA, 373
        ApEn values, 374–375
        gait parameters, 372
        Huntington's disease, 372–373
        LyE, 374, 376
        neurodegenerative disease, 372–373
        Parkinson's disease, 372–373
        treadmill speed, 373
Chaotic system
    application, 13
    differential equations, 12
    logistic equation, 11
    Lorenz equations, 13
    Lyapunov exponents, 84–87
    nonlinear system dynamics, 3
    phase space plots, 13–14
    random and periodic systems, 24
Chronic obstructive pulmonary disease (COPD)
    custom MATLAB programs, 360
    definition, 358
    functional limitations, 359
    step width time series, 360–361
Cobweb method, 8–10
COP, *see* Center of pressure (COP)
COPD, *see* Chronic obstructive pulmonary
    disease (COPD)
Corrected conditional entropy, 211
Correlation dimension
    capacity dimension, 336
    constant slope, 337–338
    COP time series, 339
    data length, 339
    formula, 331
    fractal dimension, 334–335
    Hausdorff dimension, 334
    Koch curve, 334–336
    log–log plot, 337–338
    Lorenz attractor, 337
Cross entropy algorithms, 212–213

D

Damped filter, 43
da Vinci™ surgical system (dVSS), 366,
    368–369

Detrended fluctuation analysis (DFA), 355
    ambulatory activity, 280
    fGn/fBm, 276
    long-range correlation measurement, 355
    procedure, 282–284
    upper limb movement, 281
Detrending process, 48, 276
Developmental delays (DD), 190, 345–349
DFA, *see* Detrended fluctuation analysis (DFA)
Differencing process, 48, 275
dVSS, *see* da Vinci™ surgical system (dVSS)
Dynamical systems
    bifurcation diagram, 10–12
    chaos, 3, 12–14
    continuous *vs.* discrete, 4–5
    definition, 2
    deterministic *vs.* stochastic, 3–4
    examples, 2
    growth model, 5–8
    linear systems, 5–6
    logistic map (*see* Logistic map)
    nonlinear systems, 2–3, 5–6
    phase space, 3
    set of functions, 2
    technical description, 2

E

Entropy
    approximate entropy (*see* Approximate entropy)
    arrow of time, 175
    Boltzmann entropy, 174
    classical thermodynamics, 174
    corrected conditional entropy, 211
    cross entropy algorithms, 212–213
    definition, 174–175
    Fuzzy entropy, 211
    Kolmogorov entropy, 208, 211
    Kolmogorov–Sinai entropy, 211
    Lempel–Ziv entropy, 211
    mixing, 175
    multiscale entropy (*see* Multiscale entropy)
    permutation entropy, 211–212
    randomness, 176
    sample entropy (*see* Sample entropy)
    Shannon Entropy, 175–176
    spectral entropy, 211
    statistical thermodynamics, 174
    symbolic entropy (*see* Symbolic entropy)
    visual representation, 177
    von Neumann entropy, 211

F

False nearest neighbor method
    data points, 66–67
    m-dimensional space, 66, 68–69
    percentage, 70, 76–77

Feigenbaum's number, 12
1/*f* fractal scaling phenomenon movement
    variability, 24–25
Filtering, 42–45
Fractal analysis
    ambulatory activity, 280
    coastline representation, 262–263, 265–266
    data analysis, 287–289
    data collection, 285, 287
    design, 285–286
    DFA procedure, 282–284
    Euclidean geometry, 264
    fBm, 274–276
    fGn, 274–276
    fractal dimension, 271
    "fractal tree," 271
    human gait, 277–279
    logarithmic estimation, 266–268
    paradigm shift, 289–291
    postural control, 281–282
    power law
        branches distribution, 271–272
        log–log plot, 268, 270
        negative exponent, 268–269
        positive exponent, 268
        significance of, 272–274
    probability density function, 271
    report, 289
    research journey, 285–286
    Romanesco Broccoli
        distribution, 270
        human movement, 265–266
        self-similarity, 262–263
    scaling patterns, 291–292
    Sierpinski triangle
        construction process, 263–264
        quantification, 270
    square magnification, 263–264
    state of the art, 289
    technology, 292
    upper limb movement, 280–281
Fractional Brownian motions (fBm), 274–276
Fractional Gaussian noise (fGn), 274–276
Fuzzy entropy, 211

G

Gait
    amputation
        ankle joint angle time series, 362–363
        LyE, 362
        neuromuscular system, 361–362
    COPD
        custom MATLAB programs, 360
        definition, 358
        functional limitations, 359
        step width time series, 360–361

PAD
    ankle joint angle, 357–358
    definition, 357
    LyE, 357
    phase portraits, 357, 359
    variability, 356

H

Haken–Kelso–Bunz (HKB) model, 19–21
Hausdorff dimension, 334
High-pass filter, 43
HKB model, *see* Haken–Kelso–Bunz (HKB) model

I

Iterated amplitude-adjusted Fourier transform
        (IAAFT)
    adjusted amplitude, power spectra,
        distribution, 139
    converged time series, power spectra,
        distribution, 139
    numerical example
        adjusted surrogate series, 144
        amplitude distribution, 142, 144–145
        Fourier transform, 141
        FTRandomized coefficients, 142–143
        imaginary coefficients, 142
        null hypothesis, 141
        power spectrum amplitude adjusted
            surrogate, 146
        power spectrum surrogate, 144
        real coefficients, 142
        shuffled amplitude distribution, 143
        shuffled power spectrum, 143
    original time series, power spectra,
        distribution, 138
    power spectrum preservation, 138, 140
    procedure steps, 136, 140
    shuffled time series, power spectra,
        distribution, 138

J

Jackson filter, 43

K

Koch curve, 334–336
Kolmogorov entropy, 208, 211
Kolmogorov–Sinai entropy, 211

L

Lempel–Ziv entropy, 211
Logistic map
    autocorrelation function, 312–313, 315
    chaos, 11

cobweb method, 8–10
difference equation, 7
growth curve, 7
MI, 325–326, 330
period four oscillation, 11
period two oscillation, 11
quadratic curve, 8
steady-state, 11
Lorenz attractor
coordinates, 58–59
three-dimensional graph, 58, 60
time lag values, 64–65
Lorenz system, 313–314, 316
Low-pass filter, 43
Lyapunov exponent (LyE), 113
amputation, 362
ASD, 352–353
calculation of, 83
chaotic system
aperiodic deterministic system, 84
property, 84
sensitive dependence, 84–87
convergence, 87
COP, 344–345
divergence, 85, 89
exponential decay, 87
Lorenz attractor, 87–88
MS, 350–351
PAD, 357
Parkinson's mice, 374, 376
robot-assisted laparoscopy, 368–369, 371
Rosenstein et al.'s algorithm, 100–104
spectrum of
definition, 89
directions of local instabilities, 93
principal axis of ellipsoid, 91–92
Rossler system, 89–90
three-dimensional sphere, 89, 91
time horizon, 93
volume, principal axes, 91–92
TD and DD directions, 348–349
Wolf et al.'s algorithm, 94–100
z-coordinate, 379, 381
LyE, see Lyapunov exponent (LyE)

M

MI, see Mutual information (MI)
Motor control
autism, 365–367
gait variability in stroke, 362, 364–365
robot-assisted laparoscopy
advantages, 366
API, 369
coefficient of variation, 369
definition, 366
dVSS, 366, 368–369

dynamic-dominance hypothesis, 372
LyE, 368–369, 371
needle passing task, 368
OSATS, 368
pre-to posttraining tests, 369–371
standard deviation, 369
Multiple sclerosis (MS)
ApEn, 350–351
COP, 349
definition, 349
LyE, 350–351
Multiscale entropy
calculation of
coarse-grained time series, 198–200
complexity index, 199
numerical example, 200–204
sample entropy, 198–199
uses of, 204–205
Mutual information (MI)
example, 316–317
Lorenz attractor, 72, 75
power spectrum, 78–79
time lag, 72–74, 77
time series
computation process, 318–319
joint angle for ankle, 320, 322
joint probability distributions, 319
lag k, 317–318
logistic map, 325–326, 330
Lorenz attractor, 325, 332–333
Lorenz system, 325, 331
periodic, 320–322
random, 320, 323–325, 329
Rossler system, 325–326, 330
sine wave, 325, 327–328

N

Negative natural logarithm, 191
Nonlinear analysis
definition, 112
direct application of nonlinear
measures, 112
measurement distortion, 112
surrogate methods (see Surrogate methods)
Nonlinear systems, 2–3, 5–6, 112
Nyquist sample theory, 36, 44

O

Objective structured assessment of technical skill
(OSATS), 368

P

Peabody Gross Motor Scale, 346
Peripheral arterial disease (PAD)
ankle joint angle, 357–358
definition, 357

LyE, 357
  phase portraits, 357, 359
Permutation entropy, 211–212
Postural control
  aging, 354–356
  ApEn, 345
  ASD
    COP, 352, 354
    experimental setup, 352
    LyE, 352–353
    phenotypic expressions, 351
    RMS values, 352–353
  infants
    anterior–posterior direction, 346
    ApEn, 346
    COP, 346
    DD, 345–346, 348
    dynamic stabilization, 345
    LyE, 348–349
    medial–lateral direction, 346
    Peabody Gross Motor Scale, 346
    postural sway time series,
      345–347
    RMS, 346, 348
    TD, 346
  LyE, 344–345
  MS
    ApEn, 350–351
    COP, 349
    definition, 349
    LyE, 350–351
  orientation, 344
  stability, 344
Power law
  branches distribution, 271–272
  log–log plot, 268, 270
  negative exponent, 268–269
  positive exponent, 268
  significance of, 272–274
Power spectral density analysis, 276
Pseudoperiodic surrogate (PPS) method
  application, 149
  discriminating statistics, 154–156
  embedding parameters, 149
  implementation, 121
  intercycle dynamics, 148, 151
  intracycle dynamics, 148
  knee angle kinematic time series, 152
  Lorenz attractor, 151, 153
  noise radius, 149–150
  null hypothesis of, 148
  Rossler attractor, 151, 153
  spikes, 148, 150
  state space reconstruction, 149
  surrogate series, 150–151,
    162–168
  time lag, 149

R

RANDBETWEEN function, 181
Randomized controlled trial (RTC), 290
RMS, *see* Root-mean-square (RMS)
Robot-assisted laparoscopy
  advantages, 366
  API, 369
  coefficient of variation, 369
  definition, 366
  dVSS, 366, 368–369
  dynamic-dominance hypothesis, 372
  LyE, 368–369, 371
  needle passing task, 368
  OSATS, 368
  pre-to posttraining tests, 369–371
  standard deviation, 369
Root-mean-square (RMS)
  ASD, 352–353
  infants, 346, 348
  magnitude of fluctuation, 282
Rosenstein et al.'s algorithm
  average divergence, 101
  description, 100–101
  procedure, 101–104
Rossler system
  autocorrelation function, 313–314
  MI, 325–326, 330

S

Sample entropy (SampEn)
  vs. approximate entropy, 191,
    197–198
  calculation of, 191–194
  multiscale entropy, 198–199
  parameter selection, 195–196
  sample step width time series,
    214–219
  sample time series, 219
  sampling frequency and Nyquist rate, 191
  signal-to-noise ratio, 191
  surrogate testing, 120–123
  uses of
    cardiology, 196
    climate temperature dynamics, 197
    gait and posture biomechanics, 197
    psychology/neuroscience, 197
    respiration, 196
    sepsis prediction in neonates, 197
    team synchronization, 197
    triage tool, 197
SCALMX, 96–98
Self-organization
  boids model, 15–16
  cellular automata models, 16–18
  complexity, 23–24
  definition, 15, 23

1/*f* fractal scaling phenomenon movement
  variability, 24–25
global coordination, 15
in human movement, 18–21
principle, 21
property, 15
tell-tale signs, 22–23
Shannon Entropy, 175–176, 178, 206–207
Smoothing, 42–43
Spectral analysis, 36, 38–40
Spectral entropy, 211
Spline function, 43
State-space reconstruction
  embedding dimension
    biological data, 80
    dynamic invariant, 64, 66
    false nearest neighbor method (*see* False
      nearest neighbor method)
    objects, 61
  geometric objects, 56–58
  Lorenz attractor
    coordinates, 58–59
    three-dimensional graph, 58, 60
  time lag
    autocorrelation function (*see*
      Autocorrelation function)
    average mutual information (*see* Mutual
      information)
    scalar time series, 62–64
Stationarity, 46–49, 274–275
Surrogate methods
  in biological signals, 114–118
  discriminating statistics
    selection of, 119
    tools, 114
  general procedure, 113–114
  hypothesis testing
    confidence level of inference, 119
    knee flexion/extension time series, 120–122
    parametric criterion, 119
    rank-order criterion, 120
    SampEn, 120–123
  knee joint flexion/extension angle
    original series, 157–162
    PPS surrogate series, 162–168
  linear surrogate methods
    Algorithm 0, 124–126
    Algorithm 1 (*see* Algorithm 1)
    Algorithm 2, 134–137
    IAAFT, 136, 138–140
  null hypothesis rejection, 140, 147–149
  PPS (*see* Pseudoperiodic surrogate (PPS)
    method)
Symbolic entropy
  calculation of
    median value, 205

numerical example, 206–208
threshold values, 205, 209–210
description, 178
uses of, 208

T

Three-body problem, 2
Time series
  definition, 29
  discrete *vs.* continuous, 31
  examples of, 32–34
  filtering, 42–45
  generation of, 30
  height *vs.* age, 30–31
  human movement data, 31–33
  length of, 35
  noise, 41–42
  nonstationarity, 46–49
  resolution, 45–46
  sampling frequency
    definition, 36
    frequency-domain analysis, 36
    front-to-back postural sway, 37, 39
    in human locomotion, 36
    knee joint angle, 37, 39
    Nyquist sample theory, 36
    signal, various frequencies, 37, 40
    sine and cosine waves, 36–39
    sun spot number, 37, 39
  smoothing, 42–43
  spectral analysis, 36, 38–40
  stationarity, 46–49
Typically developing (TD) infant, 346

V

Von Neumann entropy, 211

W

Wolf et al.'s algorithm
  description, 94
  procedure
    angular separation, 97–98
    data length, 98
    embedding dimension selection, 95
    embedding point selection, 95
    evolution time, 96
    exponential growth calculation, 95–96
    initial distance between vectors, 95
    local expansion/contraction rates, 98
    nearest neighboring point selection, 95
    reference and replacement trajectories, 98–99
    running average, 99–100
    SCALMX, 96–97
    time lag selection, 95